Sustainable Development Goals Series

The **Sustainable Development Goals Series** is Springer Nature's inaugural cross-imprint book series that addresses and supports the United Nations' seventeen Sustainable Development Goals. The series fosters comprehensive research focused on these global targets and endeavours to address some of society's greatest grand challenges. The SDGs are inherently multidisciplinary, and they bring people working across different fields together and working towards a common goal. In this spirit, the Sustainable Development Goals series is the first at Springer Nature to publish books under both the Springer and Palgrave Macmillan imprints, bringing the strengths of our imprints together.

The Sustainable Development Goals Series is organized into eighteen subseries: one subseries based around each of the seventeen respective Sustainable Development Goals, and an eighteenth subseries, "Connecting the Goals", which serves as a home for volumes addressing multiple goals or studying the SDGs as a whole. Each subseries is guided by an expert Subseries Advisor with years or decades of experience studying and addressing core components of their respective Goal.

The SDG Series has a remit as broad as the SDGs themselves, and contributions are welcome from scientists, academics, policymakers, and researchers working in fields related to any of the seventeen goals. If you are interested in contributing a monograph or curated volume to the series, please contact the Publishers: Zachary Romano [Springer; zachary.romano@springer.com] and Rachael Ballard [Palgrave Macmillan; rachael.ballard@palgrave.com].

Sanghmitra S. Acharya ·
Sampurna Kundu · Sampurna Singh
Editors

Paradigm Shifts in Population and Health in India

A Multidimensional Approach to SDGs

Springer

Editors
Sanghmitra S. Acharya
Centre of Social Medicine
and Community Health, School
of Social Sciences
Jawaharlal Nehru University
New Delhi, Delhi, India

Sampurna Kundu
Postdoctoral Research Fellow
in Epidemiology, Faculty of Health
and Life Sciences
University of Exeter
Exeter, United Kingdom

Sampurna Singh
Mindfield Research Services
New Delhi, Delhi, India

ISSN 2523-3084 ISSN 2523-3092 (electronic)
Sustainable Development Goals Series
ISBN 978-981-95-1718-3 ISBN 978-981-95-1719-0 (eBook)
https://doi.org/10.1007/978-981-95-1719-0

This Springer imprint is published by the registered company Springer Nature Singapore Pte Ltd.
The registered company address is: 152 Beach Road, #21-01/04 Gateway East, Singapore 189721, Singapore

Foreword

Having realized much desired goal of replacement fertility, India's population has reached a point where the population growth is largely driven by the momentum built in its age structure. The geographic heterogeneity in India with respect to gender, health, and quality of life brings in several learning opportunities, however, they pose countless challenges for population (especially youth) management. On one side, states like Tamil Nadu, West Bengal, Andhra Pradesh, etc., that are experiencing lower levels of fertility (with a total fertility rate, TFR, of 1.6 children per woman or below) and have far exceeded the sustainable development goals (SDGs) that generates new domains of population issues including aging of the population and are at a threshold of negative population growth rate in the near future as their share of working population is shrinking. At the other extreme, there are states like Uttar Pradesh and Bihar which are almost twenty years behind these states.

Most important and dynamic change when it comes to policy shift was the strategic launch of National Rural Health Mission in 2005, which marked a paradigm shift in focus from direct intervention of family planning to the health of women and children with the combination of nutrition, drinking water, and sanitation as key determinants to reach out to unreached. The outcome of this shift is seen in rapid reductions in maternal mortality and child mortality rates in the past 15 years. Going forward, there have been several positive add up and initiatives such as Poshan Abhiyan, Anaemia mukt Bharat, Ayushman, etc., to further accelerate the program outreach under the National Health Mission. These programs have strategically targeted to reduce prevailing inequalities in health as well as in social sector such as access to education, sanitation, drinking water, and nutrition.

As India completes demographic transition and moves towards a known and inevitable path in which rising burden of non-communicable diseases is further going to deepen further and the greying population will outnumber child population whose health care and supportive needs would require special targeted interventions. The emerging epidemiological conditions would require more and more specialized health care facilities and new health financing system to ensure equitable access to quality and affordable care to all. Alongside these, there are several other emerging challenges such as environmental degradation impacting millions, distress migration without any support for health, livelihood opportunities and proper shelter that impacts urban eco-system.

In this context I am delighted to learn that Prof. Sanghmitra S Acharya and her colleagues Dr Sampurna Singh and Dr Sampurna Kundu from Centre of Social Medicine and Community Health, Jawaharlal Nehru University, New Delhi, came up with timely effort of editing a book entitled "Paradigm Shifts in Population and Health in India: A Multidimensional Approach to SDGs" addressing these multi-facet aspects of the changing demography of India's population. Every paper in the book meticulously addresses the emerging challenges outlined above. The editorial team and the authors of the carefully selected papers do not need any introduction as each one of them has done excellent research work in their own specialized spaces and are known for their contributions to the subject, demography. The book addresses the achievement in the field of health including digitalization, nutrition, gender inequality, environment, and its consequences, migration, and subjects like infertility/childlessness. I am extremely happy to notice that the authors have made special efforts to ensure that the papers not only critically looks at and analyze the themes from a researcher's perspective alone, but rather, present their research findings more in the context of policy relevance for future improvements.

In view of SDG and India's global commitment to reach the last one needing any services, this book will guide the researchers to explore new domains of academic debate and at the same time will be instrumental for learning/modifying the future policies for maximum outcome. I am confident that the papers in this edited volume would facilitate the policy makers and program implementers and help them choose carefully their future strategies to both existing as well as newly emerging domains in changing spectrum of the demography of the country. I notice that the themes covered in the book would cater to multiple Ministries of Government of India and therefore it will be very pertinent to devise the way to communicate to each concerned ministry about the key policy issues that need to be addressed. Finally, the book will be helpful to the students of many disciplines beyond population scientists and will become "must have" for most of the libraries of Indian University.

Jaipur, India

Prof. F. Ram
Director (Former), IIPS, Mumbai

Contents

List of Figures

List of Tables

Introduction: Shifting Paradigm Towards Inclusive Development—From Rhetoric to Reality

1

Sanghmitra Acharya, Sampurna Kundu, and Sampurna Singh

Population, health, and development are the primary aspects to indicate the positive change in a country. India has been particularly concerned about the interconnects in the trajectory of the three in context of the inclusive measures that it mandated for itself for bringing about the change. This book provides a platform to get an insight into the processes and the outcomes towards this. It has covered the different aspects of the trajectory and its three elements, and how over time the trends and patterns have changed. Also, it endeavors to examine the inclusive measures mandated by the state in bringing about the change. Therefore, examining the inter-linkages with policies and programs, and the process of policy formulation and program implementation becomes imperative.

S. Acharya (✉)
Centre of Social Medicine and Community Health, School of Social Sciences, Jawaharlal Nehru University, New Delhi, Delhi, India
e-mail: sanghmitra.acharya@gmail.com

S. Kundu
Postdoctoral Research Fellow in Epidemiology, Faculty of Health and Life Sciences, University of Exeter, UK, Exeter, United Kingdom
e-mail: sampurna34@gmail.com

S. Singh
Senior Researcher, Mindfield Research Services, New Delhi, India
e-mail: sampurna62@gmail.com

As evident, the 2017 National Health Policy (NHP) focused on efforts and strategies to strengthen and prioritize the role of the Government in shaping health systems in all its dimensions (NHP, 2017). Investment in health, organization and financing of healthcare services, prevention of diseases and promotion of good health through cross sectoral action, access to technologies, and developing human resources continues to be the prime goal. Encouraging medical pluralism, building the knowledge base required for better health, financial protection strategies and regulation and legislation for health also become imperative for holistic health goal. The goal of universal health coverage has been the direction towards the original 'Health for ALL' Declaration of the Alma Ata in 1978. Thus, advocating health as a fundamental right, whose 'denial' would be deemed impingement on social justice enshrined in the constitutional safeguards, directly established linkages with population and becomes crucial in connecting with development. It highlights the urgency to improve the performance of health systems, as also evident in the budget of the current financial year.

For growth of a country, correlation between population, health, and development has been well acknowledged by the academia as well as policy makers. However, in India, concerns about the population growth, poor health status, especially of women and children and poor health-

S. S. Acharya et al. (eds.), *Paradigm Shifts in Population and Health in India*, Sustainable Development Goals Series, https://doi.org/10.1007/978-981-95-1719-0_1

care system have become deep rooted. There are various reasons and practices, social and cultural, which enhance the problem and many a times remain unidentified. The current available facilities are also not adequate to fulfill the health needs of the people. The current policies and program also do not address the needs of people and a large proportion of people are not even aware of the benefits from policies and programs. It has been repeatedly argued for long that expanding and strengthening the health system, policies and program can be one way out to meet health care needs of the people.

Growing population is impacting development and raising various health issues. In the first chapter on health systems in India authored by Aalok Ranjan Chaurasia, it is evident that to combat the health care needs of the people, we need to focus on two key aspects. The first is to prevent diseases and avoid premature deaths. The second is to provide treatment and cure for individuals who are suffering from specific diseases and ailments. It is the prevention of diseases and premature deaths that has a preponderance over the treatment and cure of diseases and ailments as regards to population health. He emphasizes that meeting the health care needs of the people is critically dependent upon the quality, equity, and efficiency of the health system. He further argues that for improving and making the health care system 'battle ready' to address health emergencies, it requires a comprehensive reinvigoration of the existing health system. Additional investments in the existing public health infrastructure, as being targeted through the Ayushman Bharat Health Infrastructure Mission may continue to remain inadequate.

The improved health system is envisaged to impact positively on population dynamics. A brief on long-term trends in population size, live births, and premature deaths in India and globally is given in the second chapter by Usha Ram, Prakash Kumar, and K. V. Ananya, on gendered perspectives of child mortality. They have measured two main outcome variables infant mortality rate (IMR) and under-five mortality rate (U5MR) as these are important indicators of health and are also used to document the progress in the achievement of the fourth Development Goal (*MDG-4: a commitment to reduce under-five mortality by two-thirds*) which translates into SDG 3-Good health and wellbeing, *Target 3.2-Newborn and child mortality: By 2030, end preventable deaths of newborns and children under 5 years of age*. This chapter explains trends in life expectancy at birth (LEB), infant mortality rate (IMR), and U5MR (all gender specific) for India as a whole over the past five decades (WHO, 2021). The authors also try to corroborate these changes with improvements in socio-economic and demographic context and behavioral indicators. Patterns of discrimination reflecting on inequalities in service utilization by gender, place of residence, wealth, caste, and religion, are effectively illustrated. Further, the chapter by Shilpa Jadhav Bhakare on inequity in early childhood has addressed some on the programmatic challenges in view of vulnerability pertaining to malnutrition, reproductive health, education, and employment.

This section discusses the contribution of different innovations like digitalization and mobile clinics in improving the health care infrastructure. During health emergency conditions like the recent Covid-19 pandemic, remote services like online consultation and mobile health clinics, have proven to be a boon. To overcome the challenges many innovations and developments have occurred. The mobile health clinic, for instance, evolved as an alternative strategy to provide health care services to the people primarily displaced due to wars, political upheaval, and in different emergencies like disasters where no other health facility is available to the people (MoHFW, 2015). The paper on mobile health clinics authored by Jayanti Saha establishes the connect between the health emergency conditions and alternative strategies to provide healthcare services. It gives a brief description of the history of mobile health clinic and its role during disasters and health emergencies in the Indian context.

Frontline workers and Anganwadi centers have proven to be the backbone for the health care service sector has been argued in the paper by Vaishnavi Mangal. The author explores digital tools and technologies used by community health care workers and Anganwadi workers in India for health service delivery. Anganwadi Workers are the primary workforce for the Integrated Child Development Scheme (ICDS). Exploration in the use of digital applications has helped the ground-level workforce in their service delivery; the subsequent digitization of their work has brought on both positive and negative aspects to the health services ecosystem. The chapter covers socio-technical issues around usage, practices, and the feasibility of use of digital applications among healthcare workers, and the enabling systematic support health care anganwadi workers need in their work. Although the gap between the demand and supply remains high.

The technological innovations and development have made significant contribution in the health sector. However, meeting the health outcomes in context of SDGs, is still a challenge. The chapter by Sandhya Mahapatro on unmet need for healthcare focuses on the universal health access by analyzing the National Sample Survey data. It shows how over time the unmet need has declined and the socio-economic differentials have widened. The prevalence of anemia among women, adolescents, and children is quite high, as evident from the recent NFHS-5. The chapter by Sampurna Kundu, Subhojit Shaw, Madhushree Banerjee, and Balram Paswan further evaluates nutritional anemia in association with various anthropometric, biochemical, dietary, and socio-demographic behaviors among the adolescents by using Comprehensive National Nutrition Survey (CNNS) data (2016–2018) (MoHFW, 2019). In India, micronutrient deficiencies have a significant association with anemia. The paper reveals that a good diet among adolescent girls is likely to protect against anemia in women in the reproductive age group. Women face many health issues right from the age of adolescent to old age. They experience many health complications during the reproductive span as child bearing responsibility rests on their shoulders. Repeated pregnancy due to fear of losing a child or not using any contraception many a time lead to a condition of hysterectomy.

Hysterectomy is considered one of the most common non-pregnancy-related major surgery performed on women. The chapter by Manali Swargiary, Chandrima Paul, and Sampurna Kundu aim to examine the national and state-level prevalence of hysterectomy among women aged 40 and above and understanding the association of socio-demographic factors, lifestyle habits, and pregnancy history over the individuals undergoing hysterectomy. The Longitudinal Ageing Study in India Wave-1 (2020), a nationally representative survey was used for the study. It is a cross-sectional, national survey of scientific investigation of the health, economics, and social determinants of population aging in India (LASI, 2020). The main contributor to the rural–urban differential is the number of pregnancies, wealth, social-group, and lifestyle factors. Undergoing hysterectomy is not mandatory for all cases; unless it is extremely life-threatening which needs to be made aware of along with other gynaecological morbidities.

To understand the association of population, development, and health, it becomes important to understand that health and sanitation are interrelated with educational attainment. School hygiene education aims to improve behavior by teaching appropriate hygiene practices. School Sanitation and Hygiene Education (SSHE) is globally recognized as a key intervention to promote children's right to health and a clean environment. The chapter by Shazia Farooq Fazli focused on school sanitation stems from the fact that children have a right to basic facilities such as school toilets, safe drinking water, clean surroundings, and information on hygiene.

WASH-Water, Sanitation, and Hygiene is also important to achieve the Sustainable Development Goal (SDG) 6 ensure universal access to safe drinking water, adequate infrastructure, provide sanitation facilities and encourage hygiene at every level by 2030. It is estimated that about one billion people still do not have access to safe drinking water, and today more than 2.5 billion people are still devoid of improved sanitation facility. Based on the data more than 40 percent of the population around the world is facing scarcity of water due to increase the global temperatures as a result of climate change. In India still 650 million slums population is exposed to water borne diseases and vector-borne diseases due to lack of water supply and sanitation facility. For the present micro picture of water and sanitation the next chapter by Ajit Kumar Lenka and Rajshree Chanchal discusses the condition of water supply and sanitation facilities and the hygienic practices among slums population in Bhubaneswar city.

The SDG 13 focuses on climate change and its implications. Environment and health are closely related, thus making it important to be addressed. The next chapter by Debayanti Bhowmick has discussed that climate change and wellbeing uses political ecology as a lens of analysis. In order to determine the strategic implications of policies aimed at mitigating climate change on health and wellbeing, this study reviews the phenomenon of climate change via the theoretical framework of the 'Political Ecology of Health.' While doing this, the article also considers the many discourses on wellbeing and climate change that are seen in various global places and populations.

Globally most of the countries are going through the demographic transition phase. India projects about 19% of the total population to be aged by the year 2050. Normally 60 or 65 years is considered as the starting of old age. Aging is a normal biological process that is a part of the life process. Thus, where there is continuous increase of elderly population which is the result of decrease in birth rate as well as death rate and increase in life expectancy. Increase in the elderly population is considered as a burden on the productive age groups. Thus, it becomes important to have a healthy aging. For a healthy aging the wellbeing of the elderly population also has to be looked into. Wellbeing adds to the component of increasing longevity. Wellbeing is associated with reduction in monetary burden and rise in economic contribution. Further the chapter by Trisha Mukhopadhyay and Sumanta Roy focuses on analyzing LASI data to understand the aging and wellbeing of the elderly population on the basis of various socio-economic indicators. And thus understand the scenario of population and development.

The social practices like early marriage, dropout rates from schools, domestic violence etc. are also the hinderance for the development and are common problem in the Indian population. These factors have also pushed the SDGs goals from being achieved. A case study from Maharashtra has been covered by Malika B. Mistry that spoke about the sexual exploitation of a minority religious group, that is, Muslim Naikin women. Further, this book also highlights nexus between domestic violence, women mental health and domestic violence which is presented in chapter by Sampurna Singh and Sanghmitra S. Acharya. The data shows a strong association between domestic violence on the mental health of women. In fact, during the pandemic, the jobs of women were lost, and they were overburdened with care work at home and lacked support. Families were in a distressful condition; use of alcohol has increased which trickled down on women in terms of violence. Thus, the evidence shows an increasing case of domestic violence, which has pushed the SDGs.

The next chapter by Anubhuti Jambhulkar presents the interlinkage between democracy and social wellbeing via the praxis of spirituality. Indian society since historical times has been plagued by 'graded inequality' based on caste as a governing feature of social life, and hence there is no singular social but multiple socials in India. This chapter seeks to explain the interlinkage of spirituality, *maitri* and how it can promote and sustain social wellbeing vis-a-vis democratic triad of liberty, equality, and fraternity.

As we engage with literature in health, it is important to take incognizant the mental wellbeing of populations as it is directly connected to health and development outcomes. Often in the understanding of the population, health and development trajectory, the systems analysis becomes center stage. The relevance of this connect remains incomplete without the intersecting with the issues and concerns of specific population groups such as the elderly, differently abled, adolescents, migrants, childless couples, minorities, abused women and children, marginalized groups etc., on one hand, and the industry and market on the other.

This intersection provides space for logical arguments pertaining to equity in health as it oversees social inequalities in health.

In the trajectory of system, program, and utilization, it is imperative to engage with inclusive processes towards universal coverage and catering to SDGs. Therefore, it is imperative to examine these connects and deliberate on the plausible pathways for a viable policy and its execution towards a system of health and wellbeing based on the learnings about health and health care. In doing so, it is envisaged that the thematic lens of the discourse covered in this book engages with population, health and development issues and concerns in context of the inclusive policies and measures which entail equity in health, and highlight the inequalities prevalent in access to health through all it services, resources, and outcome indicators, causing hindrance towards development. The current book endeavors to carve pathways in this direction.

References

Government of India. (2017) *National health policy.* Ministry of Health and Family Welfare.

International Institute for Population Sciences (IIPS), National Programme for, Health Care of Elderly (NPHCE), MoHFW, & Public Health (HSPH) and the University of Southern California (USC). (2020). *Longitudinal Ageing Study in India (LASI) Wave 1, 2017–18, India Report.* International Institute for Population Sciences, Mumbai. https://www.iipsindia.ac.in/lasi/

Ministry of Health and Family Welfare. (2015). *Operational guidelines for mobile medical units.* Available at: https://nhm.gov.in/New_Updates_2018/NHM_Components/Health_System_Stregthening/MMU/Mobile_Medical_Units.pdf

Ministry of Health and Family Welfare (MoHFW), G. o. I., UNICEF and Population Council. (2019). *Comprehensive national nutrition survey (CNNS). National report.* Retrieved from New Delhi.

WHO. (2021). *Life expectancy and healthy life expectancy data by WHO region.* Available from: https://apps.who.int/gho/data/view.main.SDG2016LEXREGv?lang=en

Part I

Population, Health and Development-Understanding the Intersections

2 Reinvigorating the Health System in India

Aalok Ranjan Chaurasia

Abstract

This paper argues that improving the response of the health system to meet the health care needs of Indian people and to make system 'battle ready' to address health emergencies requires a comprehensive reinvigoration of the existing health system and not just additional investments in the existing public health infrastructure as is being currently targeted. There is a need to develop a business model for strengthening the health system in the context of health system response to health care needs of the people and in terms of battle readiness of the system to deal with health emergencies. The paper presents an overview of the existing health system in India and outlines a business model for reinvigorating the health system of the country. The paper also suggests a framework for strengthening and expanding the health system, especially, the public health system in India.

A. R. Chaurasia (✉)
Mewalal Chaurasia Foundation and 'Shyam' Institute, Bhopal, Madhya Pradesh, India
e-mail: aalok@mlcfoundation.org.in

2.1 Background

Meeting the health care needs of the people is critically dependent upon quality, equity, and efficiency of the health system. In this context, weaknesses of India's health system are well-known. These weaknesses have persisted over time despite efforts to remedy them. These weaknesses have also been amply exposed during the current COVID-19 pandemic when the health system of the country was found grossly wanting to deliver services that were critical to both checking the transmission of the Novel Coronavirus that causes the COVID-19 disease and preventing premature deaths amongst those who got infected from the virus. Estimates prepared by the United Nations Population Division suggest that during the period of COVID-19 pandemic in India (2020–2021), the life expectancy at birth decreased by around 3.7 years (United Nations, 2022). This drop in the life expectancy at birth is amongst the highest in the world (Chaurasia, 2023). It is also estimated that there were around 4.3 million excess deaths in the country during this period (Chaurasia, 2023).

Concerns about the poor response of the health system to the health care needs of the Indian people are not new. It has been repeatedly argued that expanding and strengthening the health system is the only way out to meet health care needs of the people and to achieve a degree of

S. S. Acharya et al. (eds.), *Paradigm Shifts in Population and Health in India*, Sustainable Development Goals Series, https://doi.org/10.1007/978-981-95-1719-0_2

preparedness necessary to safeguard people from emerging and re-emerging diseases. The experience with COVID-19 pandemic has emphasised that the health system must always be at a constant state of 'battle readiness' to effectively combat and thwart threats to the health of the people that cannot be predicted in advance. One of the factors that have been found to be responsible for the extremely poor response of the health system in meeting the health care needs of the people in general and thwarting the challenge of the COVID-19 pandemic in particular has been the grossly inadequate public health infrastructure. The onus has, therefore, been put on the government to increase investment in health as current investment, by all accounts, remains abysmally low. The public health infrastructure is the foundation of the health system and, therefore, critical for the 'battle readiness' of the health system. It is the most critical element that determines the efficiency and effectiveness of the health system in meeting the routine health care needs of the people and in dealing with public health emergencies such as the COVID-19 pandemic. There are at least two key aspects of meeting the health care needs of the people. The first and the primary one is preventing diseases and avoiding premature deaths. The second, on the other hand, is the treatment and care of individuals who are suffering from specific diseases and ailments. It is the prevention of diseases and premature deaths that has a preponderance over the treatment of diseases and ailments as regards population health.

The Government of India has recently launched the Ayushman Bharat Health Infrastructure Mission to augment the public health infrastructure in the country (Government of India, 2021). The Mission is directed towards improving the response of the health system to health care needs of the people and to boost the 'battle readiness' of the system to effectively mitigate the challenge of health emergencies such as COVID-19 pandemic. The Mission, essentially, aims at establishing 150 thousand Health and Wellness Centres in the rural areas of selected states and in the urban areas throughout the country out of which 79 thousand are claimed to be already functioning. The Mission also aims to establish Public Health Units at the block level and Integrated Public Health Laboratories in all districts of the country. Another objective of the Mission is to establish critical care hospital blocks in all districts with a population of at least 500 thousand. The total outlay of the Mission is pegged at Rs. 64,000 crores which, actually, translates to less than Rs. 500 per person at current prices. The Mission, however, lacks a vision for the health system of the country in the context of quality, equity and efficiency of the health system that is critical to improving the response of the health system to not only the routine health care needs of the people but also to the challenge of health emergencies like COVID-19 epidemic. Public health infrastructure is only one of the many dimensions of the health system that determine health system response to health care needs of the people. It would have been in the fitness of things if the Mission would have been based on a vision of the health system directed towards improving the health system response to both visible and unforeseen health-related concerns facing the people. The Mission falls short of such an expectation.

This paper argues that improving the response of the health system to meet the health care needs of the people and to make the system 'battle ready' to address health emergencies like COVID-19 pandemic requires a comprehensive reinvigoration of the existing health system and not just additional investments in the existing public health infrastructure as is being targeted through the Ayushman Bharat Health Infrastructure Mission. There is a need to develop a business model for strengthening the health system in the context of the health system response to the health care needs of the people and in terms of the battle readiness of the system to deal with health emergencies effectively and efficiently. It is in this context that this paper presents an overview of the existing health system in India, outlines a conceptualisation or a business model that may serve as the basis for reinvigorating the health system and suggests a framework for strengthening and expanding the health system of the country.

2.2 Health System in India

The health system in India can broadly be classified into four categories as regards the delivery of health care services: (1) public health system in the rural areas; (2) private health system in the rural areas; (3) public health system in the urban areas; and (4) private health system in the urban areas. This distinction is important as the health care services delivered by the four categories of the health system are essentially different. Salient features of the four categories of the health system are summarised in Table 2.1. It is clear from the table that all the four categories of the health system do not comprehensively respond to the health care needs of the people, and they are not 'battle ready' to address health emergencies like COVID-19 epidemic at their own as critical elements necessary to effectively respond to health emergencies are missing in each category of the health system. Obviously, reinvigorating the health system is the first step towards strengthening the health system, especially in the context of its battle readiness to address health emergencies.

Table 2.1 Salient features of four categories of the health system in India

	Rural	Urban
Public	Comprises of primary health care institutions organised in hierarchical manner Covers entire rural population, at least, theoretically Follows an extension approach for thc delivery of health care services Primarily focuses upon promotive and preventive aspects of health care	Largely confined to secondary and tertiary level hospital-based care Does not cover entire urban population Follows institution-based approach for the delivery of health care services Primarily focuses on the delivery of hospital-based treatment of diseases and ailments
Private	Largely confined to dispensing services Largely unorganised and unregulated Provides clinic-based care Extremely limited coverage	Delivers services ranging from clinic-based care to highly specialised health care Very limited delivery of primary health care services Provides institution-based health care Weak regulatory mechanism

2.3 Conceptualising Health System

The health system can be conceptualised in different ways. In this paper, we argue that the health system may be conceptualised as a business model in which infrastructure is purposely created and facilities are intentionally provided to put certain processes in motion that lead to perceived or expected output. This conceptualisation or business model of the health system may be conceived as a three-layered pyramid. The first or the bottom layer of the pyramid comprises of the infrastructure necessary for setting business processes in motion. The second or the middle layer of the pyramid comprises of essential health care processes necessary to produce the desired or the expected output. Finally, the third or the top layer of the pyramid is related to the appropriateness of the output of the processes put in motion. This conceptualisation or the business model implies that the output of the health system is contingent upon both health infrastructure and facilities in place and health care processes in operation. If health infrastructure and facilities are inadequate or inappropriate then health care processes may not be efficient in terms of the appropriate outputs and, therefore, may not be capable of generating the response that is necessary to meet the health care needs of the people including health emergencies.

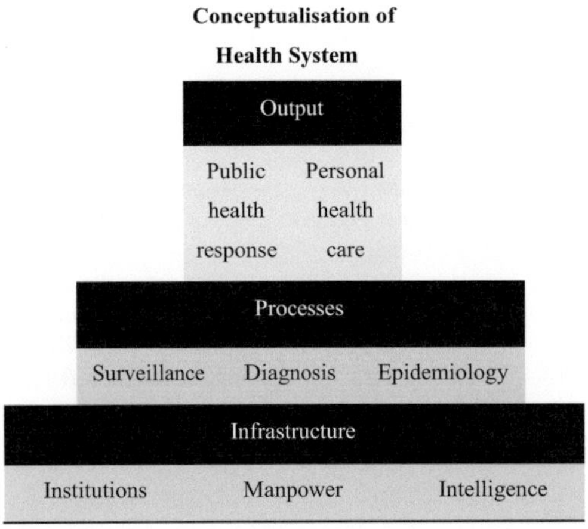

The infrastructure layer of the business model of the health system may further be conceptualised in terms of institutions, manpower, and intelligence. Similarly, the processes layer can be conceptualised in terms of surveillance, diagnosis, and epidemiology. Finally, the output layer of the business model can be conceptualised in terms of public health response and individual treatment and care. This business model argues that a certain threshold of infrastructure and processes is necessary for producing the output that is adequate and appropriate to meet the health care needs of the people. Deficiencies in either infrastructure or processes or both have a ripple effect throughout the health system and affect the health system output. This conceptualisation perceives health system as a closely inter-linked multi-layered and multi-dimensional entity. A brief overview of different layers of the health system may be illustrative to make an idea of the current state of the health system in the country.

2.4 Infrastructure

2.4.1 Institutions

India has both public and private institutions to meet the health care needs of the people. However, growth and expansion of health institutions in India has rarely followed a planned approach. There is very high rural–urban inequality in the availability of health institutions. Health institutions in the rural areas are predominantly public health institutions established following population-based norms with little consideration to disease burden. The population-based norms in the urban areas are grossly inadequate. On the other hand, establishment of private health institutions is purely arbitrary and there is very heavy concentration of these institutions in large metropolitan cities and towns. A unique feature of public health system in the rural areas is that it covers entire rural population in a hierarchical manner. This is not the case in the urban areas. One limitation of private health institutions in the urban areas is that these institutions, largely, deliver curative services at the cost of promotive and preventive dimensions of health care.

2.4.2 Manpower

Availability of manpower in public health institutions is guided by Indian Public Health Standards laid down by the Government. There is, however, little evidence about the extent up to which these standards are met in different categories of public health institutions. The population-based availability of manpower, especially, doctors and nurses, is estimated on the basis of the number of doctors registered under the Medical Council of India and the number of nurses registered under the Nursing Council of India. On the other hand, there is little idea about the health manpower norms for private health care institutions. These institutions are also supposed to follow the Indian Public Health Standards. There is, however, little information about the proportion of private health care institutions that have achieved Indian Public Health Standards.

WHO recommends that there should be one doctor for every 1000 population and three nurses for every doctor (WHO, 2021). This means that there should be 300 nurses for every 100 doctors. There is, however, little information about the nurse-doctor ratio in the health institutions of the country, either public or private. Similarly, there has never been any attempt to estimate the demand of other categories of health manpower. Health manpower planning in India remains a grossly neglected area. Creating more health institutions carries little meaning unless these are not fully and adequately staffed. Health manpower development is a time-consuming process. It is possible to establish additional health institutions within a short notice, but it is not possible to staff them through properly trained and adequately skilled manpower. The government of India has now allowed establishing new medical colleges and nursing institutions in the private sector. The government has also decided as a policy to establish a medical college in every district of the country. It is expected that establishing additional medical colleges and nursing institutions would result in increased availability of health manpower. However, the evidence is that paucity of health manpower in health institutions remains a major challenge. At the same time, there is very little knowledge about the adequacy of health manpower in private health care institutions.

2.4.3 Intelligence

The weakest component of the health infrastructure in India is the intelligence component. Intelligence is needed to provide evidence for planning and programming, monitoring, and evaluating the impact of the health system. Health intelligence also serves the foundation for developing an early warning system that may be crucial in controlling the spread of epidemic and responding to other health emergencies. The 'battle readiness' of the health care system depends, very crucially, upon the availability of specific, meaningful, accurate, reliable, and timely, or SMART, information so as to facilitate appropriate action at appropriate time. Health intelligence contributes to evidence-based decision-making. It also helps in improving the quality, equity, and efficiency of health care services. Although India has a Central Health Intelligence Bureau, by name, at the national level with field survey units at the state level, yet the role of the Bureau in providing intelligence for decision-making is limited to the compilation of selected data from different sources with little triangulation of different types of data. The existence of health intelligence system in the country is grossly inadequate to monitor population health, to identify gaps and disparities in population health and to monitor and evaluate performance of different health care interventions and programmes. Health intelligence requires combining data from different sources into a meaningful whole and transforming data into evidence and knowledge for decision-making.

2.5 Processes

The second layer of the health system comprises of processes that need to be put in motion to generate the response to the health care needs of the people. Health infrastructure, although necessary, is not sufficient to produce appropriate health system response to health care needs of the people in the absence of necessary health care processes.

2.5.1 Surveillance

Health surveillance may be defined as the continuous but systematic collection, analysis, and interpretation of health-related data and timely dissemination of these data for appropriate response of the health system to the health care needs of the people. Health surveillance may be perceived as a tool for identifying the need for health-related interventions well in time and for measuring the effect of these interventions in terms of the system response. Surveillance is critical for appropriate and timely response of the health system to the health care needs of the people.

Health surveillance may be classified further into passive surveillance and active surveillance. Active surveillance is conceived as an initiative of the health system to regularly reach out to the people to collect information related to their health conditions. Active surveillance provides the most accurate and timely information that is critical for controlling the spread of epidemics and for preventing premature deaths. Passive surveillance, on the other hand, is based on people accessing health institutions to inform about their health conditions and health needs. The appropriateness, quality, and timeliness of information from passive surveillance, however, remains doubtful as it is driven by the people and not by the health system. Experience suggests that passive surveillance contributes little to controlling epidemics and to preventing premature deaths. An active health surveillance system is necessary for appropriate health system response to health care needs of the people. In India, an active health surveillance system does not exist in its totality. The Government of India has launched an Integrated Disease Surveillance Project, but the project relies primarily on passive surveillance.

2.5.2 Diagnosis

Diagnosis includes testing. In combination with an active health surveillance system, diagnosis constitutes the first but the most critical line of defence to safeguard people from infections, diseases, and premature deaths. The weakness of the health system in India in this context has amply been highlighted during the COVID-19 pandemic. It is imperative that every health institution must have a testing and diagnosis facility as an integral component. The current scenario, however, leaves much room in this context. At the national level, it has been decided to establish a public health laboratory in every district of the country, but the progress is painstakingly slow. Out of more than 700 districts of the country, a public health laboratory could be approved in only 250 districts as of March 2017 and very little is known about how many of these are functional. There has been vast expansion of testing and diagnosis facilities in the private sector, but this expansion has virtually been confined to large metropolitan towns and cities only. In the vast rural tracts of the country, there are bare minimum testing and diagnosis facilities which hinder the appropriate health system response to the health care needs of the people.

2.5.3 Epidemiology

The third indispensable process to meet the health care needs of the people is the capacity of the system to objectively investigate the disease process including unforeseen emergence of a disease or any other health emergency or epidemiology. Epidemiology is the process of identifying the causes of health outcomes and diseases in the population. Epidemiology treats patients as community and individuals are viewed collectively. Epidemiology is defined as the scientific, systematic, and data-driven study of the frequency and pattern (distribution) and causes and risk factors (determinants) of health-related states and events (including diseases) in the population and the application of this knowledge to the control of health problems (Centers for Disease Control & Prevention, 2012). Epidemiology provides the much-needed data-driven or empirical evidence for planning and programming health care services to meet the health needs of the people. The planning and programming for health care services is directed towards putting in place the necessary infrastructure and setting in motion necessary health processes to achieve the desired output in terms of both public health response and individual treatment and care.

Epidemiological activities in India have virtually been limited to the investigation of outbreaks of diseases, especially, communicable diseases. Ideally, epidemiological services must be able to investigate and diagnose health-related problems and hazards being faced by the people that can serve as the basis for planning and programming of health care services to achieve the desired level of output. This means that epidemiological services must be proactive in nature rather than reactive in scope as is the case at present. It is imperative that epidemiological services must regularly provide the information about the health-related problems and hazards being faced by the people so that this information can constitute the basis for planning and programming health care services delivery to meet the health needs of the people. Since health-related problems and health hazards facing people are dynamic in nature, the task of investigating and diagnosing health-related problems and hazards facing people must be a regular activity of the health system.

It may also be emphasised that epidemiological services should be distinguished from the process of health surveillance. Health surveillance, whether passive or active, is limited to the observation of the health state, primarily occurrence of diseases and ailments in the community, whereas epidemiological services are dedicated to the investigation and diagnosis of the prevailing health state—health problems and health hazards facing people. The scope of epidemiology is different from that of health surveillance.

2.6 Health System Output

The health system response to health care needs of the people constitutes the output of the health system. Responding to the health care needs of the people and minimising the impact of health emergencies require leveraging both health infrastructure and health processes. The inability of the health system to effectively respond to health care needs of the people exposes the system to critical gaps in services delivery which have a negative impact on the health and well-being of the people. This negative impact, in turn, affects the efficiency of the health system. The health system response to health care needs of the people is also the public face of the health system which contributes significantly towards building the community confidence in the system.

The health system response to health care needs of the people can be divided into public health response and personal health care or individual care and treatment. Public health response is related to the health of the population, with the expression of illness found in the lives of individuals. Personal health care, on the other hand, is directed towards the individual patient, within the context of the family and the community. For the health system, the two categories of health response provide distinct yet complementary perspectives. Public health response is primarily directed towards the prevention of diseases and premature deaths. Personal health care stresses prevention, diagnosis, and treatment of ailments in individuals. Personal health care is a well-established health profession with a sharp public image whereas public health response is characterised by multiple professional identities and diffused public image. Both are complementary and reinforce each other and, in combination, decide the output of the health system. Integration of the two components of the health system output is needed to promote the overall efficiency and effectiveness of the health system and achieve gains in population health. The health system cannot effectively respond to health needs of the people by either focussing on personal health care or promoting public health action. Public health action alone cannot stop all illnesses and prevent all premature deaths just as personal health care cannot reduce health hazards facing the people.

The health system output or response to health care needs of the people may be both pro-active and reactive. A proactive response is directed towards safeguarding the entire population from different health hazards and health emergencies thereby preventing premature deaths. The reactive response waits for the people to access the health system for the treatment and cure of diseases and ailments. In the context of population health, the scope of the reactive response is, at best, limited because a large section of the population may not be able to access the health system for many reasons both endogenous and exogenous to the health system. This is particularly the case with the vulnerable and the marginalised sections of the community, although health care needs of these sections of the community, incidentally, are the most demanding. It is imperative that the health system reaches out to all people to prevent diseases and avoid premature deaths rather than waiting for the people to access the system.

There is currently little idea about the nature of the health system response to health care needs of the people. Since health care needs of the people are very diverse and dynamic in nature, it is obvious that the health system must be an adaptive system rather than a normative one so as to better respond to the health care needs of the people. One requirement to ensure that the health system is adaptive rather than normative is the regular measurement and monitoring of health system response to the health care needs of the people. Such a measurement and monitoring system is also necessary to provide an evidence-based impetus for investment in the health infrastructure and for institutionalising health care processes. Since, the health system response to health care needs of the people is the public face of the health system, improving the response must be an intrinsic goal of the health system.

2.7 Evolution of Health System in India

The evolution of the health system in India can be traced back to the Health Survey and Development Committee, also known as Bhore's Committee, constituted in 1943. The Committee recommended a long-term programme and a short-term programme of the development of health services for the people of the country (Government of India, 1946). The long-term programme proposed by the Committee comprised of establishing 150 primary units, 6 secondary units, and 1 district unit in every district of the country. This programme was based on the assumption that the average population of a district, at that time, was around 3 million. The Committee, therefore, named this long-term programme as the Three Million Plan. Under this plan, every primary unit was envisaged to have a 75 bedded hospital facility; every secondary unit was envisaged to have 200 bedded hospital facility; and every district unit was envisaged to have 2500 bedded hospital facility so that the total number of beds available in a district with a population of 3 million would have been 17,000. In other words, the Three Million Plan recommended by the Committee, when implemented, would have resulted in a bed-population ratio of 5.67 beds per 1000 population. The long-term plan was to be implemented over a period of 30–40 years.

The Health Survey and Development Committee also recommended a short-term programme which was to be implemented in a duration of 10 years. This plan envisaged establishing a primary health unit for every 40 thousand population with each unit having a dispensary with 2 emergency and 2 maternity beds; establishing a 30 bedded hospital facility for every 2 primary units over a period of 10 years; and a secondary health unit with a 200 bedded hospital facility for every 12–13 primary units. The Committee envisaged that, at the end of the short-term programme or after a period of 10 years, there would be 23 primary units each with a dispensary having 4 beds—2 emergency and 2 maternity beds—13 hospitals, each with 30 beds, 2 secondary units, one with a hospital having 200 beds, and the other having a hospital having 500 beds capacity for every 1 million population. The short-term programme, thus, aimed at a bed-population ratio of 1.18 beds per 1000 population.

After the independence in 1947, the Government of India constituted the Health Survey and Planning Committee in 1959 which is popularly known as the Mudaliar Committee (Government of India, 1962). This Committee recommended that the development of health services for the people of the country should aim at achieving the norm of 1 bed for every 1000 population. To achieve this norm, the Committee proposed that (1) there should be one 10-bedded primary health centre and three 4-bedded primary health centres for every 40 thousand population; (2) there should be one sub-district level hospital with at least 50 beds capacity; and (3) the bed strength of the district level hospital should be between 300 and 500 beds. After the Health Survey and Planning Committee or the Mudaliar Committee, the Government of India constituted Committees from time to time to recommend steps to be taken for the reorganisation, expansion and strengthening of the health system in the country to meet the health care needs of the people, but none of these Committees dealt with the issue of organisation of the health system in the context of improving the health system response to the health care needs of the people. The current evidence suggests that there is still substantial scope in improving the health system response to the health care needs of the people in the country. One implication of far from satisfactory health system in response to the health care needs of the people is that population health in India remains low by international standards as is reflected from the life expectancy at birth which is the most commonly used indicator of population health (United Nations, 2022).

The Government of India currently follows a population-based normative approach for the creation of health institutions in the country. These norms are given in Table 2.2 and are different for rural and urban areas of the country (Government of India, 2022e). In the rural areas, the norms followed by the Government of India ensure, at least in principle, universal coverage of the population through the health system which is a hierarchical system. This is, however, not the case with the norms laid down for the urban areas. It is argued that there is a very strong presence of the private health care services in the urban areas and, therefore, a health system similar to that in the rural areas is either not necessary or not desired. It is, however, well-known that a substantial proportion of the urban population of the country remains uncovered through either the government or the private health system. At the same time, there remains substantial gap between the number of health institutions required according to the norms laid down by the government of India and the number of health institutions in existence. The Government of India has also laid down public health standards for different categories of health institutions in the context of the quality of health care services (Government of India, 2022a; 2022b; 2022c; 2022d). However, there is no system in place to measure and monitor the realisation of these public health standards at the health institution level. In the absence of such a measurement and monitoring system, there is no information about the proportion of different category of health institutions in the country either in rural or in urban areas which meet the public health standards and, therefore, ensure the quality of health care services delivered through the institution. It is well-known that there are substantial gaps in terms of both quantity and quality.

The norms laid down by the Government of India for establishing health institutions in the rural areas suggest that total number of hospital beds available in a population of 120 thousand is 54–60 which implies, in principle, one hospital bed for every 2000 population. This hospital bed-population ratio is in quite contrast to WHO recommendation of 5 hospital beds per 1000 population. The WHO recommendations imply that there should be 600 hospital beds for every 120 thousand population in the rural areas of the country. On the other hand, there is no specific norm or guidelines laid down by the Government of India for establishing secondary and tertiary level public health institutions except that there is one health institution in every district which is designated as the district hospital. Establishing secondary and tertiary level public health insti-

Table 2.2 Population norms for establishing primary health care institutions in India

SN	Health institution	Population norm	Bed facility
Rural areas			
1	Health sub-centre	For every 5000 population (3000 in hilly/tribal/hard to reach areas)	No bed facility
2	Primary health centre	For every 30,000 population (20,000 in hilly/tribal/hard to reach areas)	4–6 beds
3	Community health centre	For every 120,000 population (100,000 in hilly/tribal/hard to reach areas)	30 beds
Urban areas			
1	Community health centre	For every 250,000 population (500,000 for metro cities)	30–50 beds
2	Primary health centre	For every 50,000 population	No bed facility

Source Government of India (2022e)

tutions is largely arbitrary in the country and all these institutions are located in the urban areas resulting in a big gap in the availability of hospital beds in the rural areas as compared to that in the urban areas. Similarly, most of the private health institutions are also located in the urban areas, especially, in big towns and metropolitan areas so that there is a very heavy concentration of hospital beds in large metropolitan cities and big towns while there is serious paucity of beds in the rural areas and in small urban towns. The private health system of the country is heavily biased towards the personal health care component of the health system response at the cost of public health response to health care needs of the people.

2.8 Reinvigorating the Health System

The foregoing discussions suggest that there is a strong case for a comprehensive reinvigoration of the existing health system in India. This reinvigoration must be directed towards improving the health system response to the health care needs of the people and must focus on both public health response and personal health care or individual care and treatment. Personal health care has a sharp public image, yet it is the public health response that ultimately contributes to lasting gains in population health and contributes to the 'battle readiness' of the health system in meeting health emergencies such as the COVID-19 epidemic. In this context, it is proposed to adopt a hospital beds-based approach of reinvigorating India's health system. This approach is based on two cardinal principles. The first is that the reinvigoration of the health system should be based on the bed-population ratio. The second, on the other hand, is that health institutions should be as near to the people as possible. This principle was laid down by the Health Survey and Development Committee or the Bhore's Committee that was constituted way back in 1943.

The World Health Organization recommends that there should be 5 beds for every 1000 population, 1 doctor for every 1000 population or for every 5 beds, and 3 nurses per doctor (WHO, 2021). According to these norms, total hospital bed requirement in India is around 7 million assuming a projected population of 1392 million in 2023 (Government of India, 2020). Against this normative requirement, the actual number of beds available in the country are not known, although it is estimated that there are around 1.90 million hospital beds in the country—0.71 million in the public sector and 1.19 million in the private sector (Kapoor et al., 2020). This means that there is a shortage of more than 5 million hospital beds in the country with reference to the norm of 5 beds per 1000 population recommended by the World Health Organization. It is also estimated that around 70% of the available hospital beds are concentrated in large metropolitan towns and cities which implies that there is very significant distribution inequality in the hospital beds that are currently available in the country. This also means that any effort to reinvigorate the health system in the country should not only focus on increasing the number of hospital beds but must also address the very strong inequality in the distribution of hospital beds that currently persists in the country. Addressing this distribution inequality is the key to realise the second cardinal principle of reinvigorating the health system.

In other words, the foregoing calculations suggest that an additional 5 million hospital beds need to be created in the country to meet the norms recommended by the World Health Organization. This is a tall order and requires a massive expansion of health institutions. The National Health Policy 2017 of the country (Government of India, 2017) aims at universal access to good quality health care services through increasing access, improving quality, and lowering the cost of health care delivery but is conspicuously silent about the need of creating additional hospital beds which is imperative to achieve the goal of universal access to health care. The hospital bed-population ratio in India is currently very low by international standards. According to the estimates prepared by the World Health Organization, there were only 0.53 hospital beds per 1000 population in India in 2017 compared to more than 4.3 hospital beds per 1000 population in China and more than 4.1 hospital beds per 1000 population in Sri Lanka (WHO, 2021). Obviously, the hospital bed-population ratio in the country is grossly inadequate to realise the goal of universal access to good quality health care as emphasised in the National Health Policy 2017.

One approach to reinvigorating the health system in India may be based on the principle of increasing the availability of hospital beds in the country to achieve the norms laid down by the World Health Organization. This approach is justified in view of the demographic and epidemiological transition that the country is undergoing. Fertility in India has now decreased below the replacement level which implies that the population of the country will increasingly get older. On the other hand, the share of the non-communicable and degenerative diseases in the disease profile of the country is increasing. This means that the demand for the institution-based health care to meet the health needs of the people will increase in the coming years. The universal access to health care also demands that the inequality in the distribution of health institutions is decreased substantively so that the institution-based health care is available as near to the people as possible. In this context, creation of additional hospital beds in the country must also take into consideration the rural–urban distribution of population and the distribution of the urban population across different size class towns in the country.

Most of the population of the country lives in the rural areas. According to the population projections prepared by the Government of India, it is estimated that around 490 million or around 35% population of the country lives in the urban areas as defined at the time of 2011 population census while the remaining 65% population lives in more than 600 thousand villages as identified at the 2011 population census. The urban population of the country is very highly unequally distributed across different size class towns. However, it is estimated that more than 70% of the health institutions in the country are located in big cities and large metropolitan towns and majority of these health institutions are in the private sector. The result is that a large section of the population living in the rural areas, especially the poor and the marginalised ones, does not have access to health facilities to meet its health care needs. This unequal distribution of health institutions has implications for the health of the population and needs to be corrected in any reinvigoration of the health system.

The hospital bed-based approach of reinvigorating the health system will require both creation of new health institutions and expansion of existing ones. The increase in the number of health institutions is necessary for increasing the number of hospital beds as there is a limit to the number of beds that may be made available in a health institution. Moreover, increasing the number of health institutions is also necessary to realise the second cardinal principle of reinvigorating the health system which emphasises that the health institutions must be as near to the people as possible so that they are easily accessible. Easy accessibility of the health institution is one of the necessary requirements for the use of health care services available at the institution.

An astute distribution of hospital beds, therefore, is the first requirement for reinvigorating the health system. The first consideration in this direction is the distribution of hospital beds between public health institutions or the health institutions owned by the government and private health institutions. Health care services available through the private health institutions are available only at a cost and are concentrated in big cities and large metropolitan areas. These institutions, in general, provide curative health care services at the cost of preventive and promotive health care services. The accessibility of private health institutions to the people, especially, the poor and the marginalised ones is therefore limited.

It is, therefore, proposed that the number of hospital beds required in India according to the norms recommended by the World Health Organization should be distributed between public and private health institutions in 2:1 ratio. There should be around 4.7 million hospital beds in the public health institutions and 2.3 million hospital beds in the private health institutions. Hospital beds in public health institutions should be distributed equally between rural and urban areas so that there should be around 2.35 million hospital beds in rural public health institutions in around 2.35 million beds in urban public health institutions. Hospital beds in the urban areas should be distributed further across different size class towns according to the proportionate distribution of the urban population. Table 2.3 summarises the proposed distribution of hospital beds in the country. To realise the proposed distribution of hospital beds in the public health institutions, there is a need of increasing the number of hospital beds in the existing public health institutions and, at the same time, creating new public health institutions. Given the number of additional hospital beds required to meet the recommendations laid down by the World Health Organization, it is imperative that new public health institutions must be established, especially in the rural areas of the country. At present, there is a wide gap between the bed-population ratio in the urban areas and the bed-population ratio in the rural areas of the country. Similarly, bed-population ratio varies widely within the urban areas, across different size class towns. The reinvigoration of the public health system in the country must address the highly distorted distribution of hospital beds that currently exists in the country.

It is in the above context; the following framework is proposed for increasing the number of hospital beds in the existing public health institutions and for establishing new public health institutions to improve the hospital bed-population ratio in the country and to balance the distribution of hospital beds across urban and rural areas and across different size class towns in the urban areas:

1. Expand all existing Sub Health Centres and Primary Health Centres into Gram Panchayat Health Institution with at least 5 hospital beds. At present, there are 161,829 Sub Health Centres and 31,053 Primary Health Centres in the rural areas of the country (Government of India, 2022e). Sub Health Centres do not have hospital beds at present while the number of hospital beds in the Primary Health Centres ranges between 6 and 10.
2. Establish a public health institution having at least 5 hospital beds in all those Gram Panchayats which, currently, do not have a public health institution. This will make sure that every Gram Panchayat of the country (approximately 300 thousand) has a public health institution of its own with at least 5 hospital beds to meet the health needs of the people of the Gram Panchayat.
3. Every Gram Panchayat Health Institution will have at least 1 Health Officer and 3 Nurses as recommended by the World Health Organization.
4. Increase the number of beds in the existing Community Health Centres to at least 50 hospital beds in every Community Health Centre. At present, there are 6064 Community Health Centres in the country (Government of India, 2022e). These Community Health Centre would serve as the first referral unit (FRU) to the Gram Panchayat Health Institutions.
5. Establish a Community Health Centre with at least 50 hospital beds in all those development blocks of the country which, currently, do not have a Community Health Centre to serve as the first referral point for the grass roots level Gram Panchayat Health Institutions.
6. Every Community Health Centre must have at least 10 doctors and 30 Nurses as recommended by the World Health Organization.
7. Increase the number of hospital beds in every district hospital of the country to 500 beds. The district hospital would serve as the second referral unit for Community Health Centres and Gram Panchayats health institutions. The district hospital should have at least 100 doctors and 300 Nurses. The district hospital may be attached to the district medical college to serve as the teaching hospital also. The Government of India has already launched a scheme to establish a medical college in every district of the country.
8. Establish at least one public health institution in every urban local body of the country. The number of beds in the public health institution of the urban local body should be in proportion to the population of the urban local body. Urban local bodies are usually divided further into municipal zones and municipal

Table 2.3 Proposed distribution of hospital beds in India to comply with the norms recommended by the World Health Organization

Institution	Beds		Doctors		Nurses	
	Number	%	Number	%	Number	%
Public	4,485,000	64.0	897,000	64.0	2,691,000	64.0
Rural	2,235,000	31.9	447,000	31.9	1,341,000	31.9
Gram panchayat	1,500,000	21.4	300,000	21.4	900,000	21.4
Janpad panchayat	360,000	5.1	72,000	5.1	216,000	5.1
District panchayat	375,000	5.4	75,000	5.4	225,000	5.4
Urban	2,250,000	32.1	450,000	32.1	1,350,000	32.1
Class I	500,000	7.1	100,000	7.1	300,000	7.1
Class II	500,000	7.1	100,000	7.1	300,000	7.1
Class III	650,000	9.3	130,000	9.3	390,000	9.3
Class IV	370,000	5.3	75,000	5.4	225,000	5.4
Class V	200,000	2.9	40,000	2.9	120,000	2.9
Class VI	30,000	0.4	5000	0.4	15,000	0.4
Private	2,515,000	35.9	503,000	35.9	1,509,000	35.9
Total	7,000,000	100.0	1,400,000	100.0	4,200,000	100.0

Source Author

zones are further divided into municipal wards for administrative and development purposes. In those urban local bodies where there are more than one municipal zones, a public health institution may be established in every municipal zone depending upon the population in the zone.

9. The remaining hospital beds required to comply with the recommendations of the World Health Organization may be created in the private sector.

Table 2.3 summarises the proposed distribution of hospital beds in the country. Almost one third of the hospital beds will be available in the public health institutions in the rural areas of the country while another one third will be available in the public health institutions in the urban areas which means that around two-third of the total hospital beds in the country will be available in the public health institutions. The remaining one third of beds will be available in the private health institutions.

Table 2.3 also gives the number of doctors and the number of nurses required as recommended by the World Health Organization. Provision of the adequately trained and skilled manpower as per the norms laid down by the World Health Organization is critical for the effective utilisation of hospital beds. If the manpower is inadequate either in numbers or in skill, hospital beds will remain largely unutilised or under-utilised as is the case at present. It is, therefore, imperative that any effort to increase the number of hospital beds must invariably be associated with the effort to make the necessary manpower available so that hospital bed facility is optimally and effectively utilised. There is little sense in augmenting the hospital bed facility without meeting the recommended health manpower requirements.

In the above context, it may be pointed out that Government of India has already launched a centrally sponsored scheme of establishing a medical college with an intake capacity of 100 in every district of the country (Government of India, no date). The scheme is currently limited to under-served districts. In order to meet the health manpower requirements of the proposal of increasing the number of hospital beds to meet the WHO norms, it is suggested that the scheme of the Government of India may be extended to all districts which do not currently have a medical college. Moreover, medical colleges to be established under the scheme should not be restricted to training only doctors but should also be engaged in the training of nurses. Establishment of a medical college, in every district, it is expected, will be able to meet the health manpower requirement of the health institutions, especially, the public health institutions in the district.

The last and the most crucial requirement of increasing the number of hospital beds to meet the WHO standards is the mobilisation of financial resources. In this context, it is proposed that a specific proportion (ideally 6%) of the allocation to the state government by the central government and to Panchayats by the state government may be marked exclusively for increasing the number of hospital beds and associated physical and other infrastructure in the public health institutions while the capital cost of creating new public health institutions may be shared by the central government and the state government. Other innovative and time trusted approaches may also be used to generate financial resources for increasing the number of hospital beds. One such approach is the Patient Welfare Committee (*Rogi Kalyan Samiti*) which has been introduced under the National Rural Health Mission. At present, the Patient Welfare Committee is constituted in every public health institution of the country. It is suggested that a pool of resources may be created out of the funds generated by Patient Welfare Committees in every district and these funds may be used for increasing the number of hospital beds.

2.9 Conclusion

The public health care delivery system that currently exists in India was conceptualised more than 50 years ago when infectious and parasitic diseases were the primary cause affecting the health of the people. The scenario has now changed significantly and non-communicable, degenerative disease are the primary cause affecting the health of the population. It is obvious that, with the epidemiological transition, the public health care delivery system must also evolve. This has, however, not happened in India, although the need of such an evolution has repeatedly been emphasised in different policy documents. The need of reinvigorating the health system in India is also justified from the observation that, by international standards, the health of the people of the country remains poor as reflected from the low rank of the country in the life expectancy at birth in relation to other countries of the world.

This paper proposes a hospital beds-based approach of reinvigorating the public health care delivery system in India with the objective of meeting the hospital bed-population norms recommended by the World Health Organization. The approach outlined in the paper calls for increasing the number of hospital beds in the existing public health institutions and creating new public health institutions so as to achieve a balanced distribution of hospital beds which, currently, happens to be highly skewed. The essential idea of the approach outlined in the paper is that the health facilities must be as near to the people as possible so as to make them efficient as well as effective.

References

Centers for Disease Control and Prevention. (2012). *Introduction to epidemiology*. Atlanta, Georgia, Centres for Disease Control and Prevention.

Chaurasia, A. R. (2023). Seventy years of mortality transition in India 1950–2021. *Indian Journal of Population and Development, 3*(1), 1.

Government of India. (no date). *Guidelines for centrally sponsored scheme establishment of new medical colleges attached with existing district/referral hospitals.* New Delhi, Government of India, Ministry of Health and Family Welfare, Medical Education Division.

Government of India. (1946). *Report of the health survey and development committee.* Manager of Publications.

Government of India. (1962). *Report of the health survey and planning committee.* Manager of Publications.

Government of India. (2017). *National health policy.* New Delhi, Ministry of Health and Family Welfare.

Government of India. (2020). *Population projections for India and states 2011–2036.* New Delhi, Ministry of Health and Family Welfare, National Commission on Population.

Government of India. (2021). *Operational guidelines for PM Ayushman Bharat health infrastructure mission.* New Delhi, Ministry of Health and Family Welfare.

Government of India. (2022a). *Indian public health standards. Sub-district hospital and district hospital* (Vol

I). New Delhi, Ministry of Health and Family Welfare, National Health Mission.

Government of India. (2022b). *Indian public health standards. Community health centre* (Vol II). New Delhi, Ministry of Health and Family Welfare, National Health Mission.

Government of India. (2022c). *Indian public health standards. Health and wellness centre-primary health centre.* Vol III. New Delhi, Ministry of Health and Family Welfare, National Health Mission.

Government of India. (2022d). *Indian public health standards. Health and wellness centre-sub health centre* (Vol IV). New Delhi, Ministry of Health and Family Welfare, National Health Mission.

Government of India. (2022e). *Rural health statistics 2021–22.* New Delhi, Ministry of Health and Family Welfare. Statistics Division.

Kapoor, G., Hauck, S., Sriram, A., Joshi, J., Schueller, E., Frost, I., Balasubramanian, R., Laxminarayan, R., & Nandi, A. (2020). State-wise estimates of current hospital beds, intensive care unit (ICU) beds and ventilators in India: Are we prepared for a surge in COVID-19 hospitalizations? *MedRxiv.* https://doi.org/10.1101/2020.06.16.20132787

United Nations. (2022). *World population prospects 2022 revision.* New York, Department of Economic and Social Affairs. Population Division.

WHO. (2021). *Hospital beds (per 10000 population).* Geneva, World Health Organization, Global Health Observatory. https://www.who.int/data/gho/data/indicators/indicator-details/GHO/hospital-beds-(per-10-000-population)

3 An Investigation into India's Experience in Reducing Child Mortality: A Gender Perspective

Usha Ram, Prakash Kumar, and K. V. Ananya

Abstract

India surpassed China and became the most populated country recently. The population of India is expected to further grow for several decades before it stabilizes. The recent past has shown remarkable improvements in socio-economic development indicators for India, yet, they are far from satisfactory levels. India's health care service provisions, particularly in the public sector, continues to face challenges in terms of both access and quality. India is one of the few countries where gender plays a vital role for one's socio-economic and health outcomes. Thus, India's overall achievement in improving the health of its people is certainly laudable; however, it becomes essential to learn whether these benefits are shared equally across population subgroups. Between 1950 and 2020, India's population grew from 357 million to 1396 million; a nearly 300% rise in 7-decades, with an increase from a total of 15.7 million to 23.1 million annual live births during the same time. The childhood mortality has reduced substantially: infant mortality rate reduced substantially from 181.2 in 1950 to 26.6 per 1000 live births in 2020, and the under-5 mortality rate, reduced from around 300 in 1950 to 32.6 per 1000 live births in 2020. In 1950, a newborn in India, on an average, lived 41.7 years which rose to 70.2 years in 2020. Along with this progress in mortality reductions, household's living conditions and other socio-economic development indicators have also shown laudable improvements; 95% of the households in 2019–21 have access to improved source of drinking water and 69% had access to basic sanitation services. Women's literacy rate increased from only 2 in every 5 women aged 15–49 literate in 1992–93 to 4 in every 5 women in 2019–21 and total fertility rate declined from 3.4 children per women to 2.0 during the same period. Over 85% of the mothers received antenatal care from a skilled provider(s) in 2019–21, substantial increase from 50% in 1992–93. The institutional delivery increased from about one-quarter in 1992–93 to 89% in 2019–21. Early initiation of breastfeeding has risen more than four-folds and exclusive breastfeeding has risen by one and a half times and at the same time, the coverage of full immunization has increased to more than three-quarters in 2019–21. There has been consistent improvement in the mortality indicator as well as socio-economic and health care utilization, however, gender differential is persistent, mostly to the

U. Ram (✉) · P. Kumar · K. V. Ananya
International Insitute for Population Sciences, Deonar, Mumbai, India
e-mail: usharamagrawal@gmail.com

S. S. Acharya et al. (eds.), *Paradigm Shifts in Population and Health in India*, Sustainable Development Goals Series, https://doi.org/10.1007/978-981-95-1719-0_3

disadvantage of female children, and this is regardless of time period.

3.1 Introduction

The United Nation's latest global population projections suggest that India surpassed the population of mainland China in April 2023 (United Nations, 2022a, 2022b) and became the most populous country with respect to population. Further, the same projections suggested that India will continue to experience positive population growth for several decades in future. This implicates both opportunities as well as challenges in all areas of life—from socio-economic to public health for India. Most of the socio-economic development indicators for India, although suggest improvements in the recent past, however, they are far from satisfactory levels (Balarajan et al., 2011; Paul et al., 2011). Additionally, India health care service provisions, particularly in the public sector, continues to face challenges in terms of both access and quality (Rao et al., 2011).

India is one of the few countries where gender plays a vital role for one's socio-economic and health outcomes. The recently published Global Gender Gap Report (World Economic Forum, 2023) tracked the progress of countries in economic participation and opportunity, educational attainment, health and survival and political empowerment based on the current state and evolution of gender parity. According to the report, India ranked at 127th place out of 146 countries. In health and survival, India slipped further down to 142nd place only above Qatar, Vietnam, China and Azerbaijan. Thus, India's overall achievement in improving the health of its people is certainly laudable; however, it becomes essential to learn whether these benefits are shared equally across population subgroups. In other words, it needs to be understood if these improvements have systematically been less fruitful for a particular gender or group.

Given not so conducive socio-economic context, India has achieved impressive reductions in mortality of its people in general and that of its infants and children in particular. Similar to other Asian nations, although India started its health transition at a low life expectancy at birth (LEB) around 24.8 years in 1920s, however, it increased to 62 years by the end of the century (Riley, 2005). The average life expectancy of the global population was 73.3 years in 2019 (WHO, 2021). The latest estimates of the Registrar General of India (RGI, 2014–18) indicated that the average life expectancy at birth was 69.4 years during 2014–18. According to the 2019 World Development Indicators data (WDI, 2021), India was only ahead of Pakistan and Afghanistan in terms of life expectancy at birth among South Asian countries. Further, there is a significant difference among and between national populations, distinction by sex and place of residence (Borah, 2021). Crimmins et al. (2019) compared life expectancy at birth in 198 countries between 1960 and 2016 and noted that unlike past, female now live longer than the males resulting in greater number of women in the population at the older ages. India witnessed this scenario, rather recently, in 1983 when for the first time its female life expectancy at birth exceeded that of males (Office of Registrar General, 2022; 55.7 versus 55.4 years). Nonetheless, Borah (2021) found that the mortality declines at younger ages have benefitted Indian males more than the females.

India has shown remarkable declines in the under-5 mortality rate (U5MR) and was successful in meeting the Millennium Development Goals for child mortality in 2015. For example, nationally, the sample registration system (SRS) India estimated U5MR of 208 deaths per 1000 live births in 1971 and 101 in 2000 (Office of Registrar General, 1982, 2003). This translated into an annual average reduction of 4% in three decades. The past decade has witnessed an accelerated pace of reduction in child mortality in India. For example, the U5MR nationally declined to 59 in 2010 from 32 in 2020 (Office of Registrar General, 2012, 2022). Similar to the child mortality, the infant mortality rate (IMR) in India also showed remarkable progress over the years. The IMR declined from 129 infant deaths per 1000 live births in 1971 to 68 in 2000 and further to

28 in 2020 (Office of Registrar General, 2003, 2022). However, the declines in child mortality is not similar across population subgroups or geographies. The improvements varied by socio-economic indicators including gender, place of residence, and regions or states.

India is one of the few countries where mortality levels among girl children is higher than that for the boys (Chao et al., 2018; Murthi et al., 1995; Ram et al., 2013). For example, Ram et al. (2013) found that out of 597 districts, there were 303 districts in India where mortality at ages 1–59 months was higher among girl children compared to the male children. The study further observed that these districts found in almost all states including progressive state like Kerala. Guilmoto et al. (2018) estimated that there are around excess of 18.5 under-5 mortalities among girls per 1000 live births than boys in 2000–2005) Further, the study also noted excess female mortality to be widespread and identified in 90% of India's districts, of which northern states of Uttar Pradesh, Bihar, Rajasthan, and Madhya Pradesh accounted for two-thirds of the total excess in female under-5 deaths.

Biological gender alone has nothing or minimal effect on the health or the mortality outcomes (Crimmins et al., 2019; Vlassoff, 2007). In the absence of gender-based discriminatory practices where both boys and girls are provided equal access to resources including food and healthcare, newborn boys are at a biological disadvantage of experiencing higher mortality (Sawyer, 2012). Yet, in several populations girl children are at greater disadvantages in terms of mortality outcome.

India is known as a pro-male biased patriarchal society by far (Bannerji, 2016; Singh et al., 2022). The gendered social norms expose girl children in extremely vulnerable situations for survival. This happens through a variety of reasons ranging from gender-based inequalities in healthcare access and utilization, breastfeeding practice (including initiation to intervening and duration of breastfeeding), negligence in treatment seeking for illness and immunization, unfair food allocation and dietary practices and so on even during infancy and childhood. Several studies (Arokiasamy, 2007; Fledderjohann et al., 2014; Mishra et al., 2004) have documented that the full immunization coverage rates were higher among boy children than the girl children in India. They further noted clear evidence of gender-based biases in the feeding practices with higher rate of breastfeeding among boy children than the girl children. Fledderjohann et al. (2014) observed that girl children, on average, were breastfed for almost half a month fewer than boys. Not only this, they also noted that if the older sibling was a female child, the second-born girl children had almost a month shorter duration of breastfeeding than boys. The study also revealed that the girl children were relatively less likely to consume fresh milk and breast milk.

Several other studies (Bose, 2011; Jose, 2017; Maitra & Rammohan, 2011; Pande, 2003) also pointed out these discriminatory practices against the girl children in the allocation of supplemental foods, including milk, meat, fish, and eggs and the prevalence of malnutrition—mainly stunting and underweight at national and state levels. The study by Mishra et al. (2004) revealed an interesting fact that discrimination against girls in exclusive breastfeeding had in fact benefitted the girl children since continued exclusive breastfeeding among boys even after 6 months resulted in the higher prevalence of diarrhea. Thus these differential gendered practices towards boy and girl children have long-term implications for their health and future development which go beyond childhood. Girls being less prioritized in allocating nutritious food can also have adverse effects on their physical and cognitive development, perpetuating a cycle of gender inequality and reduced life opportunities (Martins, 2011).

A systematic review of literature from South Asia (Ismail et al., 2019) found that treatment seeking rates for newborn females are lower than the newborn males; and in fact, parents are willing to pay more and seek care from health providers perceived to be of good quality for the treatment of son's illness than the sick girl newborn. Similar findings favoring boys with regard to the health treatment seeking behavior was found in many studies, especially for nutritional status and acute illness (Arokiasamy, 2007; Mishra et al., 2004).

These gender-based discriminatory practices are not restricted to post-birth situations alone. For example, Jha et al. (2011) found that the practice of pre-natal sex selection and sex selective abortions in India have increased notably. This has resulted in a skewed child male–female ratio in India in favor of earlier (Jha et al., 2006).

Over the years, various child health initiatives and policy interventions have been implemented in India to improve child health outcomes including the launch of National Rural Health Mission (NRHM) in 2005 (now known as the National Health Mission—NHM), Reproductive, Maternal, Newborn, Child, and Adolescent Health (RMNCH + A) approach, Janani Suraksha Yojana (JSY), and so on (Bhushan et al., 2023; Bora et al., 2019; Ram et al., 2023). However, whether these efforts have resulted in tangible improvements in addressing gender bias in child health outcomes is questionable. Given this perspective, through this study, we seek to assess gender disparities in child mortality over the years thoroughly, shed light on the factors driving these disparities and identify persistent challenges that hinder the achievement of equal opportunities for child health and survival, regardless of gender.

3.2 Data and Methods

For the current research, we primarily utilized three data sources: The World Population Prospect estimates and projections of the United Nations (United Nations, 2022a, 2022b), Economic survey of India (Ministry of Finance, 2023), and five rounds of National Family and Health Survey (International Institute for Population Sciences (IIPS) and ICF, 2021).

The latest revision of United Nation (UN) World Population Prospect (WPP) (Revision 2022) is the twenty-seventh edition of the official UN population estimates and projections (United Nations, 2022a, 2022b). It is prepared by the Population Division of the Department of Economic and Social Affairs of the UN Secretariat. The revision 2022, provides the comprehensive set of population and demographic estimates and projection from years 1950 to 2100 for 237 countries or regions. This latest edition has utilized the results of 1758 national population censuses conducted between 1950 and 2022, vital registration systems and 2890 nationally representative sample surveys. The UN population estimates are widely used for the calculation of many development indicators used by the United Nations system including indicators used to monitor the progress to achieve SDGs. This was the first incident where the estimates of all the demographic indicators are provided by single age and sex for 1-year interval. We have compiled data on population (as on July 1), number of live births, life expectancy at birth, infant mortality rate (IMR), under-5 mortality rate (U5MR) and sex ratio at birth (SRB) from the UN-WPP 2022. The Economic survey of India was used to assess the change in the per-capita income of the population in India over time.

The changes in the levels of associated socio-economic and demographic indicators have been examined using data from the five rounds of National Family and Health survey, a nationally representative survey implemented by International Institute for Population Sciences, Mumbai conducted during 1992–93 (NFHS1), 1998–99 (NFHS2), 2005–06 (NFHS3), 2015–16 (NFHS4) and 2019–21 (NFHS5). The NFHS surveys are a nationally representative household survey. The surveys use a multistage stratified sampling design. Except for the first round of NFHS, all the rounds collected information from ever married women aged 15–49 years of age. The sample size in each round was increased to have more reliable and realistic estimates of the indicator. While the first three rounds of the NFHS (NFHS1, NFHS2 and NFHS3) were implemented at the state level, the NFHS4 and NFHS5 were implemented at the district level. The NFHS data provides array of information related to household characteristics, population composition and characteristics, fertility, family planning, morbidity and treatment seeking behavior, mortality, nutrition, child health, reproductive health, etc. We have used NFHS data in mainly two ways: estimation of indicators related to household wellbeing; and indicators related to gender differential. The detailed information on these surveys can be found at (https://rchiips.org/nfhs/index.shtml).

Additionally, we have calculated a few more indicators including India's share in global numbers for population size, livebirths, infant deaths, and under-5 deaths to assess the improvements and female advantage/disadvantage with respect to selected indicators of feeding practices, immunization and treatment seeking behavior of childhood illnesses.

3.3 Results

Table 3.1 presents trends in estimated population and live births of India for one and a half century (1950–2100) with an interval of 10 years. In the same table we also present life expectancy at birth, infant and child mortality including the gender gap for India for the same years. Additionally, we have included sex ratio at birth and share of female deaths in all deaths during infancy and childhood. The data is presented in two panels. The first panel gives the data for the past 7-decades (1950–2020) and the second panel gives the same for 2030–2100.

3.3.1 Period 1950–2020

Between 1950 and 2020, India's population grew from 357 million to 1396 million; a nearly 300% rise in the past 7-decades. India recorded a total of 15.7 million annual livebirths in 1950 and showed an upward trend until 2000, reaching 28.6 million. The number started to decline and reached 23.1 million annual livebirths in 2020. India is one of the few countries that had consistently showed a sex ratio at birth (SRB) skewed in favor of male babies. Until 1990, the SRB in India remained around 105–107 male births per 1000 female births, before reaching 110 in 2000 and 2010. The 2020 showed an improvement as the SRB declined to 108. Until 2010, share of female deaths during infancy and childhood revolved close to 50%, however, it declined to 48.7% for each in 2020.

The childhood mortality has also revealed tremendous improvement over the years. The infant mortality, defined as death among newborn before celebrating first birthday per 1000 livebirths, reduced substantially from 181.2 in 1950 to 67.8 in 2000 and further to 26.6 in 2020. Similarly, the under-5 mortality rate, defined as death among newborn before celebrating fifth birthday per 1000 livebirths, reduced markedly from close to 300 in 1950 to 91.5 in 2000 and further to 32.6 in 2020. It is important to note that the male children have huge survival advantage over their female counterparts during the infancy and childhood in India. Nonetheless, the male advantage is reducing over time. For example, for every 1000 livebirths in India, compared to the male babies, on an average, additional 8.6 and 15.6 female infants and children, respectively, died in 1950. This gender gap, reduced to 6.3 and 9.6 deaths per 1000 live births during infancy and childhood, respectively, in 2000 and less than 1 death per 1000 livebirths in 2020.

In 1950, a newborn in India, on an average, lived 41.7 years which rose to 62.7 years in 2000 and further to 70.2 years in 2020. However, the average life expectancy at birth differed notably for male and female newborn, mostly to the disadvantage of the later. For example, until 1970, a male newborn in India lived an average of 1.3–1.8 years longer than the female newborn in the same year. Nonetheless, post 1970, the female disadvantage for the first time turned into female advantage as the female life expectancy at birth exceeded by 0.2 years than that of males in 1980. This female advantage has been widening since then reaching 3.2 years in 2020.

3.3.2 Period 2020–2100

In April 2023, India's population reached 1425.8 million making it the most populous country in the world surpassing China's population (1425.7 million; United Nations, 2022a, 2022b). India as a nation is expected to experience positive population growth until 2060 before it starts declining in 2070 reaching 1529.9 million by the end of

Table 3.1 Trends in population size, livebirths, share of female deaths in all infant and under-5 deaths, infant and under-5 mortality rate (per 1000 live births) and life expectancy at birth (in years) and gender gap, India (1950–2100)

Year	Population (in million)	Livebirths (in million)	Share of female deaths in total deaths during*		IMR (per 1000 live births)		U5MR (per 1000 live births)		Life expectancy at birth (in years)	
			Infancy	Childhood	Person	Excess female mortality*	Person	Excess female mortality*	Person	Female disadvantage*
Panel: 1950–2020										
1950	357.0	15.7	49.9	50.3	181.2	8.6	283.7	15.5	41.7	−1.8
1960	446.0	19.0	49.9	50.1	158.2	7.3	242.5	13.0	45.2	−1.4
1970	557.5	22.0	49.7	49.9	141.7	5.8	213.5	10.2	48.2	−1.3
1980	696.8	25.2	49.6	49.8	115.2	5.5	168.1	9.2	53.6	0.2
1990	870.5	27.7	49.7	49.9	89.8	5.0	126.1	8.1	58.7	1.7
2000	1059.6	28.6	50.0	50.4	67.8	6.3	91.5	9.6	62.7	1.9
2010	1240.6	26.6	50.0	50.3	45.2	4.2	58.1	6.0	66.9	3.3
2020	1396.4	23.1	48.7	48.7	26.6	0.6	32.6	0.8	70.2	3.2
Percentage (%) change										
1950–2000	196.8	82.8	0.2	0.2	−62.6		−67.7		50.2	
2000–2020	31.8	−19.1	−2.8	−3.3	−60.8		−64.3		11.9	
1950–2020	291.1	47.8	−2.5	−3.2	−85.3		−88.5		68.1	
Panel: 2030–2100										
2030	1515.0	22.5	45.8	46.0	18.5	−2.0	23.2	−2.3	73.7	3.5
2040	1611.7	20.9	43.9	44.3	12.7	−2.5	16.0	−2.8	75.9	3.8
2050	1670.5	19.2	43.5	44.0	9.2	−1.9	11.6	−2.2	77.9	3.8
2060	1695.3	18.1	44.4	45.0	7.1	−1.2	8.9	−1.3	79.7	3.6
2070	1690.2	16.9	46.0	46.6	5.6	−0.6	7.0	−0.6	81.5	3.2
2080	1654.9	15.5	47.9	48.6	4.5	−0.2	5.6	−0.0	83.1	2.6
2090	1597.9	14.6	49.3	50.1	3.8	0.1	4.6	0.3	84.6	2.3
2100	1529.9	13.6	50.1	51.0	3.2	0.2	3.9	0.4	86.0	2.1
Percentage (%) change										
2020–2050	19.6	−17.2	−10.7	−9.7	−65.5		−64.5		11.0	
2050–2100	−8.4	−29.2	15.3	16.0	−65.0		−66.1		10.4	
2020–2100	9.6	−41.4	3.0	4.8	−87.9		−88.0		22.5	

Source UN world population prospects, 2022
* Authors calculation

the century in 2100. The decline in annual birth is to continue in future as well reaching 13.6 million in 2100. The SRB is likely to reach international level of 105 in next 2 decades or so and maintain it in future. The country is expected to achieve the SDG U5MR goal of 25 per 1000 livebirths a couple of years before 2030 and fall into single digit circa mid-century. Similar trends are expected for infant mortality. Nonetheless, female disadvantage in mortality during infancy and childhood is expected to continue until 2070 before equalizing or taking a marginal lead. The life expectancy at birth (LEB) is estimated to cross 75 years' mark in 2040 and 85 years by the end of the century. The female advantage in LEB is expected to maintain the levels observed during 2010 or later (3.2–3.8 years during 2030–70) before reaching 2.1–2.3 years at the end of the century.

3.3.3 Female and Male LEB in India and World (1950–2100)

Comparison of gender-specific life expectancy at birth for India with the levels estimated globally since the 1950s suggest that Indian female had been at a huge disadvantage (Fig. 3.1 and Annexure 1). On an average, in the 1950, while a female newborn in world lived nearly 4 years longer than the newborn male, in India, they lived nearly 2 years shorter than the male newborn, suggesting an absolute disadvantage of 6 years. This female disadvantage in average life years lived by the Indian female newborn continued until 1980 before turning in favor of females matching global trend. However, the difference remains at around 2-years. For example, in 2000, globally females had advantage of nearly 4 years as against of just 2 years in India. By 2020, while Indian females live a little more than 3 years longer than the males, nonetheless, globally this difference was well over 5 years. The UN projections until 2100 show that this difference is likely to remain in future as well.

Likewise, comparison of infant and childhood mortality for boy and girl children show that the India girl children have huge disadvantage in survival during these ages since 1950s (Fig. 3.2 and Annexure 1). For example, in 1950, for every 1000 livebirth, an additional of 15.5 children below 5 years and 8.6 under the age one died than the male children. However, the female disadvantage in infant and child mortalities in India is closing over the years and very soon as the mortality levels for female during the infancy and childhood are likely to fall below the projected levels for male infants and children similar to the patterns observed globally.

3.3.4 India's Share in Global Population, Births, and Deaths

In 1950, one in every 7 people in the world was an Indian (Table 3.2). This number reached below 6 people during 2000 and expected to remain around this until 2060 before rising above 6 in subsequent decades. With regard to livebirths, one in every 6 births occurred in 1950 in the world was from India and this declined to less than 5 in 2000. This number started rising post 2000 reaching once again at 6 in 2020 and further expected to rise above 7 by mid-century and 8 or higher four decades later in 2090. India accounted for almost 21% and 23% of all global infant male and female deaths, respectively, in 1950. This share rose to 28% and 30%, respectively, in 1980 and started to decline thereafter. India's share reduced to about 15% of global male infant deaths and 17% of female infant deaths in 2020. This reduction is further expected to accelerate in future as by 2100, India's share in globally will be 3.4% and 5.6% for male and female infant deaths, respectively. Similar trends are seen for deaths among children below 5-years. India's share in global under-5 male deaths was a little over 20% in 1950 which reduced to below 16% in 2020. The corresponding numbers for female under-5 deaths are 22.6% and 15.7%, respectively. By the end of century, India is expected to have 3% of male under-5 global deaths and 5.1% of female under-5 global deaths.

3.3.5 Living Conditions and Socio-economic Context

To understand the contextual changes in India's socio-economic and development indicators including maternal health service utilization, we have compiled selected indicators for the past three decades (1992–2021) using data from five rounds of the national family health surveys implemented in 1992–93, 1998–99, 2005–06, 2015–16, and 2019–21 and other data sources. The same are presented in Table 3.3. The per-capita income for India compiled from the economic survey of India, measured as per-capita Gross National Income (GNI), has risen from 7690 INR during 1992–93 to 86,659 INR during 2019–20. Notably higher proportion of India's population now live in the urban areas than previously. About 28% of the surveyed people during

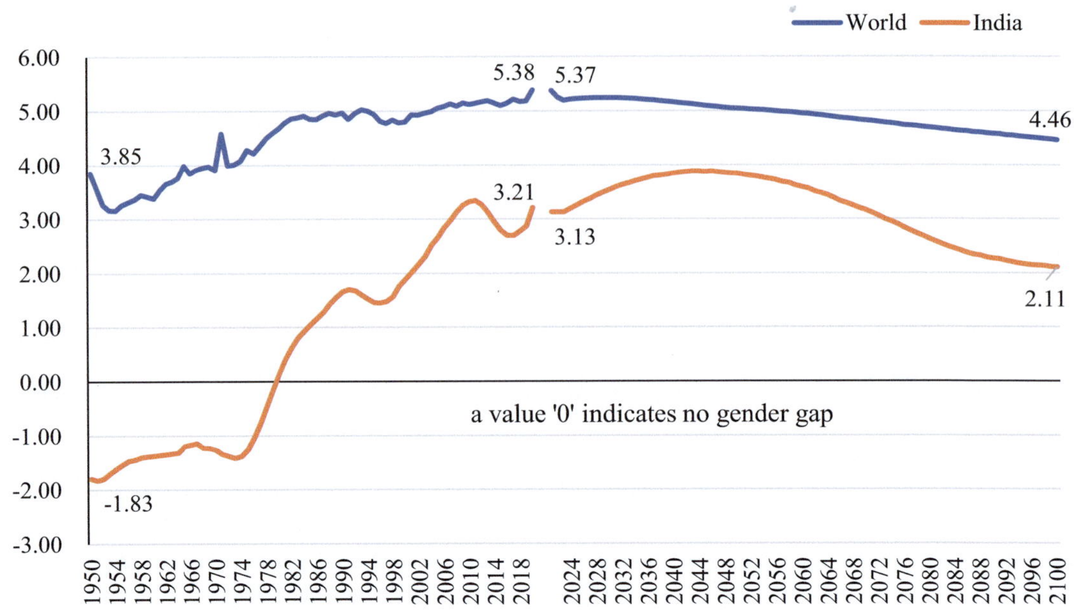

Fig. 3.1 Comparison of trends in gender gap for female and male life expectancy at births (in years), World and India (1950–2100)

the 1990s lived in urban areas which increased to slightly higher than 33% in 2019–21.

Over 95% of the households had access to improved source of drinking water, and 69% had access to basic sanitation services in 2019–21. Although about 19% of the households in 2019–21 reported that they go for open defecation, their proportion has consistently declined over the past three decades as nearly 70% of the households in the early 1990s practiced open defecation. Women's literacy rate has shown remarkable improvement over the past 30-years. For example, only 2 in every 5 women aged 15–49 in 1992–93 were literate, defined as ever attended school or could read either all or part of a sentence. The percentage of literate women improved to 3 in 2005–06 and further to 4 in 2019–21. Just about one-quarter of the households in 1992–93 had one or more women aged 15–49 years who had completed 10 or more years of education which increased to close to 50% in 2005–06. The percentage of such households increased to two-thirds in 2019–21.

3.3.6 Fertility and Contraceptive Use

The fertility levels in India have shown dramatic reduction over the past 2–3 decades. The total fertility rate (TFR, average number of children per woman) declined from 3.4 children per women to 2.0 during 1992–93 and 2019–21; a reduction of 1.4 children per woman. Between 1992–93 and 2005–06, the median age at first marriage among women aged 20–49 years rose by 0.8 years from 16.4 to 17.2 years. However, past 15 years (2005–06 to 2019–21) witnessed sharper rise in the median age at first marriage, the data also showed notable increase in the use of modern contraceptive methods among the currently married women. The rate of use of any modern contraceptive method rose from 22% during 1992–93 to around 49% in 2005–06 and further to 57% in 2019–21. Besides, use of modern spacing methods to space between two subsequent births too has shown improvements over the analysis period. For example, only 6% of

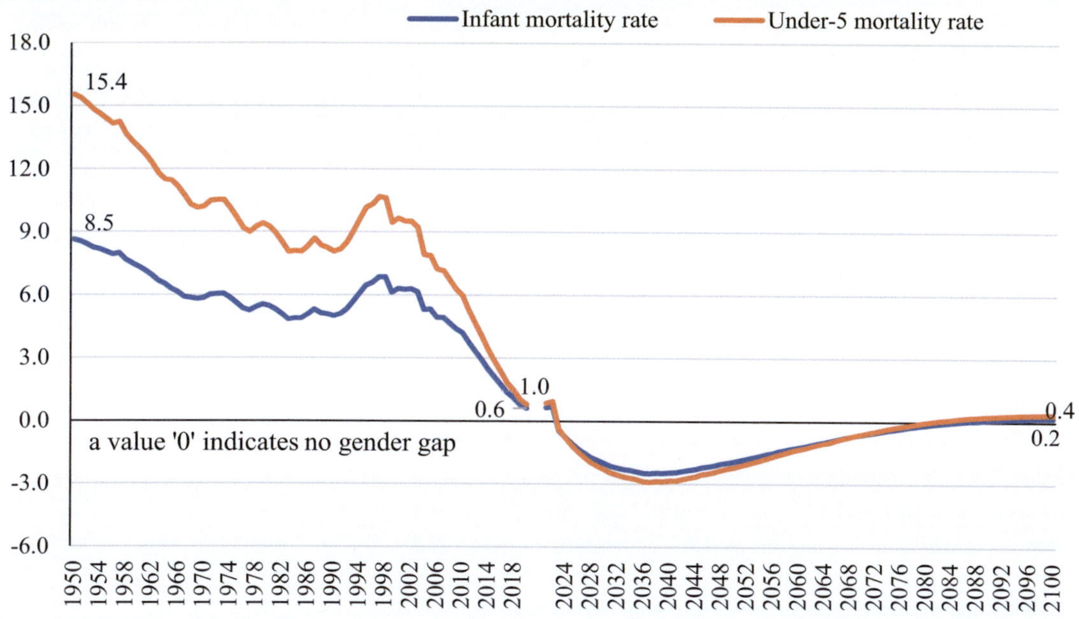

Fig. 3.2 Trends in gender differential in infant and under-5 mortalities per 1000 live births, India (1950–2100)

Table 3.2 India's share in the global population, livebirths, infant and under-5 deaths among male and female children, 1950–2100

Year	Population	Livebirths	Infant deaths		Under-5 deaths	
			Male	Female	Male	Female
Panel: 1950–2020						
1950	14.3	17.0	20.5	22.6	20.3	22.6
1960	14.8	18.5	20.7	22.6	19.3	20.9
1970	15.1	17.8	24.4	26.8	24.6	27.0
1980	15.7	19.9	27.2	29.9	27.2	29.9
1990	16.4	19.4	25.7	28.7	25.1	28.2
2000	17.2	21.4	25.5	29.1	24.2	27.8
2010	17.8	18.8	21.4	24.7	20.1	23.4
2020	17.8	17.1	15.2	17.1	14.0	15.7
Panel: 2030–2100						
2030	17.7	16.5	12.4	13.5	11.3	12.3
2040	17.5	15.1	9.4	10.1	8.4	9.1
2050	17.2	14.1	7.2	8.1	6.4	7.3
2060	16.8	13.9	6.0	7.4	5.3	6.6
2070	16.4	13.2	5.0	6.7	4.4	6.0
2080	15.9	12.6	4.1	6.2	3.6	5.6
2090	15.3	12.5	3.7	5.9	3.3	5.4
2100	14.8	12.2	3.4	5.6	3.0	5.1

Authors calculation using UN world population prospects, 2022 data

Table 3.3 Trends in selected socio-economic and development indicators and coverage of maternal health services, India (1992–93 to 2019–21)

Indicators	1992–3	1998–9	2005–6	2015–6	2019–21
Per-capita income (as per per-capita gross national income)$	7690	15,881	28,067	83,003	86,659
Population living in urban areas (%)	27.6	27.7	32.6	34.9	33.2
Households with improved source of drinking water (%)	94.4	80.2	88.5	94.0	95.9
Households with basic sanitation service (%)	23.3	29.2	29.1	48.5	69.3
Households using open defecation (%)	69.7	63.7	55.3	38.9	19.4
Women aged 15–49 years ever been to school or can read full or part of sentence (%)	38.9	47.0	60.2	73.7	78.9
Households with one or more women aged 15–49 years completed 10 or more years of education (%)	26.4	41.3	47.6	62.8	66.4
Total fertility rate (TFR, average number of children per woman)	3.4	2.9	2.7	2.2	2.0
Median age at first marriage among women aged 20–49 years	16.4	16.7	17.2	19.0	19.2
Proportion of women aged 20–24 years married before age 18 (%)	61.6	59.2	47.4	26.8	23.3
Currently married women using any modern contraceptive method (%)	22.3	42.9	48.5	47.8	56.5
Currently married and non-pregnant women using any modern spacing method (%)	6.1	7.4	11.0	12.3	19.2
Ever married women aged 15–49 years sterilized after having one or two daughters only (%)	2.1	2.6	3.7	5.5	5.8
Ever married women aged 15–49 years who were anaemic (%)	–	54.9	55.3	53.1	57.0
Children under-5 years who were anaemic (%)*	–	73.8	69.7	59.3	69.0
Children under-5 years who were stunted (%)*	51.5	53.7	48.0	38.4	35.5
Children under-5 years who were wasted (%)*	17.5	28.0	19.8	21.0	19.3
Child's birth size and weight					
Children who were smaller than average size at birth for gestational age (%)	21.4	22.9	21.3	12.6	11.2
Children who weighed less than 2.5 kg at the time of birth (%)	24.1	21.4	20.3	16.4	17.0
Maternal and child health service utilization					
Women who registered their pregnancy in first trimester (%)	24.9	33.2	44.3	58.7	70.2
Women who received antenatal care from skilled provider (%)*	50.1	59.7	73.2	79.3	85.1
Women who received full antenatal care (%)**	27.4	43.2	21.4	24.3	34.2
Institutional births out of all births (%)*	25.5	33.7	38.7	78.9	88.6
C-section births out of all births (%)*	2.5	7.1	8.5	17.2	21.5
Mother or child received one more postnatal check-up within 48 h of birth (%)	–	13.4	38.3	67.4	82.8
Children aged 12–23 months who were fully immunized (%)	35.4	39.4	43.5	62.0	76.4

Notes CPR stands for contraceptive prevalence rate; PNC for Postnatal care

$ Gross national income (per-capita) at constant price was taken from the economic survey of India (respective years)

* Livebirths in the 3 years preceding the survey is considered for 1997–8 (NFHS 2) and livebirths in 4 years preceding the survey is considered for 1992–3 (NFHS 1)

** In 1992–3 (NFHS1) and 1997–8 (NFHS2) women received IFA tablets/syrups is considered, since the number of days information is not there the currently married and non-pregnant women used any modern spacing method in 1992–93 which increased steadily to 11% in 2005–06 and nearly doubled to a little over 19% in 2019–21. Percentage of ever married women aged 15–49 years who were sterilized after 'only one or two daughters' increased from a meagre 2% in 1992–93 to 4% in 2005–06 and further to 6% in 2019–21. In other words, percentages of women adopting sterilization after only one or two daughters have nearly tripled during the past 3-decades.

3.3.7 Prevalence of Anaemia and Nutrition

In 1998–99, 55% of the women aged 15–49 years interviewed were anaemic. The percentages of anaemic women has remained somewhat similar or increased marginally to 57% in 2019–21. The nutritional status of the children, however, has shown improvement. Almost three-quarters of the children under 5 years of age were anaemic in 1997–98 which declined to 69% in 2019–21. The percentage of under-5 children who were stunted declined from 51.5% in 1992–93 to 48% in 2005–06 and 35.5% in 2019–21. However, the percentage of under-5 children who were wasted remained somewhat similar at around 18–19% during the analysis period. About one-fifth (21%) of the mothers in 1992–93 perceived their child to be smaller than the average for the gestational age. The proportion of such mothers has declined over the period reaching 11.2% in 2019–21.

Similarly, prevalence of low birth weight babies (newborn who weighed less than 2.5 kg at the time of birth) also declined from 24 to 17% between 1992–93 and 2019–21.

3.3.8 Maternal and Child Health Service Utilization

At the outset, it may be pointed out that all indicators used to assess coverage of maternal and child health service utilization have shown tremendous improvements over the analysis period. The data suggests that over 85% of the mothers received antenatal care from a skilled provider(s) in 2019–21, substantial increase from 50% in 1992–93. The data further reveals gain in percentages of mother who received full antenatal care (defined as mother who received 4 or more ANC visits, one or more TT Injections, consumed 100 or more IFA tablets/syrup when pregnant with the youngest surviving child). For example, fewer than one-quarter of mothers in 1992–93 had received full ANC. Number of such mothers increased to 31% in 2019–21. Only about one-quarter of mothers reportedly delivered their youngest surviving child in a health facility in 1992–93. The share of institutional deliveries increased to about 40% in 2005–06 and is currently at 89% in 2019–21. C-section delivery rate (percentage of c-section in all births) has increased many folds from only 2% in 1992–93 to 17.2% in 2015–16, reaching the WHO indicated c-section rates. In 2019–21, more than one-fifth of all births were c-section births. Only about 13% of either mother or newborn received a postnatal check-up within 48 h of birth in 1992–93. Percentage of mother-newborn who had a postnatal check-up jumped to 38% in 2005–06. Currently, close to 83% of mothers-newborn received their postnatal health check-up within 48 h of birth in 2019–21. The full immunization coverage among the children aged 12–23 years has more than doubled from 35% in 1992–93 to 44% in 2005–06 reaching 76% in 2019–21.

Table 3.4 presents trends in breastfeeding and feeding practices, immunization coverage and treatment seeking behavior for ill children overall and by gender in India over past three decades' period.

3.3.9 Breastfeeding Practices

While early initiation of breastfeeding has risen more than four-folds and exclusive breastfeeding has risen by one and a half times in the past three decades, pre-lacteal feeding has reduced to one-fourth the levels observed in 2005–06. Concurrently, the proportion of children below two years of age who received age appropriate breastfeeding

Table 3.4 Trends in levels of and gender gap in initiation of breastfeeding, pre-lacteal feeding, exclusive and age-appropriate breastfeeding, feeding/dietary practices, immunization, and prevalence and treatment seeking behavior for diarrhea, fever, and symptoms of acute respiratory infections among children and gender gap, India (1992–93 to 2019–21)

Indicator	Coverage levels					Gender gap (male–female indicator)				
	1992–3	1998–9	2005–6	2015–6	2019–21	1992–3	1998–9	2005–6	2015–6	2019–21
Breastfeeding practices										
Newborn was initiated breastfeeding within 1 h of birth (%)	9.3	16.0	23.1	41.5	41.4	0.12	0.24	0.04	−0.03	0.14
Newborn received a pre-lacteal feed (%)	–	–	57.7	21.1	15.5	–	–	−0.12	0.12	1.13
Children below 6 months exclusively breastfed (%)	43.3	46.8	46.4	54.9	63.7	–	–	1.15	2.46	−1.12
Children below 2 years received age appropriate breastfeeding (%)	56.2	58.1	67.7	65.8	63.2	–	–	1.53	1.10	0.96
Food/dietary practices for children aged 6–23 months										
Fed solid/semisolid food (%)	56.4	68.1	84.7	75.1	74.6	0.35	−1.66	0.63	−0.34	0.42
Fed milk/other milk products (%)	43.1	52.3	54.6	51.2	53.2	3.85	3.27	3.53	2.10	1.57
Fed a minimum diverse food (%)	–	–	12.8	19.8	23.6	–	–	−0.05	−0.55	0.14
Fed minimum meal frequency (%)	–	–	40.9	35.9	38.8	–	–	−0.22	1.16	−0.86
Fed a minimum acceptable diet (%)	–	–	8.3	9.6	11.4	–	–	0.42	0.30	0.13
Children aged 12–23 months who were fully immunized (%)	35.4	39.4	43.5	62.0	76.4	2.59	2.19	3.85	0.12	0.97
Prevalence and treatment for diarrhea among children										
Prevalence of diarrhea (%)	4.8	19.2	9.0	9.2	7.3	0.40	0.50	1.10	0.60	0.60
Sought advice/treatment (%)	65.4	70.6	68.1	76.8	76.2	3.73	2.57	2.11	2.15	1.09
Sought treatment within a day (%)	–	–	39.5	54.5	54.6	–	–	3.95	0.16	−0.14
Sought treatment from public health facility (%)	24.8	19.5	18.1	23.9	31.2	−1.73	1.32	2.21	−2.05	−1.11
Sought treatment from private health facility (%)	70.4	72.9	78.6	69.9	66.5	3.02	0.19	−2.55	2.89	1.12

(continued)

Table 3.4 (continued)

Indicator	Coverage levels					Gender gap (male–female indicator)				
	1992–3	1998–9	2005–6	2015–6	2019–21	1992–3	1998–9	2005–6	2015–6	2019–21
Prevalence and treatment for fever among children										
Prevalence of fever (%)	20.2	29.5	14.9	12.9	13.2	1.70	1.80	−1.10	1.00	1.10
Sought advice/treatment (%)	72.7	53.5	77.4	81.0	79.8	6.06	6.34	3.44	1.67	1.28
Sought treatment within a day (%)	–	–	45.4	58.0	58.4	–	–	2.77	1.22	1.94
Sought treatment from public health facility (%)	23.7	18.6	15.2	22.8	27.2	−0.22	2.18	−1.23	−1.94	−1.17
Sought treatment from private health facility (%)	72.3	73.8	83.0	71.7	70.1	1.25	−0.06	2.06	2.24	1.71
Prevalence and treatment for symptoms of ARI among children										
Prevalence of ARI (%)	6.5	19.3	5.8	2.7	2.8	1.20	2.80	0.40	0.40	0.50
Sought advice/treatment (%)	78.2	70.9	74.9	85.4	56.3	3.69	5.19	5.49	4.97	2.64
Sought treatment within a day (%)	–	–	39.4	57.6	38.5	–	–	0.13	5.20	2.14
Sought treatment from public health facility (%)	24.4	19.8	13.0	22.5	28.1	−2.58	1.96	4.78	−0.85	−0.54
Sought treatment from private health facility (%)	71.8	71.9	85.5	72.8	68.7	4.66	0.07	−4.16	1.62	1.83

has also improved over the years. In the early 1990s, one in 10 mothers initiated breastfeeding to their newborn within the first 1 h of birth. This increased to more than 2 in 10 in 2005–06 reaching more than 42% in the recent years. In addition, much fewer mothers now give a pre-lacteal feed to their newborn than mothers did in the early 2000s; 58% of mothers gave a pre-lacteal feed to their newborn in 2005–06 which reduced to less than 16% in 2019–21. Further, prevalence of exclusive breastfeeding among children below 6 months has increased from 43 to 64% between 1992–93 and 2019–21.

3.3.10 Food/Dietary Practices

The mothers were asked to recall and report food items they fed to their child in the past 24 h preceding the survey date. The results show that proportion of children aged 6–23 months who were fed solid/semi solid food increased from 56% in 1992–93 to 85% in 2005–06, however, this has shown a decline in the recent years (75% in 2019–21). About half of the children were given milk or milk products and this share has more or less remained unchanged during the analysis period. More children now receive a minimum diverse food than previously. For example, percentage of children given a minimum diverse food nearly doubled from 13% in 2005–06 to 24% in 2019–21. The percentage of children who were given a minimum meal frequency in the past 24 h has remained at around 40% during the past 15 years. Similarly, the proportion of children who received a minimum acceptable diet has increased only marginally over the past 15 years; from 8.3% in 2005–06 to 11.4% in 2019–21.

3.3.11 Immunization Among Children

In 1992–93, a little over one-third of the children aged 12–23 months received full immunization, defined as children who received one dose of BCG, three doses of DPT, three doses of polio vaccine (excluding polio 0 given at birth) and one dose of measles/MCV. Their share increased to close to 44% in 2005–06. The recent data shows that more than three-quarters of the children had been fully vaccinated in 2019–21.

3.3.12 Treatment Seeking for Ill Children

The information is available for children under five years of age who suffered from diarrhea, fever and showed symptoms of acute respiratory infections (ARIs) during the past 2-weeks preceding the survey and the treatment seeking behavior when child suffered from these illnesses. About 7% of children reportedly suffered from diarrhea and 13% from fever and about 3% experienced one or more symptoms of ARI during the past 2-weeks in 2019–21. The treatment seeking for ill children is rising over the past three decades as more and more mothers reported that they sought advice/treatment from a health facility for their ill child; more than three-quarters of mothers in 2019–21 did this. It is encouraging to note that more and more mothers sought treatment for their ill child within a day (ranging from 40–45% in 2015–16 to 55–58% in 2019–21 for diarrhea and fever). In case of ARI symptoms, 78% of mothers sought advice/treatment from a health facility in 1992–93 which increased to 85% in 2015–16. Similarly, mothers who did so within a day too rose from 39 to 58% during the same time. Although significantly higher proportions of the mothers sought treatment for ill child from a private health facility, however, their share is declining over the analysis period. Relatively, more mothers now go to a public health facility for treating their ill child. In the early 1990s, around 24–25% of mothers sought treatment from a public health facility when child suffered from diarrhea or fever or ARI symptoms. The percentages of mothers seeking treatment from a public health facility increased to 27–31% in 2019–21.

3.3.13 Female Disadvantage in Feeding and Treatment for Illness

The analysis suggests a strong gender gradient in terms of these practices, mostly to the disadvantage of female children, and this is regardless of time period. Further, the gender gaps either remained at similar levels or are closing rather slowly. For example, irrespective of analysis period, slightly higher percentage of mothers reported initiating breastfeeding within first hour of birth, gave a pre-lacteal feed or age appropriate breastfeeding to the male newborn/child than the females. On the other hand, marginally higher percentages of mothers with children below 6 months of age reported exclusive breastfeeding female children than the male children in 2019–21. Similar patterns may be seen with respect to other indicators including minimum diverse food, meal frequency and acceptable diets. In the 1990s, an additional 3–4% of mothers reported that they gave milk or milk products to their male child than the mothers of female children. However, this seemingly has reduced to about 2% in the recent times. Likewise, an additional 3% male children received full immunization than the female children in 1992–93 which has reduced to about 1% in 2019–21.

Similar female disadvantage is seen in case of treatment seeking practices for childhood illness.

Generally speaking, compared to the female children with the same illness, slightly higher percentage of male children received treatment or prompt treatment within a day. At the same time, while more female children were taken to a public health facility for treatment of illness, more male children received treatment from a private health facility when suffered from diarrhea, fever, or ARI.

3.4 Discussions and Conclusions

This paper assesses India's progress in overall, early childhood as well as gender disparities in mortality over time and looked at improvements in well documented socio-economic development indicators that influence mortality outcomes. The paper identifies persistent challenges India continue to face in achieving equal opportunities for overall and childhood survival. The population health and equity is a powerful indicator to measure the level of the development of a population. Over the past seven decades, India has made significant progress in reducing its overall mortality and more specifically during the infancy and childhood, yet people and children of India continue to be disadvantaged when compared with the global average. The life expectancy at birth (LEB) in India has improved over the years, however, it is only after the 1980 that Indian females started to experience longer survival compared to males matching the global gender trend. Until 1980, Indian females had an absolute disadvantage of nearly 6-years compared to their global counterparts. Further, the gender-specific crossover of LEB and higher female LEB in India was mainly due to the gains at older ages and also the mortality declines at younger ages have benefitted Indian males more than the females (Borah, 2021).

India has successfully achieved the under-5 mortality rate MDG and is expected to achieve the SDG well before 2030 nationally. As a matter of fact, India's progress in reducing child mortality was faster than the decline observed globally, more specifically in the past two decades (Bhushan et al., 2023; Ram et al., 2023). India's share in global child deaths has reduced and is expected to reduce further; from a major contributor (one-fifth in 1950) of global child deaths to 14% in 2020. India's share is expected to reach 3–5% by 2090. This reduction has been substantial for both male and female children, nonetheless, share of female deaths is relatively higher suggesting lower female to male deaths ratio for India compared to the world. Lower female to male death ratio suggests that the difference between female and male deaths is higher for world than India and also suggest that there is scope of further improvement in the female mortality as the females tends to have lower childhood mortality and better life expectancy.

Along with this progress in mortality reductions, India in the past three decades, have witnessed encouraging improvements in the household's living conditions and other socio-economic development indicators. For example, more households now have access to basic amenities such as electricity, safe drinking water, improved sanitation, clean fuel for cooking and live in pucca houses than previously. The literacy rates and educational attainments among women have increased, age at marriage for girls have risen alongside elevated levels of women who now own bank/post office accounts. These improvements have crucial role in influencing lives/life of women and girl children. We observe that women and girl children now have increased opportunities than previously for a better education, employment, decision-making and access and utilization of various services, within as well as outside the homes.

Gender alone does not affect health outcomes, if boys and girls are provided equal access to resources such as food and healthcare, newborn boys are at a biological disadvantage of high mortality (Sawyer, 2012), however, its interplay with other social determinants of health does. A few social evils such as practice of female early/forced marriages, dowry, honor killing, and gender biased sex selection are a few of such practices that show how Indian girl children and women are subjected to systematic discrimination through their lives. Generally speaking, India is a gender-governed society in which men, by far, control almost all social, political, religious, economic and cultural institutions and women are confined to the stereotype roles. Not only this, Indian men have elevated access compared to women, especially at younger ages with respect to access to food, health care utilization, education, and financial access (Aurino, 2017; Basu, 1989). Poverty, social class, religion, caste, education, place of residence, and so on, differentially and profoundly influence child health outcomes based on gender. Mayer (1999) documented that the differences in the care of sons and daughters in South Asia stem from parents' perception where sons are seen as assets and daughters as liabilities. However, Murthi et al. (1995) noted that the districts in India showed less bias against the girl children if more female participated in the labor force.

Similarly, increased educational attainment alongside increased work participation has delayed age at marriage for girls in India which reduces fertility levels (Ram & Ram, 2021), on one hand, and greater utilization of maternal and child health care services including immunization among children, on the other. These have been shown as important factors associated with reduced levels of infant and child mortality as well as reduced gender gaps in child survival (Rutstein, 2000). Using data for 175 countries, Gakidou et al. (2010) estimated that of 8·2 million deaths in children below age 5 years averted between 1970 and 2009 globally, 4·2 million (51·2%) could be attributed to increased educational attainment of the women in the reproductive ages. Additionally, improvements in educational levels also influence mortality levels indirectly. Use of improved source of water and sanitation are more among educated households/families where both mortality as well as morbidities among children are lower. Improved sanitation, for example, lowers chances of diarrhea and fever (Kumar & Vollmer, 2013). Günther and Fink (2011) estimated that full household coverage with water and sanitation infrastructure could lead to an absolute reduction of 2.2 million annual child deaths in the developing world and save around 65–80% of annual per-capita gross domestic product (GDP). Scaling up the coverage of piped water and improved sanitation to 95%, could result into averting 43,352 diarrheal episodes and 68 diarrheal deaths per 100,000 under-5 children per year, compared with the baseline (Nandi et al., 2017).

India has shown improvement in health care utilization, however, inequalities related to socio-economic status, geography, and gender are persistent (Balarajan et al., 2011). The substantial reduction in childhood mortality might be attributed to increased uptake in maternal and child health services especially among marginalized group of rural and poor population (Bhushan et al., 2023; Ram et al., 2023). The authors further observed increase in the uptake of MCH services with quality. Nonetheless, variation in mortality and uptake of MCH services across states persist.

Breastfeeding and feeding practices have shown sharp improvements in India with narrowing gender gap in feeding practices. Compared to exclusively breastfed infants aged 0–5 months, all-cause mortality was higher in children who were predominantly or partially breastfed and were not breastfed at all (Sankar et al., 2015). A recent study (Mal & Ram, 2023) found that early initiation of breastfeeding within 1 h after birth increased rapidly from 25 to 42% during 2005–06 and 2019–21, and the pre-lacteal feeding practice declined from 57 to 15% during the same period. The study further noted that an early breastfeeding initiation is associated with lower neonatal mortality, whereas pre-lacteal feed is not harmful compared to late breastfeeding initiation. The benefit of improved breastfeeding practices goes beyond childhood mortality reduction. Duration of breastfeeding is found to influence fertility levels negatively. Maternal undernutrition contributes to 800 000 neonatal deaths annually through small for gestational age births; stunting, wasting, and micronutrient deficiencies and are estimated to cause over 3 million child deaths annually (Bhutta et al., 2013). The study further noted that 90% coverage of nutrition interventions would reduce under-5 mortalities by 15%. The complementary feeding too has shown improvements.

The study notes improvement in the full immunization coverage as well as reduction in gender gap in it for boys and girls over time in India. Several studies have documented the reduction of childhood mortality with increased coverage of full immunization (Corsi et al., 2009; Rutstein, 2000). The World Health Assembly in 2012 adopted the Decade of Vaccines Global Vaccine Action Plan 2011–2020 to prevent millions of deaths by providing more equitable access in all communities (Bustreo et al., 2015).

It will not be out of context to bring in the importance of conditional cash transfer (CCT) schemes which have been found to be very effective in promoting utilization of health care and bridge gender gap globally. The CCTs further reduces child mortality (Krishnan et al., 2014; Rasella et al., 2013). Especially over the past one and a half decade, India has launched several important interventions particularly aiming to reduce persistent higher maternal and childhood mortality as well as to eliminate gender differentials in health care service utilization. For example, two major cash incentive schemes: '*Janani Suraksha Yojana* (JSS)' and *Janani Sishu Suraksha Karyakram* (JSSK)' have been instrumental in increasing the uptake of institutional delivery and hence has brought the pregnant women to hospital especially the marginalized population (Lim et al., 2010; Marie Ng et al., 2014; Gupta et al., 2012). Many gender-specific policies and programs focusing on the welfare and development of women has also helped in bridging the gender gap in child mortality and lower female mortality in recent times. Policies/government schemes for welfare of girl child, like *Bati Bachao Beti Padhao, Sukanya Samriddhi Yojna, Balika Samridhi Yojana*, might have changed the perception and attitude of population towards girl child (Baruah et al., 2013; Sinha & Yoong, 2009).

Although the present paper is restricted to the gender-specific childhood survival, as a country of huge diversity, the differentials in childhood mortality in India go beyond the biological stratifier. For example, children belonging to the disadvantaged castes (scheduled castes/tribe and other backward classes) experience a lower survival probability before age five (Dommaraju et al., 2008; Ghosh, 2012). While women with lower educational attainment may lead in reduced health literacy and delayed decision-making on healthcare for themselves and their children; having an educated or employed mother can result in improved child survival, specifically by following good childcare practices, maintaining hygiene, utilizing of health service etc. Basu and Stephenson (2005); Iqbal et al. (2018) and Bora et al. (2019) found that in contrast to a child born in a highly educated and affluent family of privileged caste residing in the urban areas, children born into a poor family of marginalized caste in rural residence, mother with less than elementary education are at high risk of dying before celebrating their fifth birthday.

References

Arokiasamy, P. (2007). Sex ratio at birth and excess female child mortality in India: Trends, differential and regional patterns. In *Watering the neighbor's garden: The growing demographic female deficit in Asia* (pp. 49–72). CICRED.

Augsburg, B., & Rodríguez-Lesmes, P. A. (2018). Sanitation and child health in India. *World Development, 107*, 22–39.

Aurino, E. (2017). Do boys eat better than girls in India? Longitudinal evidence on dietary diversity and food consumption disparities among children and adolescents. *Economics and Human Biology, 25*, 99–111.

Balarajan, Y., Selvaraj, S., & Subramanian, S. V. (2011). Health care and equity in India. *The Lancet, 377*(9764), 505–515.

Bannerji, H. (2016). Patriarchy in the Era of Neoliberalism: The Case of India. *Social Scientist, 44*(3/4), 3–27. http://www.jstor.org/stable/24890241

Baruah, J., Rajkonwar, A., Medhi, S., & Kusre, G. (2013). Effect of conditional cash transfer schemes on registration of the birth of a female child in India. *South East Asia Journal of Public Health, 3*(1), 30–35.

Basu, A. M. (1989). Is discrimination in food really necessary for explaining sex differentials in childhood mortalit? *Population Studies, 43*(2), 193–210. https://doi.org/10.1080/0032472031000144086

Basu, A. M., & Stephenson, R. (2005). Low levels of maternal education and the proximate determinants of childhood mortality: A little learning is not a dangerous thing. *Social Science and Medicine, 60*(9), 2011–2023.

Bhushan, H., Ram, U., Scott, K., Blanchard, A., Kumar, P., et al. (2023). Making the health system work for 25 million births annually: Drivers of the notable decline in maternal and newborn mortality in India. *BMJ Global Health, 9*, e011411.

Bhutta, Z. A., Das, J. K., Rizvi, A., Gaffey, M. F., Walker, N., Horton, S., Webb, P., Lartey, A., & Black, R. E. (2013). Evidence-based interventions for improvement of maternal and child nutrition: What can be done and at what cost? *The Lancet, 382*(9890), 452–477.

Bora, J. K., Raushan, R., & Lutz, W. (2019). The persistent influence of caste on under five mortality: Factors that explain the caste based gap in high focus Indian states. *PLoS ONE, 14*(8), Article e0211086. https://doi.org/10.1371/journal.pone.0211086

Borah, G. (2021). Gender gap in life expectancy in India and role of age groups: A comparison between before and after male–female life expectancy at birth crossover. *PLoS ONE, 16*(12), Article e0260657. https://doi.org/10.1371/journal.pone.0260657

Bose, S. (2011). The effect of women's status and community on the gender differential in children's nutrition in India. *Journal of Biosocial Science, 43*(5), 513–533. https://doi.org/10.1017/S002193201100006X

Bustreo, F., Okwo-Bele, J. M., & Kamara, L. (2015). World Health Organization perspectives on the contribution of the Global Alliance for Vaccines and Immunization on reducing child mortality. *Archives of Disease in Childhood, 100*(Suppl 1), S34–S37.

Chao, F., You, D., Pedersen, J., et al. (2018). National and regional under-5 mortality rate by economic status for low-income and middle-income countries: A systematic assessment. *The Lancet Global Health, 6*, e535-47 12.

Corsi, D. J., Bassani, D. G., Kumar, R., Awasthi, S., Jotkar, R., Kaur, N., & Jha, P. (2009). Gender inequity and age-appropriate immunization coverage in India from 1992 to 2006. *BMC International Health and Human Rights, 9*(1), 1–12.

Crimmins, E. M., et al. (2019). Differences between men and women in mortality and the health dimensions of the morbidity process. *Clinical Chemistry, 65*(1), 135–145. https://doi.org/10.1373/clinchem.2018.288332

Dommaraju, P., Agadjanian, V., & Yabiku, S. (2008). The pervasive and persistent influence of caste on child mortality in India. *Population Research and Policy Review, 27*, 477–495.

Fledderjohann, J., Agrawal, S., Vellakkal, S., Basu, S., Campbell, O., Doyle, P., Ebrahim, S., & Stuckler, D. (2014). Do girls have a nutritional disadvantage compared with boys? Statistical models of breastfeeding and food consumption inequalities among Indian siblings. *PLoS ONE, 9*(9), Article e107172. https://doi.org/10.1371/journal.pone.0107172

Gakidou, E., Cowling, K., Lozano, R., & Murray, C. J. (2010). Increased educational attainment and its effect on child mortality in 175 countries between 1970 and 2009: A systematic analysis. *The Lancet, 376*(9745), 959–974.

Ghosh, R. (2012). Child mortality in India: A complex situation. *World Journal of Pediatrics, 8*, 11–18.

Guilmoto, C. Z., Saikia, N., Tamrakar, V., et al. (2018). Excess under-5 female mortality across India: A spatial analysis using 2011 census data. *The Lancet Global Health, 6*, e650–e658.

Günther, I., & Fink, G. (2011). *Water and sanitation to reduce child mortality: The impact and cost of water and sanitation infrastructure (March 1, 2011)*. World bank policy research working paper no. 5618. Available at SSRN: https://ssrn.com/abstract=1799842

Gupta, S. K., Pal, D. K., Tiwari, R., Garg, R., Shrivastava, A. K., Sarawagi, R., Patil, R., Agarwal, L., Gupta, P., & Lahariya, C. (2012). Impact of Janani Suraksha Yojana on institutional delivery rate and maternal morbidity and mortality: An observational study in India. *Journal of Health, Population, and Nutrition, 30*(4), 464.

International Institute for Population Sciences (IIPS) and ICF. (2021). *National family health survey (NFHS-5), India, 2019–21: Mizoram*. Mumbai: IIPS.

Iqbal, N., Gkiouleka, A., Milner, A., Montag, D., & Gallo, V. (2018). Girl's hidden penalty: Analysis of gender inequality in child mortality with data from 195 countries. *BMJ Global Health, 3*, Article e001028. https://doi.org/10.1136/bmjgh-2018-001028

Ismail, S. A., McCullough, A., Guo, S., Sharkey, A., Harma, S., & Rutter, P. (2019). Gender-related differences in care-seeking behaviour for newborns: A systematic review of the evidence in South Asia. *BMJ Global Health, 4*(3), Article e001309. https://doi.org/10.1136/bmjgh-2018-001309

Jayachandran, S., & Kuziemko, I. (2011). Why do mothers breastfeed girls less than boys? Evidence and implications for child health in India. *The Quarterly Journal of Economics, 126*(3), 1485–1538.

Jha, P., Kesler, M. A., Kumar, R., Ram, F., Ram, U., Aleksandrowicz, L., et al. (2011). Trends in selective abortions of girls in India: Analysis of nationally representative birth histories from 1990 to 2005 and census data from 1991 to 2011. *Lancet, 377*, 1921–1928.

Jha, P., Kumar, R., Vasa, P., Dhingra, N., Thiruchelvam, D., & Moineddin, R. (2006). Low male-to-female sex ratio of children born in India: National survey of 1·1 million households. *Lancet, 367*, 211–8 26.

Jose, S. (2017). Decomposition of gender differential in malnutrition in Indian children. *Journal of Social and Economic Development, 19*, 299–322. https://doi.org/10.1007/s40847-017-0047-x

Koenig, M. A., & D'Souza, S. (1986). Sex differences in childhood mortality in rural Bangladesh. *Social Science and Medicine (1982), 22*(1), 15–22. https://doi.org/10.1016/0277-9536(86)90303-5

Krishnan, A., Amarchand, R., Byass, P., Pandav, C., & Ng, N. (2014). "No one says 'No'to money"—A mixed methods approach for evaluating conditional cash transfer schemes to improve girl children's status in Haryana, India. *International Journal for Equity in Health, 13*(1), 1–10.

Krishnan, A., Dwivedi, P., Gupta, V., Byass, P., Pandav, C. S., & Ng, N. (2013). Socioeconomic development and girl child survival in rural North India: Solution or problem? *Journal of Epidemiology and Community Health, 67*(5), 419–426.

Kumar, S., & Vollmer, S. (2013). Does access to improved sanitation reduce childhood diarrhea in rural India? *Health Economics, 22*(4), 410–427.

Lim, S. S., Dandona, L., Hoisington, J. A., James, S. L., Hogan, M. C., & Gakidou, E. (2010). India's Janani Suraksha Yojana, a conditional cash transfer programme to increase births in health facilities: An impact evaluation. *The Lancet, 375*(9730), 2009–2023.

Mayer, P. (1999). India's falling sex ratios. *Population and Development Review, 25*(2), 323

Maitra, P., & Rammohan, A. (2011). The link between infant mortality and child nutrition in India: Is there any evidence of a gender bias? *Journal of the Asia Pacific Economy, 16*(1), 81–110.

Mal, P., & Ram, U. (2023). First 72-hours after birth: Newborn feeding practices and neonatal mortality in India. *PLoS ONE, 18*, e0292353.

Martins, V. J., Toledo Florêncio, T. M., Grillo, L. P., Franco, M. D. C. P., Martins, P. A., Clemente, A. P., Santos, C. D., Vieira, M. D. F. A., & Sawaya, A. L. (2011). Long-lasting effects of undernutrition. *International Journal of Environmental Research and Public Health, 8*(6), 1817–1846. https://doi.org/10.3390/ijerph8061817

Ministry of Finance. (2023). *Economic survey 2022–23*. Economic Division, Department of Economic Affairs, Ministry of Finance, Government of India, New Delhi, January 2023. https://www.indiabudget.gov.in/economicsurvey/doc/echapter.pdf

Mishra, V., Roy, T. K., & Retherford, D. (2004). Sex differentials in childhood feeding, health care, and nutritional status in India. *Population and Development Review, 30*(2), 269–295. https://doi.org/10.1111/j.1728-4457.2004.013_1.x

Murthi, M., Guio, A.-C., & Dreze, J. (1995). Mortality, fertility, and gender bias in India: A districtlevel analysis. *Population and Development Review, 21*, 745–782.

Nandi, A., Megiddo, I., Ashok, A., Verma, A., & Laxminarayan, R. (2017). Reduced burden of childhood diarrheal diseases through increased access to water and sanitation in India: A modeling analysis. *Social Science and Medicine, 180*, 181–192.

Ng, M., Misra, A., Diwan, V., Agnani, M., Levin-Rector, A., & De Costa, A. (2014). An assessment of the impact of the JSY cash transfer program on maternal mortality reduction in Madhya Pradesh, India. *Global Health Action, 7*(1), 24939.

Office of Registrar General of India. (1970–75, 1981–85, 2014–18). *SRS-based abridge life tables of India and the major states*. New Delhi: Registrar General of India.

Office of Registrar General of India (RGI). (2020). *Sample registration system statistical report 2020*. Office of the Registrar General & Census Commissioner, New Delhi, India.

Office of The Registrar General of India; Census Commissioner. (1982).*Sample registration system: Statistical report 1970-75. Ministry of Home Affairs*, Government of India, New Delhi, June 6, 1982.

Office of The Registrar General of India; Census Commissioner. (2003).*Sample registration system: Statistical report 2000. Ministry of Home Affairs*, Government of India, New Delhi, August 2003.

Office of The Registrar General & Census Commissioner. (2022). *Sample registration system: Statistical report 2020*. Ministry of Home Affairs, Government of India, New Delhi, September 2022.

Pande, R. P. (2003). Selective gender differences in childhood nutrition and immunization in rural India: The role of siblings. *Demography, 40*(3), 395–418. https://doi.org/10.1353/dem.2003.0029

Paul, V. K., Sachdev, H. S., Mavalankar, D., Ramachandran, P., Sankar, M. J., Bhandari, N., Sreenivas, V., Sundararaman, T., Govil, D., Osrin, D., & Kirkwood, B. (2011). Reproductive health, and child health and nutrition in India: Meeting the challenge. *The Lancet, 377*(9762), 332–349.

Ram, U., Jha, P., Ram, F., et al. (2013). Neonatal, 1–59 month, and under-5 mortality in 597 Indian districts, 2001 to 2012: Estimates from national demographic and mortality surveys. *The Lancet Global Health, 1*, 219–226.

Ram, U., Ramesh, B. M., Blanchard, A., Scott, K., Kumar, P., et al. (2023). A tale of two exemplars: The maternal and newborn mortality transitions of two state clusters in India. *BMJ Global Health, 9*, e011413.

Rao, M., Rao, K. D., Kumar, A. S., Chatterjee, M., & Sundararaman, T. (2011). Human resources for health in India. *The Lancet, 377*(9765), 587–598.

Rasella, D., Aquino, R., Santos, C. A., Paes-Sousa, R., & Barreto, M. L. (2013). Effect of a conditional cash transfer programme on childhood mortality: A nationwide analysis of Brazilian municipalities. *The Lancet, 382*(9886), 57–64.

Riley, J. C. (2005). The timing and pace of health transitions around the world. *Population and Development Review, 31*(4), 741–764.

Rutstein, S. O. (2000). Factors associated with trends in infant and child mortality in developing countries during the 1990s. *Bulletin of the World Health Organization, 78*(10), 1256–1270.

Sankar, M. J., Sinha, B., Chowdhury, R., Bhandari, N., Taneja, S., Martines, J., & Bahl, R. (2015). Optimal breastfeeding practices and infant and child mortality: A systematic review and meta-analysis. *Acta Paediatrica, 104*, 3–13.

Sawyer, C. C. (2012). Child mortality estimation: Estimating sex differences in childhood mortality since the 1970s. *PLoS Medicine, 9*(8), Article e1001287. https://doi.org/10.1371/journal.pmed.1001287

Singh, A., Chokhandre, P., Singh, A. K., et al. (2022). Development of the india patriarchy index: Validation and testing of temporal and spatial patterning. *Social Indicators Research, 159*, 351–377. https://doi.org/10.1007/s11205-021-02752-1

Sinha, N., & Yoong, J. (2009). *Long-term financial incentives and investment in daughters: Evidence from conditional cash transfers in North India* (February 27, 2009). RAND Working Paper No. WR-667. Available at SSRN: https://ssrn.com/abstract=1354883 or https://doi.org/10.2139/ssrn.1354883

Stewart, C. P., Iannotti, L., Dewey, K. G., Michaelsen, K. F., & Onyango, A. W. (2013). Contextualising complementary feeding in a broader framework for stunting prevention. *Maternal and Child Nutrition, 9*, 27–45.

Subramanian, S. V., Nandy, S., Irving, M., et al. (2006). The mortality divide in India: The differential contributions of gender, caste, and standard of living across the life course. *American Journal of Public Health, 96*, 818–825.

United Nations. (2022a). *World population prospects 2022: Summary of results.* Department of Economic and Social Affairs, Population Division, UN DESA/POP/2022/TR/NO. 3.

United Nations. (2022b). *World population prospects 2022, online edition.* Department of Economic and Social Affairs, Population Division, United Nation. Downloaded from: https://population.un.org/wpp/Download/Standard/Mortality/

United Nations Inter-agency Group for Child Mortality Estimation (UN IGME). (2023). *Levels & trends in child mortality: Report 2022, estimates developed by the United Nations inter-agency group for child mortality estimation.* United Nations Children's Fund.

Usha, R., & Ram, F. (2021). Demographic transition in India: Insights into population growth, composition, and its major drivers. *Oxford Research Encyclopaedia on Global Public Health.* https://doi.org/10.1093/acrefore/9780190632366.013.223

Vlassoff, C. (2007). Gender differences in determinants and consequences of health and illness. *Journal of Health, Population, and Nutrition, 25*(1), 47.

WDI, Life Expectancy at Birth, Total (Years). Washington, DC: World Bank. World Bank [cited June 18, 2021]. Available from: https://data.worldbank.org/indicator/SP.DYN.LE00.IN

WHO. (2021). *Life expectancy and healthy life expectancy data by WHO region.* Available from: https://apps.who.int/gho/data/view.main.SDG2016LEXREGv?lang=en

World Economic Forum. (2023). *Global gender gap report 2023: Insight report, June 2023.* World Economic Forum. Geneva. https://www3.weforum.org/docs/WEF_GGGR_2023.pdf?_gl=1*1qu2rmu*_up*MQ..&gclid=CjwKCAjwqZSlBhBwEiwAfoZUIJUOKkoaDZT7xfneA7y8_XYZuJqDL3QFq57ozVBnt7RPNa03piehnBoChisQAvD_BwE. Accessed on July 7, 2023

Inequity in Early Childhood in India: Addressing Challenges

4

Shilpa Jadhav-Bhakare

Abstract

This article highlights the intersectional vulnerabilities faced by children, with a particular focus on those of migrant workers residing in urban slum-like settlements. Drawing on data from NFHS-5 (2019–20), it presents the layered discrimination rooted in the socio-economic disenfranchisement of their parents. Grounded in the capabilities approach, this article argues for robust state support for quality care in early childhood. Absence of such foundational support leads to corrosive capability failures, undermining children's long-term development and well-being. State-sponsored child care empowers women in the informal sector by enabling them to work, earn, and attain social recognition. This, in turn, generates a multiplier effect on child health and nutrition. The article throws light on the implementation of social protection schemes that are nominally universal, requiring to fulfill certain eligibility criteria resulting in exclusion of the most vulnerable. It calls for a recalibration of policy frameworks to recognize migrant workers' children as rightful claimants of inclusive welfare. In conclusion, it proposes actionable pathways to embed child-centric equity within social policy.

4.1 Introduction

While passing by jhuggis draped in blue and yellow tarpaulin sheets, we often notice children playing in tattered clothing. However, we choose to ignore the trail of thoughts to suppress the discomfort they evoke and redirect attention toward seemingly more practical concerns of our lives. It is deeply troubling that society has not only neglected the welfare of the marginalized children but has also normalized their plight to the extent that it no longer provokes collective concern. The normalization of the impoverished conditions of marginalised childeren is so deeply ingrained that it rarely elicits meaningful discussion in mainstream media or academic-social platforms questioning the status quo. We live in a world of inequality, and India is no exception, but, the compounded effects of structural injustice and layered neglect have rendered the lives of many children precarious and vulnerable. While childhood is inherently imbued with innocence, but one wonders, if these children would understand the fragmented and half hearted interventions for them, would they be able to smile and continue playing? The barriers they face are generational, foreclosing the possibility of a dignified

S. Jadhav-Bhakare (✉)
Jamnagar, India
e-mail: shilpabhakare@gmail.com

S. S. Acharya et al. (eds.), *Paradigm Shifts in Population and Health in India*, Sustainable Development Goals Series, https://doi.org/10.1007/978-981-95-1719-0_4

life marked by freedom and opportunity. The onus lies on society to intervene decisively and it is for us to act now. Failure to do so risks perpetuating a cycle of deprivation and confronting us with the uncomfortable truth that their futures may be irreparably compromised.

India has enacted legislations and policies aimed at safeguarding children's rights, including the Right to Food, the Right to Education, large scale Integrated Child Development Services (ICDS), and a comprehensive child protection framework. These initiatives reflect a rights-based approach to early childhood development, rooted in the principles of the United Nations Convention on the Rights of the Child (UNCRC). This framework emphasizes the recognition of young children as rights holders and calls for the respect of their agency as active participants within families, communities, and society at large (UNICEF, 2006). In alignment with the global Education for All movement and the Dakar Framework for Action (2000), the Government of India pledged to 'expand and improve comprehensive early childhood care and education' (ECCE).

However, to transform abstract rights into tangible realities, a robust theoretical foundation and actionable policy frameworks are imperative. This article draws on the capabilities approach articulated by Martha Nussbaum and Amartya Sen, advocating for first-order state support to ensure quality early childhood care for all children, regardless of socio-economic background. The first section examines persistent disparities in health indicators across social groups, drawing primarily from NFHS-5 (2019–20) and other national surveys. While it is well-established that Dalit and tribal children consistently lag behind in key health metrics, the normalization of such inequality remains deeply concerning. The second section highlights the intersectional vulnerabilities of children, with particular focus on those of migrant workers, who are disproportionately affected by inadequate social protection mechanisms in urban slum-like environments. The third section underscores the intrinsic value of women's empowerment, while also emphasizing its demonstrable impact on child nutrition outcomes, an essential consideration for advancing the development agenda. The success of instrumentalist advocacy hinges on translating feminist scholarship into policy discourse, which necessitates quantifying the claims of gender equity and empowerment (Kabeer, 2002). The final section outlines a way forward, offering recommendations for revisiting and strengthening policies aimed at the most vulnerable populations.

The developmental outcomes of young children are shaped by a constellation of interrelated factors spanning multiple sectors, making them acutely susceptible to the consequences of social policy failures. Within the framework of the Capability Approach, Dixon and Nussbaum (2012) advocate for assigning special priority to children's rights, offering two principal justifications. The first is the vulnerability principle, which recognizes children's heightened susceptibility due to their legal and economic dependence on adults, as well as their intrinsic physical and emotional fragility. The second is the cost-effectiveness principle, which argues that the marginal cost of safeguarding children's rights is so low that failure to do so constitutes a direct affront to their dignity; moreover, it is far more economically efficient to uphold these rights for children than for adults. Sen (1993) defines capability as 'a person's ability to do valuable acts or reach valuable states of being,' representing the range of alternatives a person can choose to do or become. Sen's capability approach is a moral framework, proposing that social arrangements should be primarily evaluated according to the extent of freedom people have to promote or achieve the functioning they value. In this light, the widespread capability deprivation among children is not only a profound moral failure but also a poor economic choice, undermining both human development and societal progress.

The inaugural Human Development Report by the United Nations Development Programme (UNDP) aptly called people as the real wealth of a nation. It emphasized that the fundamental objective of development is to foster an enabling environment in which individuals can lead long, healthy, and creative lives (UNDP,

1990). Although this principle appears self-evident, it is frequently overshadowed by the dominant focus on material accumulation and financial growth. In contrast to physical or financial capital, scholars have increasingly argued that human capital should be recognized as a defining form of twenty-first-century wealth. Expanding educational opportunities, therefore, must be viewed as a powerful equalizing instrument to address the widening disparities in wealth and opportunity (Majumdar, 2020). Among the most critical dimensions of human development is Early Childhood Care and Education (ECCE), which profoundly influences physical and cognitive development, as well as long-term economic prospects. However, unequal access to nutrition, education, and care during these formative years perpetuates a deeply entrenched landscape of inequality. While the notion of an 'early start' in learning is widely embraced among India's upper socio-economic strata, there remains an urgent need to ensure equitable early childhood opportunities for all children, regardless of background. In this context, even as child rights advocacy gains momentum, targeted attention to the most vulnerable children is essential to bridge the gaps left by fragmented and insufficient policy interventions.

4.2 Who Are the Most Vulnerable Children in Our Country?

In the Global Hunger Index 2025, India ranked 102nd out of 123 countries and dissimilarity index by the Economic and Social Commission for Asia and the Pacific (ESCAP, 2022) shows that in India, inequality is highest in pandemic preparedness, tertiary education, clean fuel, secondary education, basic sanitation, and early childhood education. The study about Global Hidden Hunger Index which was calculated as an average of three deficiencies (Zinc, Vit-A and iron) in preschool children by Muthayya et al. (2013), showed India ranked 8th and has been in the company of Sub-Saharan African countries and Afghanistan. However, international indices create an uncomfortable stir in national media and sometimes, survey methodologies and data interpretations are criticized. Panagariya (2013) notably challenged the assertion that India's malnutrition rates were worse than those of Sub-Saharan Africa, contending that such comparisons were based on flawed measurement techniques. The methodology for Global Hunger Index was criticized sharply and systematically ,disregarding scholarly wisdom about grave consequences of childhood malnourishment (Desai, 2022; Mukhopadhyay & Chakraborty, 2023). Gillespie (2013), among others, argued that dismissing the burden through methodological critiques risks obscuring the lived realities of millions of children and undermines the urgency of policy responses. This discourse highlights the critical need for methodological rigor, transparency, and contextual sensitivity in assessing child health outcomes. While highlighting that the gaps in child heights between the social groups in India are two to three times greater than the India-Sub-Saharan African child height gap, Deshpande and Ramachandran (2021) argue that the question 'Why are Indian children shorter than African children' needs to be rephrased to 'why are the gaps in child height between social groups within India so high?' The matter of concern should be understanding who these children are and how to reach out to them.

NFHS-5 (2019–20) shows that dalit and tribal children are the most deprived while suffering from undernutrition. The SC and ST children are at the bottom of the indicators, and there is a wide gap in the nutrition status of children in low wealth quintile with those in high wealth quintile. The self-explanatory tables are presented (Tables 4.1, 4.2, 4.3 and 4.4).

Poverty is an overarching phenomenon and can explain malnutrition but, it should not stop us from questioning structural compulsions. The unfortunate part of India's story about malnutrition is the status quo of discrimination. The descriptive analysis of NFHS-3 done by Thorat and Sadana (2009) also showed that for all indicators of health status, the situation of the SCs and STs is much worse than other groups. The results also indicated that even for individuals with a similar standard of living and education level, the health status

Table 4.1 Malnutrition in under-5 children by background factors: caste/tribe

Category	Height for age % below-3 SD	Height for age % below-2 SD	Weight for height % below-3 SD	Weight for height % below-2 SD	Weight for age %-3 SD	Weight for age %-2 SD
Scheduled caste	17.1	39.2	7.7	19.7	11.5	35.1
Scheduled tribe	18.7	40.9	9.4	23.2	14.6	39.5
Other backward class	14.3	34.8	7.4	18.9	10.2	31.2
Other	12.8	30.1	7.3	17.5	8.8	27
Don't know	16	40.2	7.7	21.5	10.5	36.8

Table 4.2 Malnutrition in under-5 children by background factors: wealth quintile

Wealth quintile	Height for age % below-3 SD	Height for age % below-2 SD	Weight for height % below-3 SD	Weight for height % below-2 SD	Weight for age %-3 SD	Weight for age %-2 SD
Lowest	21.8	46.1	8.6	22.5	15.4	43.1
Second	16.9	39.7	7.9	19.9	11.7	35.6
Middle	13.7	34.4	7.3	18.4	9.6	30.3
Fourth	10.7	28.1	7.2	17.7	7.5	25.4
Highest	9.1	22.9	7	16.2	6.7	20.1

Table 4.3 Anemia in children aged 6–59 months by background: caste/tribe

Anemia status by hemoglobin level				
Category	Mild 10–10.9 g/dl	Moderate 7–9.9 g/dl	Severe < 7 g/dl	Any anemia
Scheduled caste	29.2	37.8	2.5	69.5
Scheduled tribe	29.8	40.4	2.2	72.4
Other backward class	28.7	34.6	1.9	65.2
Other	30.1	33.7	1.9	65.8
Don't know	28.7	43.2	1.4	73.3

Table 4.4 Anemia in children aged 6–59 months by background: wealth quintile

Anemia status by hemoglobin level				
Wealth quintile	Mild 10–10.9 g/dl	Moderate 7–9.9 g/dl	Severe < 7 g/dl	Any anemia
Lowest	30.1	39.6	1.9	71.5
Second	30	37.2	2.1	69.3
Middle	29.2	35.7	2.2	67.1
Fourth	28.1	33.8	2.3	64.2
Highest	28.6	31.9	2	62.6

of SCs and STs is lower than their higher caste counterparts.

4.3 The Vicious Cycle of Anemia and Social Disadvantage

When we seek answers to why large sections of Scheduled Castes (SC), Scheduled Tribes (ST), and economically weaker populations continue to lag behind their counterparts, a critical pattern emerges: mothers from these communities are disproportionately worse off. Their health status during pregnancy and motherhood plays a pivotal role in shaping outcomes for the next generation. Anemia stands out as a debilitating factor. For a woman to survive pregnancy, childbirth, and thrive through her motherhood years, adequate iron levels are essential. Yet, the data reveals a worsening trend: anemia among women increased from 53% in NFHS-4 (2015–16) to 57% in NFHS-5 (2019–21). These figures are not just statistics; they reflect systemic inequities. SC, ST, and poor women face compounded disadvantages that perpetuate a cycle of poor health and limited opportunities for their children. It may seem too apparent to mention that for a woman to live a full life and contribute to the family, community, and country, she should be a healthy adult. Her anemia can have an adverse impact not only on her well-being but also on the child she will be rearing. The prevalence of severe anemia remains disproportionately high among women from Scheduled Tribes (ST), Scheduled Castes (SC), and economically disadvantaged groups. This pattern underscores the persistence of an intergenerational cycle of anemia, which can only be disrupted through a comprehensive focus on maternal health, particularly during pregnancy and lactation and the effective implementation of iron and folic acid (IFA) supplementation programs.Notably, women from SC, ST, and low-income households are more reliant on the Integrated Child Development Services (ICDS) for essential maternal and child health interventions. Paradoxically, despite being the primary beneficiaries, these groups often face substandard service provision. The normalization of inadequate services in programs designed for marginalized populations reflects a broader pattern of institutional neglect. This calls for a critical re-evaluation of program design, accountability mechanisms, and equity-focused resource allocation to ensure that the most vulnerable are not left behind (Tables 4.5, 4.6).

Discrimination against Dalits has metamorphosed over time from overt, open, and accepted norms to subtle, invisible, hidden, and 'unaccepted' behavior (Acharya, 2010). In a study of Dalit Children in Selected Villages of Gujarat and Rajasthan, she found that almost always (98% times), the AWWs serve food to the Dalit children at the end. The part of the report explaining the universe of the Dalit children during childhood and how Dalit children perceive discrimination is thought-provoking and calls for sensitization of grassroots-level providers about the corrosive behavior patterns. Ethnographic study in Gujarat's four villages by Nakkeeran et al. (2020) revealed that critical elements of caste-based organizations of social life which permeate the structure and function of the Anganwadi center (AWC)/Supplementary nutrition program (SNP). The SNP fails because the groups that have the greatest need for its services have the least representation in almost every aspect of the program. They further note that the composition of each Anganwadi Center is more or less a microcosm of the village divided along caste and community lines. The established social differentiation and hierarchy is preserved and reproduced as the dominant groups maintain exclusivity for a privileged position in terms of greater access to better-run AWCs, with staff from the same or an acceptable community background than the 'lower' or minority groups. Alternatively, dominant affluent groups may even create or access institutions parallel to AWCs state-funded or private in order to maintain their distinct caste identities (Nakkeeran et al., 2020). The Integrated Child Development Services (ICDS) scheme is among India's most expansive flagship social welfare programs, with significant potential to improve maternal and child health and early childhood development. However, its implementation has faced persistent challenges over the decades, and field observations often reveal infrastructural constraints such as limited

Table 4.5 Anemia in (15–49) by background: caste/tribe and wealth quintile

Background chracterstic	Mild (11–11.9g/dl)1	Moderate (8–10.9g/dl)2	Severe (<8g/dl)3	Any anemia (<12g/dl)4
Caste/tribe				
Scheduled caste	25.5	30.5	3.2	59.2
Scheduled tribe	26.4	35.2	3	64.6
Other backward class	25.3	26.8	2.5	54.6
Other	26.1	27.9	2.3	56.4
Don't know	26.7	32	2.9	61.7
Wealth quintile				
Lowest	27.2	33.7	2.8	63.7
Second	26.4	30.3	2.9	59.5
Middle	25.4	28.5	3	56.9
Fourth	24.8	26.9	2.6	54.4
Highest	24.5	24.5	2	51

Table 4.6 Anganwadi support during pregnancy and breastfeeding by background: caste/tribe

Caste/tribe	No services	Supplementary food	Health check-ups	Health and nutritional education
Mother received from an AWC during pregnancy				
Scheduled caste	26.3	70.4	66.9	62.6
Scheduled tribe	21	77.2	72.6	70.1
Other backward class	29.9	66.4	63.9	59.9
Other	39.1	57.8	53.9	51.3
Don't know	41.1	55.6	48.3	43.5
Mother received from an AWC while breastfeeding2				
Scheduled caste	31.2	66.7	61.1	58.8
Scheduled tribe	24.2	74.7	68.6	67
Other backward class	33.8	63.9	59.1	56.8
Other	42.8	55.1	50	48.4
Do not know	44.6	53.5	42.2	39.8

space, modest facilities, and basic food provisions at Anganwadi centers. These limitations can affect the overall experience and effectiveness of service delivery. Furthermore, Anganwadi workers who serve as the backbone of the program have limited access to capacity-building opportunities and educational resources. These factors collectively hinder the program's ability to deliver quality early childhood education and holistic care.

4.4 'Invisible' Children of Migrant Workers and Urban Slums

The harshest impact of Covid-19 was on migrant workers, who also became 'visible' to the rest of us for the first time while they walked hundreds of kilometers from inhospitable workplaces toward their homes. Due to class, caste, and linguistic divide, migrant workers generally live precarious lives, away from the middle class or policymakers' imaginations. Most of these workers are from lower strata in terms of caste, wealth and are compelled to move in search of livelihood. As Indian social protection policies are essentially designed for stable residents, by default, migrant workers get excluded. Due to the lack of a political voice of their own, this evident and layered exclusion is easily ignored at all levels.

Migration impacts children and women tremendously but, they remain peripheral to the state's imagination of migration on account of being poorly captured in employment and migration statistics. A significant component of India's migration story would be under wraps if we do not pay attention to vulnerabilities of children. Census 2011 enumerates 93 million migrants in the 0–19 years age group: 40% of whom migrate to urban areas, and 14% move across state borders (Naik et al., 2022). Temporary migration of different social groups varied considerably, with very high among scheduled tribes, i.e., 45.2 per 1000. It is 24.8 scheduled castes and 19.5 other backward classes, and 12.2 others per 1000 (Keshri & Bhagat, 2012). While in some cases, the whole family migrates, in other cases, the children are left behind at the origin with their relatives. In both cases, these children lead difficult lives without a parental presence in their native place or without any pre-primary education or nutrition intervention at the destination. Analyzing the National Sample Survey (NSS) 2007–08, Naik et al. (2022) estimate that about 54% of migrant children move with adult members of their household, 36% are left behind in rural areas while their parents move away for work, and about 10% are unaccompanied migrants.

A study across five Indian states assessing the portability of social protection and services for children affected by migration by UNICEF and Center for Policy Research (2021) found that social protection in India is embedded within contrasting logics of universalization and eligibility. Even elements such as education and health that purport universal access are, in practice, only accessible if eligibility criteria such as domicile/residence are met. Additionally, under India's federal structure, social protection schemes are split between Central and state governments. While the thrust of Central schemes is inclusionary, state schemes have different criteria of inclusion. The policy designs by central government usually take years to understand the implementation issues and then course correction.

Now, where the migrant workers choose (or are compelled to) to live in the city also impacts health-education accessibility. Bhan and Jana (2015) argue that specific patterns of spatial inequality determine where diverse urban residents can live in a city region. These patterns affect mobility, asset values, infrastructure, housing, etc. and determine narratives of the 'center' and 'periphery,' shaping belonging and citizenship. Spatial inequality is a dimension of overall inequality, which includes not only economic inequality, but inequality in social, educational, and other sectors of development such as housing, transport, sanitation, electricity and other basic amenities (Kundu & Banerjee, 2018) Water pumps, sewage, and electricity poles are looked at as means of inclusion into the legitimacy fold. These mundane objects and infrastructural interventions entail a firmer grip on citizenship rights by groups otherwise excluded from it (Harms, 2015). However, there is no acknowledgment of the existence of such spaces and people in official policies. In many instances, these settlements are not officially recognized as 'legal,' and their residents are perceived as lacking legitimate claims to the city. As a result, local municipal bodies often do not consider themselves obligated to extend basic services to these populations, further entrenching their marginalization and invisibility within urban governance frameworks.

Public investment in improved sanitation and access to clean water can significantly impact malnutrition compared to modest increments in a household's income. Unprivileged populations face a higher risk due to the general standard of living pushing them toward increasing morbidity. Desai and Throat (2013) call it 'geography as destiny.' The children who live in a poor neighborhood, which invariably has sanitation, water, and environmental issues, are subjected to disease burden leading to further undernourishment. The children migrating with their parents end up living in such under-resourced and unhygienic slums without access to any ICDS Anganwadis. Institutions for social protection are more accountable in rural areas compared to urban areas, where maximum migrant workers live. Designed as a universal scheme for nutrition, health, and development needs of children under 6 years of age, pregnant women, and nursing mothers, ideally, every child up to the age of 6 years, regardless of location or other identities, should be enrolled in Anganwadi. In reality, due to inadequate centers in the area where migrants live and a considerable distance from existing Angawadis, unawareness, and lack of sensitivity about the needs of migrant families, ICDS is not entirely accessible to these children. According to a study by the National Institute of Urban Affairs (NIUA, 2016), about 90% of migrant children did not have access to ICDS or any facilities at the worksite, 65% suffered from various communicable diseases, while 80% did not have access to education and 40% worked as child labor.

This gets reflected in child nutrition outcome indicators of urban area. Corresponding to the rural edge in reducing child malnutrition, a reflection of village-centric interventions—the diminishing urban nutrition advantage has also been fuelled by urban population Growth (Choudhary, 2022). In 2015–16, the prevalence of stunting, underweight, and wasting among children aged 0–5 years in urban India was lower than in rural India, but Choudhary draws attention to the decline in urban India was less than that in rural areas. The trend continues in NFHS-5 (2019–21) as the nutrition status of urban children is not improving at the desired pace (Tables 4.7 and 4.8).

The exclusion of migrant children is also due to the marginalized status of their parents. Not only do these families live in abject poverty, but they also face three critical types of exclusion, those related to identity, eligibility, and location. Migrants lack official identity documents that allow them to identify and register themselves as beneficiaries of schemes at their destination (Srivastava, 2020). Even seemingly inclusive policies that heavily rely on digital technology may not always translate into desired results. 'A new technology of governing spreads through social networks that reaffirm established patronage relations and posits prior recognition in the systems of power as a precondition for inclusion in the system' (Rao, 2013). Rogaly and Thieme's (2012) case study sheds light on processes of exclusion, inequality and differentiation, unequal power geometries, and social topographies and how workers use their own agency to seek to avoid the experience of humiliation and indignity in employment relations. The architecture of our social protection program is based on the assumption of rural and settled citizens. Unlike established citizens with documents, people who move from other areas cannot be easily absorbed into the new bureaucratic system, which makes the families marginalized.

Migrant families are socially and politically disfranchised through the ideals of a sedentary citizen subject (Mander et al., 2019). Similar idea about the 'school child' who would attend all classes on all days in clean uniforms leads to the exclusion of many children from the education system, which begins at the pre-primary level. Reasons for exclusion range from faulty design of the policy, sedentary imagination of policymakers, implementation failure, to unawareness among 'targeted beneficiaries'. The deep-rooted perception among service providers about either 'unwillingness' or lethargy about education is another form of discrimination. 'Despite migrant parents' willingness and aspirations for their children's education, their nowhere locations in the discourse of development and education place them at odds with the 'free' and 'open-to-all' framework of educational inclusion in India' (Ranjan, 2021). In principle, the critical components of children's welfare like accessibility to ICDS, Health and Education services are universally accessible, but mere declarations do not ensure barrier-free and equal access to all.

Table 4.7 Malnutrition in children under 5 years age: by residence

	NFHS-5 (2019–21)		NFHS-4 (2015–16)		
Measure of nutrition	Urban	Rural	Urban	Rural	Total
Height-for-age1					
Percentage below-3 SD	12.6	16	12	17.9	16.3
Percentage below-2 SD2	30.1	37.3	31	41.2	38.4
Weight-for-height					
Percentage below-3 SD	7.6	7.7	7.5	7.4	7.4
Percentage below-2 SD2	18.5	19.5	20	21.4	21
Weight-for-age					
Percentage below-3 SD	9.1	11.2	8.2	12.1	11
Percentage below-2 SD2	27.3	33.8	29.1	38.3	35.7

Table 4.8 Anemia in children aged 6–35 months: by residence

	NFHS-5 (2019–21)		NFHS-4 (2015–16)	
Anemia status by hemoglobin level	Urban	Rural	Urban	Rural
Mild (10.0–10.9 g/dl)	29	29.3	26.8	28.2
Moderate (7.0–9.9 g/dl)	33.1	36.9	27.5	29.7
Severe (<7.0 g/dl)	2.2	2.1	1.6	1.5
Any anemia (<11.0 g/dl)	64.2	68.3	55.9	59.4

4.5 Women Empowerment: One Step Forward and Two Steps Back?

Women's empowerment as the expansion in women's ability to make strategic life choices is valuable on intrinsic grounds, and prioritizing programs to improve the status of women is undoubtedly essential. However, the instrumental value of women's empowerment is also significant. There is evidence of the positive association between women's autonomy, earnings, decision-making, and mobility with greater investment in education, health, and nutrition leading to economic growth in the long term (Malapit & Quisumbing, 2015; Smith & Haddad, 2000). Gender equality has a multiplier effect on many areas of development, including health and nutrition (Pratley, 2016; Carlson, 2015; Cunningham et al., 2015; Richards et al., 2013; Levendosky et al., 2001). A higher level of gender discrimination is associated with a higher level of acute and chronic undernutrition (Muncha, 2012). In Indian context, women's empowerment indicators have advanced considerably and there is tangible change in some areas. Tremendous improvement in percentage of women's bank accounts (53% in NFHS-4 to 78% in NFHS-5) is an excellent example of how the government's thrust on certain standpoints can transform the status.

The prevalence of severe anemia remains disproportionately high among women from Scheduled Tribes (ST), Scheduled Castes (SC), and economically disadvantaged groups. This pattern underscores the persistence of an intergenerational cycle of anemia, which can only be disrupted through a comprehensive focus on maternal health, particularly during pregnancy and lactation and the effective implementation of iron and folic acid (IFA) supplementation programs. Notably, women from SC, ST, and low-income households are more reliant on the Integrated Child Development Services (ICDS) for essential maternal and child health interventions. Paradoxically, despite being the primary beneficiaries, these groups often face substandard service provision. The normalization of inadequate services in programs designed for marginalized populations reflects a broader pattern of institutional neglect. This calls for a critical re-evaluation of program design, accountability mechanisms, and equity-focused resource allocation to ensure that the most vulnerable are not left behind.

4.5.1 Women's Education, Work, and Child Care

A cross-country analysis estimates that improvements in women's status account for 11.61% of global reductions in the proportion of underweight children, and improvements in women's education secondary enrolments account for 43.01% of global reductions in the proportion of underweight children. Taken together, the two indicators accounted for over half of the reductions in children underweight (Smith & Haddad, 2000). However, in the Indian context, it seems like a missed opportunity because, despite a considerable emphasis on '*Beti Bachao-Beti Padhao,*' only 41% of women have 10 or more years of Schooling (NFHS-5, 2019–20). Girls' education directly influences marriage age and the age she becomes pregnant. Young maternal age has inherent biological risk, and the mother is not equipped with the proper knowledge for much-needed care for herself and the child. There are 23.3% of women aged 20–24 years married before age 18 years and 6.8% of women aged 15–19 years who were already mothers or pregnant at the time of the survey.

Girls dropping out of school has socio-cultural aspects, but if educational opportunities translate into employment, there is enthusiasm to spend more years in school-college. Subsequently, women's decisions regarding work are influenced by the availability of support by employer and family. Indian women are obviously reluctant to join workforce as according to NFHS-5, 25.4% of women undertook paid work in the last 12 months, and there is only a marginal rise from 24.6% (NFHS-4). Women's work and child nutrition are complex issues. There is no straightforward relationship, especially in a poor household where the woman is burdened with earning work, child care, and chores. Studies have shown that women's 'Triple Roles' lead to time poverty, which impacts child health outcomes (Saabneh, 2016). Therefore, it becomes all the more important that poor women get support for child care.

Crucial care behaviors like breastfeeding and feeding young children, hygiene and health practices, food preparation and storage, and psychosocial stimulation depend on resources for caregiving (Begin et al., 1999; Smith & Haddad, 2000). Proper nutrition, stimulation, and care during the first 1000 days of life (from conception to the second birthday) have a profound impact on the child's ability to grow, learn, and rise out of poverty and, in the process of shaping society's long-term stability, and prosperity (Mobile Creche Report, 2020). The support for mothers during pregnancy, lactation, and child-rearing is determined by their status, resulting from the interplay of macro-level political-economic factors and micro socio-cultural family dynamics. Women's ability to access and allocate resources, along with access to information and agency decisions for better household food security, is linked to their education and earning capacity.

As per the Social Security Code 2020, maternity benefits are for women working in an organized sector and those working in a setup of 10 or more workers. Most women work in the informal sector where the employer is not bound to give paid leave of 26 weeks and creche service, etc. We are aware many legal entitlements are not translated in reality, but, in this case, its ironic that even legally, women working in back breaking work in informal sector are excluded from maternity related provisions. Nevertheless, extreme poor women cannot afford not to go to work, and most of these women resume work while they are still weak. These mothers are already lagging in health indicators including hemoglobin levels, so the new-born infants are usually low birthweight with lower immunity. There is mental stress for any new mother under challenging circumstances affecting her health and the child's health. Children suffer silently when state-supported creches are almost non-existent while their mothers battle on many fronts.

4.6 Recommendations and the Way Forward

Recent policy initiatives such as Poshan Abhiyan, Swachhta Mission, Sarva Shiksha Abhiyan, and Naari Shakti reflect the government's ambitious commitment to inclusive development. While these programs are laudable in intent, their success hinges not on slogans or symbolic gestures but on the nuanced understanding of ground-level implementation challenges. For instance, schemes like One Nation One Ration have the potential to benefit marginalized populations, yet an over-reliance on digital infrastructure may inadvertently exclude those without access or literacy. It is imperative that policy design remains rooted in ethical reflection and social empathy. Gandhiji's talisman, urging us to recall the face of the poorest and weakest before making any decision, offers a timeless compass for evaluating the real-world utility of such interventions. In this light, rhetoric must be matched by responsive governance, contextual sensitivity, and participatory mechanisms that ensure no one is left behind.

4.6.1 Children as Right Holders

Young children are not passive recipients of care but active rights holders. Given their cognitive, physical, and emotional vulnerabilities, it is incumbent upon both the state and society to safeguard their rights with urgency and compassion. The marginal cost of fulfilling these rights is relatively low, making the failure to prioritize them not just a policy oversight but a profound moral lapse—especially in contexts where resource scarcity is not the primary constraint. Early childhood care and development (ECCD) form the bedrock of lifelong learning and well-being. Education, recognized as a foundational capability, enables the expansion of other capabilities essential for human flourishing. When ECCD is neglected, it leads to corrosive consequences that reverberate across generations. In a country marked by structural inequalities and fragmented social protection systems, the imperative to break the intergenerational cycle of disadvantage is both ethical and strategic. Child care must be reframed as a public good, not a private burden. Prioritizing the disadvantaged child should be elevated to a socio-political agenda, guiding policy design, budgetary allocations, and community action. Such a shift demands not only institutional commitment but also a collective moral imagination, one that sees every child as a citizen with entitlements, not merely as a future economic contributor.

4.6.2 Acknowledging, Understanding, and Addressing Discrimination

Addressing inequities requires deliberate and sustained efforts. Caste-based discrimination remains a deeply entrenched social reality in many parts of India. When such discrimination is widespread yet absent from the official policy discourse, it risks not only being perpetuated but also inadvertently reinforced through programmatic silence. It is naïve to assume that development interventions can achieve their intended outcomes without first establishing a robust protective environment and confronting the structural roots of exclusion. Mass awareness campaigns must be launched to challenge discriminatory norms and foster inclusive attitudes. Sensitization of frontline workers, such as Accredited Social Health Activists (ASHAs) and Anganwadi Workers (AWWs) is essential to ensure that service delivery is equitable and respectful. Furthermore, adequate representation from Dalit and tribal communities within the workforce can enhance trust and accountability. Expanding the reach of Anganwadi centers in marginalized localities is another critical step toward ensuring that early childhood services are accessible to those who need them most. Ultimately, equity must be embedded not just in rhetoric but in the design, implementation, and monitoring of social programs. A rights-based, inclusive approach, grounded in social justice and community participation can help dismantle intergenerational disadvantage and build a more just and compassionate society.

4.6.3 Support the Migrant Children-Wherever They Go

While the Integrated Child Development Services (ICDS), along with health and education schemes, are designed to be universally accessible, the assumption that 'free' and 'open to all' equates to equitable access is deeply flawed. Structural barriers like social, economic, and geographic continue to impede the most marginalized, particularly during the critical early years of a child's life. Despite the proliferation of innovative interventions such as residential schools, the foundational period from birth to six years remains insufficiently prioritized in policy and practice. To fulfill the transformative potential of ICDS, sustained and strategic investment is essential. This includes upgrading physical infrastructure, expanding and training human resources, and integrating contextually relevant pedagogical tools, especially in underserved and remote communities. Such efforts are not merely technical adjustments but moral imperatives, given the long-term impact of early childhood development on educational attainment and life outcomes. Moreover, the persistent gap between ICDS's stated objectives and its on-ground delivery must be openly scrutinized and brought into the realm of political accountability. The program's sedentary design fails to accommodate the lived realities of migrant workers, whose mobility, extended work hours, and lack of social support systems render static service models ineffective. It is imperative to reimagine ICDS as a dynamic, responsive, and inclusive system. This includes learning from and scaling up successful NGO-led innovations that have demonstrated adaptability and community engagement. Ultimately, making ICDS reliable and equitable is not just a policy upgrade, but it is a long-overdue commitment to the rights and dignity of every child, especially those born into disadvantage.

4.6.4 Making Underserved Neighborhoods Better

This analysis underscores the urgent and differentiated needs of underprivileged children, whose health and well-being are severely compromised by deficits in safe drinking water, open defecation practices, and poor hygiene conditions. These deprivations are not incidental but systemic, disproportionately affecting children in informal settlements and slum areas. Despite the universal rhetoric of rights and entitlements, the lived realities of these children reveal persistent gaps in access to basic services. A critical shift in policy is required, one that explicitly acknowledges the legitimacy of even officially unrecognized settlements and ensures their inclusion in sanitation and public health planning. The current exclusionary frameworks not only violate the principles of equity but also perpetuate cycles of disadvantage. Urban development schemes must extend their focus beyond metropolitan centers to tier-II and tier-III cities, where the coverage of basic amenities in slum areas remains alarmingly inadequate. While the enthusiasm surrounding the Smart Cities reflects a forward-looking vision, it must be tempered with a commitment to inclusive urbanism. Development should not come at the cost of invisibilizing the urban poor or displacing them from their socio-cultural ecosystems. A balanced approach demands that poor neighborhoods be integrated into the urban fabric, not as peripheral zones but as legitimate spaces deserving of investment, dignity, and voice. In this context, child-centric urban planning becomes a moral and developmental imperative. Prioritizing sanitation, water access, and hygiene in marginalized areas is not merely a technical fix but a foundational step toward realizing children's rights and breaking the intergenerational transmission of poverty and exclusion.

4.6.5 Inclusive Policies for Migrant Workers

Inclusive policy design for migrant workers remains a pressing concern in India's welfare architecture. Children of migrant workers often experience layered discrimination, not only due to their socio-economic status but also because of the disenfranchised and transient identity of their parents. The COVID-19 pandemic exposed these vulnerabilities starkly, offering a moment of reckoning to recalibrate policies with greater empathy and inclusion. In a welfare state, the insistence on documentary proof for identity, eligibility, and location as prerequisites for accessing social security schemes must be critically examined. Such requirements, while administratively convenient, systematically exclude the most marginalized—those who lack stable housing, formal employment, or consistent access to public services. The launch of the One Nation One Ration Card (ONORC) scheme is a step toward portability of food entitlements through the Public Distribution System (PDS). However, while the scheme promises access across states, its impact on reducing malnutrition remains limited. The quality, quantity, and nutritional adequacy of food provided must be addressed alongside logistical access. Political invisibility compounds the social exclusion of migrant workers. The non-portability of voting rights renders them electorally insignificant, stripping them of a voice in shaping policies that directly affect their lives. Migrant workers are often undervalued both at their place of origin and at their destination, caught in a liminal space where neither community fully claims responsibility for their welfare. While logistical challenges to enabling mobile voting exist, they are not insurmountable, especially in an era marked by digital innovation and expanding e-governance infrastructure.

4.6.6 When Women Flourish, Everyone Benefits

Despite incremental progress, India continues to grapple with deeply entrenched patriarchal norms that constrain women's education, delay their entry into the workforce, and reinforce early marriage practices. These issues are interlinked and cannot be addressed in isolation. Without proactive and sustained state support, structural transformation in gender equity remains elusive. Public policy must recognize that empowering women is not merely a social goal, but it is a developmental imperative with far-reaching consequences for families, communities, and the nation. Addressing anemia among women, especially adolescent girls and mothers, is one such critical intervention. It is not just a health concern but a matter of social justice. Anemia undermines women's productivity, learning capacity, and maternal health, perpetuating cycles of disadvantage. Targeted, community-based strategies, such as nutrition supplementation, awareness campaigns, and regular screening must be scaled up with urgency. Equally important is the recognition that while families are the primary unit of child care, they cannot be the sole providers, especially for women in the unorganized sector who need and want to work. State-supported quality crèche services are essential to enable women's economic participation. Such services not only allow women to earn income but also confer respect, autonomy, and social status. The ripple effect of a mother's income, enhanced food security, better health, and educational outcomes for children cannot be overstated. A phased conversion of existing Anganwadi centers into Anganwadi-cum-crèches, particularly in urban slums and underserved rural areas, is a pragmatic and equitable step forward. The defunct status of the Crèche Scheme highlights the need for renewed commitment and innovation. A robust service delivery mechanism under the Integrated Child Development Services (ICDS), with adequate staffing, infrastructure, and monitoring, can serve as a cornerstone for supporting working mothers and advancing gender equity. Ultimately, when women flourish, families thrive, and societies prosper. Investing in women's health, education, and child care is not a peripheral concern—it is central to building a just and inclusive India.

References

Acharya, S. S. (2010). *Access to health care and patterns of discrimination: A study of dalit children in selected villages of Gujarat and Rajasthan*. Working paper series. Indian Institute of Dalit Studies and UNICEF. Retrieved from https://idsn.org/wpcontent/uploads/2017/10/IIDS__Access_to_Health_Care_and_Patterns_of_Discrimination.pdf

Begin, F., Frongillo, E. A., & Delisle, H. (1999). Caregiver behaviors and resources influence child height-for-age in rural Chad. *The Journal of Nutrition, 129*(3), 680–686. https://doi.org/10.1093/jn/129.3.680

Bhan, G., & Jana, A. (2015). Reading Spatial Inequality in Urban India. *Economic and Political Weekly, 50*(22), 50(22). http://www.jstor.org/stable/24482492

Carlson, C. J., Kordas, K., & Murray-Kolb, L. E. (2015). Associations between women's autonomy and child nutritional status: A review of the literature. *Maternal and Child Nutrition, 11*(4), 82–452. https://doi.org/10.1111/mcn.12113

Choudhary, N. (2022). *COVID-19 as an opportunity to engage with urban malnutrition challenge* (Vol. 57). USA: Economic and Political Weekly (Engage). Retrieved from https://www.epw.in/engage/article/covid-19-opportunity-engage-urban-malnutrition

Cunningham, K., Ruel, M., Ferguson, E., & Uauy, R. (2015). Women's empowerment and child nutritional status in South Asia: A synthesis of the literature. *Maternal and Child Nutrition, 11*(1), 1–19. https://doi.org/10.1111/mcn.12125

Desai, S., & Throat, A. (2013). Beyond the great Indian nutrition debate. *Economic and Political Weekly, XLVIII*(7), 18–22. https://www.researchgate.net/publication/286886442_Beyond_the_great_Indian_nutrition_debate

Desai, S. (2022, May 2). *Global hunger index: A lesson in how not to measure hunger*. The Indian Express. Global Hunger Index: A lesson in how not to measure hunger | The Indian Express

Deshpande, A., & Ramchandran, R. (2021). *The missing piece of the puzzle: Caste discrimination and stunting*. Center for Economic Data and Analysis. Retrieved from https://ceda.ashoka.edu.in/the-missing-piece-of-the-puzzle-caste-Discrimination-and-stunting/

Dixon, R., & Nussbaum, M. C. (2012). Children's rights and a capabilities approach: The question of special priority. *Cornell Law Review, 97*(3), 549–595. http://SCholarship.law.cornell.edu/clr/vol97/iss3/3

ESCAP. (2022). *SDG progress report 2022: Transforming economies, realizing rights, and accelerating progress in Asia and the Pacific*. United Nations Economic and Social Commission for Asia and the Pacific. Retrieved from https://www.uneSCap.org/sites/default/d8files/knowledge-products/ESCAP-2022-FG_SDG-Progress-Report.pdf

Gillespie, S. (2013). Myths and realities of child nutrition. *Economic and Political Weekly, 48*(34), 64–67. Retrieved from https://www.im4change.org/siteadmin/tinymce/uploaded/Myths_and_Realities_of_Child_Nutrition.pdf

Government of India. Ministry of Health and Family Welfare. (2019). National Family Health Survey (NFHS-5), 2019–20: India fact sheet. http://rchiips.org/nfhs/NFHS-5Reports/NFHS-5_INDIA_REPORT.pdf

Harms, A. (2015). *Off the grid: Environmental degradation and citizenship at the margins*. Crossroads Asia Working Paper Series, No. 27. https://bonndoc.ulb.uni-bonn.de/xmlui/bitstream/handle/20.500.11811/162/Crossroads_Asia_Working_Paper_27_Harms_Off_the_Grid.pdf?sequence=1&isAllowed=y

Kabeer, N. (2002). Resources, agency, achievements: Reflections on the measurement of women's empowerment. *Development and Change, 30*(3), 435–464. https://doi.org/10.1111/1467-7660.00125

Keshri, K., & Bhagat, R. B. (2012). Temporary and seasonal migration: Regional pattern, characteristics and associated factors. *Economic and Political Weekly, 47*(4), 81–88. http://www.jstor.org/stable/41419769

Kundu, D., & Banerjee, A. (2018). Migration, caste and marginalised sections inequality in the coverage of basic services in urban India. *Economic & Political Weekly, 53*(2). https://www.researchgate.net/publication/322734325_Migration_caste_and_marginalised_sections_Inequality_in_the_coverage_of_basic_services_in_Urban_India

Levendosky, A. A., Bermann, G., & Sandra, A. (2001). Parenting in battered women: The effects of domestic violence on women and their children. *Journal of Family Violence, 16*(2), 171–192. https://doi.org/10.1023/A:1011111003373

Majumdar, M. (2020, January 25). Democratic politics should be concerned with early childhood education. *Economic and Political Weekly (Engage), 55*(4). https://www.epw.in/engage/article/democratic-politics-should-be-concerned-early

Malapit, H. J., & Quisumbing, A. R. (2015). What dimensions of women's empowerment in agriculture matter for nutrition in Ghana? *Food Policy*, 52, 54–63. https://doi.org/10.1016/j.foodpol.2014.11.002 (Malapit and Quisumbing, 2015)

Mander, H., Roy, I., Jain, P., Raman, R., Ray, R. G., Bhattacharya, A., & Siddiqi, U. J. (2019). Stolen citizenship, stolen freedoms: Locating the rights of India's circular labor migrants. *ESClavages & Post-eSClavages*, 1. http://journals.openedition.org/slaveries/610

Ministry of Women and Child Development. (2015). *Rajiv gandhi national creche scheme for the children of working mothers*. Retrieved from https://wcd.nic.in/sites/default/files/Revised%20RGNCSSCheme_210515.pdf

Mobile Creches. (2020). *State of young children in India*. London: Routledge. https://doi.org/10.1080/00094056.2021.2000274

Mukhopadhyay, P., & Chakraborty, R. (2023). The politics of child undernutrition data in India. *Economic and Political Weekly, LVIII*(17). Retrieved from https://www.epw.in/journal/2023/17/commentary/politics-child-undernutrition-data-india.html

Muncha, N. (2012). *Enabling and equipping women to improve nutrition*. Bread for the World Institute. Briefing Paper No. 16. Washington, DC. https://www.bread.org/sites/default/files/downloads/briefing-paper-16.pdf

Muthayya, S., Rah, J. H., Sugimoto, J. D., Roos, F. F., Kraemer, K., & Black, R. E. (2013). The global hidden hunger indices and maps: An advocacy tool for action. *PLoS ONE, 8*(6), Article e67860. https://doi.org/10.1371/journal.pone.0067860

Naik, M., Lahiri, A., Kaushik, U., & Manish. (2022). A case for functional social protection portability to address vulnerabilities of migration-affected children. *Economic and Political Weekly, 57*(44–45). Retrieved from https://www.epw.in/engage/article/case-functional-social-protection-portability

Nakkeeran, N, et al. (2020). Recasting food. *CASTE/A Global Journal on Social Exclusion, 1*(1), 1–16. https://doi.org/10.26812/caste.v1i1.6. Accessed 19 Dec. 2022.

NIUA with Support from Bernard van Leer Foundation. (2016). *Status of children in urban India, Baseline Study 2016*. Retrieved from https://smartnet.niua.org/sites/default/files/resources/statusl.pdf

Panagariya, A. (2013). Does India really suffer from worse child malnutrition than sub-Saharan Africa? *Economic and Political Weekly, 48*(18), 98–111. Retrieved from http://www.jstor.org/stable/23527314

Pratley, P. (2016). Associations between quantitative measures of women's empowerment and access to care and health status for mothers and their children: A systematic review of evidence from the developing world. *Social Science and Medicine, 169*, 119–131. https://doi.org/10.1016/j.socSCimed.2016.08.001

Ranjan, V. (2021). Migrant children and 'free' education in India. *Economic and Political Weekly, LVI*(48). https://publications.azimpremjiuniversity.edu.in/id/eprint/4243

Rao, U. (2013). Biometric marginality: UID and the shaping of homeless identities in the city. *Economic and Political Weekly, 48*(13), 71–77. http://www.jstor.org/stable/23391467

Richards, E., Theobald, S., George, A., Kim, J. C., Rudert, C., Jehan, K., & Tolhurst, R. (2013). Going beyond the surface: Gendered intrahousehold bargaining as a social determinant of child health and nutrition in low- and middle-income countries. *Social Science and Medicine, 95*, 2433. https://doi.org/10.1016/j.socSCimed.2012.06.015

Rogaly, B., & Thieme, S. (2012). Experiencing space-time: The stretched lifeworlds of migrant workers in India. *Environment and Planning a: Economy and Space, 44*(9), 2086–2100. https://doi.org/10.1068/a44493

Roy, I. (2016). *Enhancing mobility: Political and social rights for circular labor migrants*. International Growth Centre. Retrieved from https://www.theigc.org/publication/enhancing-mobility-political-and-social-rights-for-circular-labour-migrants/

Saabneh, A. (2016). The association between maternal employment and child survival in India, 1998–99 and 2005–06. *Asian Population Studies, 13*, 1–19. https://doi.org/10.1080/17441730.2016.1239412

Sen, A. (1993). *Capability approach and social justice in education* (E. U. Melanie Walker, Ed.). Palgrave Macmillan New York. https://doi.org/10.1057/9780230604810

Smith, C. L., & Haddad, L. (2000). *Explaining child malnutrition in developing countries: A cross-country analysis*. IFPRI. https://books.google.co.in/books?hl=en&lr=&id=cFvJ39bkNikC&oi=fnd&pg=PR4&dq=Smith,+C.+L.,+%26+Haddad,+L.+(2000).+Explaining+child+malnutrition+in+developing+countries:+A+cross-country+analysis.+IFPRI.&ots=U1RjSUD8ZE&sig=8DnoRD-sjGPPLDjw7PcX04jnH4w#v=onepage&q&f=false

Srivastava, R. (2020). *Vulnerable internal migrants in India and portability of social security and entitlements*. Centre for Employment Studies Working Paper Series, Institute for Human Development. http://www.ihdindia.org/Working%20Ppaers/2020/IHD-CES_WP_02_2020.pdf

Thorat, S., & Sadana, N. (2009). Discrimination and children's nutritional status in India. *IDS Bulletin, 40*(4), 74–83. https://doi.org/10.1111/j.1759-5436.2009.00055.x

UNICEF. (2006). *The state of the world's children 2006: Excluded and invisible*. UNICEF. https://www.unicef.org/media/84806/file/SOWC-2006.pdf

UNICEF. (2021). *Assessing the portability of social protection and services for children affected by migration: A study across five Indian states*. Center for Policy Research. https://www.unicef.org/india/documents/assessing-portability-social-protection-and-services-children-affected-migration

United Nations Development Programme. (1990). *Human development report 1990*. https://doi.org/10.18356/7007ef44-en

World Education Forum. (2000). *The Dakar framework for action: Education for all* (Dakar, Senegal) World Education Forum; The Dakar Framework for Action: Education for All: meeting our collective commitments (including six regional frameworks for action); 2000 (right-to-education.org)

Part II
Innovations in Healthcare

5 Disaster and Health Emergencies: The Indispensable Mobile Health Clinics

Jayanti Saha

Abstract

The mobile health clinic is an alternative strategy to provide health care services to the people primarily displaced due to wars, political upheaval, and in different emergencies like disasters where no other health facility is available to the people. The purpose of the study is to give a brief description of the history of the mobile health clinic and its role during disaster and health emergencies in the Indian context. This study shows that mobile health clinics emerged during the Second World War. Depending on the geographical condition, the types of mobile health clinics differ across the country. Over the period, it is found that when fixed health care delivery gets disrupted during disasters or impaired at the time of pandemic mobile health clinics are deployed to reach those affected people to provide primary care. This paper underlines the pressing need to prepare for the future to handle any public health emergencies by expanding the use of the MHCs and their services through integration into the health care delivery system as it has the potential to address the primary health care needs of the population at the time of public health emergencies.

5.1 Introduction

The Declaration of Alma-Ata stated that access to primary health care is the right of all the population and to achieve the goal of health for all (World Health Organization, 1978). Primary health care integrates care, prevention, promotion, and education to meet the health needs of all patients in the community. But still, in the twenty-first century, a substantial proportion of population are deprived of access to primary health care services across the world. Therefore, the Mobile Health Clinic (MHC) became a popular model developed over the period to provide primary health care services to underserved populations. The mobile health clinic is a customized vehicle reaching the doors of vulnerable communities living not only in rural areas but also in urban slums (Hill et al., 2012). Over the period, mobile health clinics are also found to be the authentic strategy to provide health services to the people primarily displaced due to wars, political upheaval, and in different emergency situations like disaster where no other alternative healthcare is available to the people (World Health Organization, n.d.). Basically, mobile health clinic ensures to meet the health care needs of the marginal-

J. Saha (✉)
Centre of Social Medicine and Community Health, Jawaharlal Nehru University, Delhi, India
e-mail: jysaha5@gmail.com

S. S. Acharya et al. (eds.), *Paradigm Shifts in Population and Health in India*, Sustainable Development Goals Series, https://doi.org/10.1007/978-981-95-1719-0_5

ized section of the society through removing the geographical barriers to access health care (Yu et al., 2017). Its fundamental aim is to connect marginalized sections of society with the mainstream health system of the country (Khanna & Narula, 2016). It helps to achieve health equity by improving the health outcomes of the disadvantaged population of society by providing preventative, screening, curative, diagnostic, and mental health (Oriol et al., 2009). It plays a significant role to address both acute and chronic conditions using the patient-centered approach (Fils-Aimé et al., 2018). This paper has attempted to give a brief description of the history of the mobile health clinic in India and its role during disaster and health emergencies.

5.2 Types of Mobile Health Clinics

There are various types of mobile health clinics such as mobile vans, camels, boats and helicopters to reach the hard-to-reach population in hilly areas, deserts, and islands (Ahmed et al., 2019; Post, 2017; United Nations Office for the Coordination of Humanitarian Affairs, 2010; National Health Mission Tripura., n.d.). These types of MHC varied by the nature of the physical characteristics of the geographical region and climatic condition. For instance, the boat or floating clinic is operated in the riverine islands, wetlands, marshy delta, and inland sea coast (Ahmed et al., 2019; Ahuja, 2022). In the Loreto region due to the presence of the Amazon River and its tributaries, health services are delivered through a customized ship to the communities living in the interior parts. Similar pieces of evidence are observed in the southern part of Myanmar, Congo, Burundi and Tanzania, the *char* in Bangladesh and India where health services are provided through boat clinics (Ndayizigamiye & Maharaj, 2016; Kojima et al., 2017; ReliefWeb, 2017; Neke et al., 2018; Specchio dei tempi, n.d). Camel clinics are used in the desert because their large footpads make it easier to navigate on stony and sandy roads (United Nations Office for the Coordination of Humanitarian Affairs, 2010). Likewise, primary healthcare services are provided through mobile vans in Rajasthan to the tribal people residing in inaccessible desert villages (National Health Mission Rajasthan, n.d.). In the mountainous region, motorcycles are used because of ultra-rugged terrain and poor road connectivity for visiting rural and remote communities living on hill slopes, forests, and river banks regularly. The motorcycles are used to collect the sample from far-flung villages and send it back to the laboratories for testing HIV/AIDS and associated tuberculosis (Spoth, 2008). Helicopter is one of the vehicles which are used rarely to serve the hard-to-reach underserved tribal population in undulating hilly and forest covered villages of North and Dhalai districts of Tripura in India where people have no health care facilities. In this region, the health teams visit the designated village to serve sites to provide health care services like immunization, antenatal, postnatal care, awareness campaign on hygiene and other health related issues (National Health Mission Tripura, n.d.).

5.3 Types of Services Provided by Mobile Health Clinics

It is a well-known fact that mobile clinics cannot meet static health centers in terms of consistency of care and variety of services, but it can offer essential health services with adequate efficacy in settings where permanent health centers are not available (Peters et al., 2014). Depending on the degree of economic and infrastructure development and disease burden of the country the type of services offered by mobile health clinics differs. In developing and underdeveloped countries generally, mobile health clinics are used to deliver primary care, preventive health screenings, chronic disease management, dental care, reproductive health care, and mental health care (Fils-Aimé et al., 2018). But in developed countries like Australia, Canada, New Zealand, and the United States of America, it was observed that along with a wide range of general primary care some specialty care such as breast cancer screening and ophthalmology services are also provided (Beks et al., 2020; Trivedi et al., 2022; Williams et al., 2019; "How do mobile health clinics improve access to healthcare", n.d.). Based on the disease burden of the country the mobile health clinic also facilitates services like for example African countries and India with a high burden of HIV have provision of its testing services in the MHC, in the same manner, hyperlipidemia is one of the highly prevalent chronic diseases in the USA because of that in many MHC of USA blood cholesterol screening are conducted (Geoffroy et al., 2014; Kojima et al., 2017; Rousseau et al., 2021). Similarly, evidence has been found that during the monsoon season, the burden of vector-borne disease increase as a result of this MHC extended its service and included malaria and dengue testing ("Dhanvantari Raths," 2020). Tuberculosis is a major public health issue in India, but because people in remote areas lack access to TB treatment, mobile health clinics are deployed to diagnose and treat the underserved risk population (The Hindu, n.d.).

5.4 Target Population of Mobile Health Clinics

Mobile health clinics facilitate health care services particularly to the geographically isolated, socially deprived, and vulnerable population. This is because these particular groups of populations have resided in remote and hard-to-reach areas that have unavailability of services in the vicinity and lack of transportation facilities. Therefore, to reach out to these populations MHCs are widely used to address their health care needs. By removing transport, financial and cultural barriers it reduces access related barriers to the static healthcare provision of the community, and it is considered linguistically and culturally appropriate care (Guruge et al., 2010). Thus, besides the general population the MHC emphasizes targeting low income, minority groups, tribal populations, children, pregnant women, adolescent girls, tea gardeners,displaced populations, elderly people, homeless people, migrant workers, LGBTQIAP+, etc. (Caires, 2017; Kojima et al., 2017; Kumar et al., 2020; Whelan et al., 2010; Yu et al., 2017; Government of Assam, n.d.; HelpAge India, n.d.; Patient Engagement Hit, n.d.; "The Hans foundation", n.d.).

5.5 Source of Funding for Mobile Health Clinics

The World Health Organization with the help of its partners deploys mobile health clinics to reach the underserved population without access to health services (World Health Organization, 2019). The mobile health clinics are funded by international organizations, governments, and non-profit organizations. But majorly philanthropy is the primary source of funding for mobile clinics (Malone et al., 2020). NGOs across the globe play a vital role to acquire funds and provide services through mobile clinics in remote locations. As a part of corporate social responsibility, mobile health clinics are launched across the underserved areas of the country. Before the NRHM the MHCs were operated by the state in tribal districts. But after the launch of NRHM, it has expanded its opportunity to avail funds for MHCs to "take health care to doorsteps of the public in rural areas, especially in the underserved tribal areas" (Nandi et al., 2017). The National health policy 2017 emphasizes the importance of Mobile Medicals Units (MMUs) to increase the outreach of health services to the tribal and socially vulnerable population groups with the active involvement of NGOs (Ministry of Health and Family Welfare, n.d.). Like for instance the Hindustan Petroleum Corporation Limited with the help of local NGOs runs seven mobile medical vans in the states of Andhra Pradesh, Bihar, Jammu and Kashmir, Jharkhand, Odisha, Maharashtra, and Rajasthan. Since 2008, the Centre for North East Studies and Policy Research (C-NES), an NGO, has been delivering health care services in these hard-to-reach locations using boat clinics under a public–private partnership (PPP) agreement with the National Health Mission (CSRBOX Desk, 2017). In Kenya, the Communities Health Africa Trust (CHAT), a non-governmental organization, has stepped in to assist in the transportation of medication to rural places using camels (United Nations Office for the Coordination of Humanitarian Affairs, 2010).

5.6 History of Mobile Health Clinics in India

Mobile health clinic in India has its own historical development process. At the very beginning of the Second World War, Baron Dominique Jean Larrey, a French surgeon and military doctor came up with the idea of a mobile army surgical hospital to provide immediate lifesaving treatment to soldiers on the battlefield and deploy them to the military hospitals (All India Women's Conference, n.d.). In India, a British woman named Hilda Seligman introduced a mobile clinic because after staying for a long period of time in India she had observed the distressful condition of rural and tribal women and children, hence decided to found a fund known as "Skippo" in 1945. Using that fund a mobile medical van was custom-built in the United Kingdom and offered to the All India's Women Conference (AIWC) to reach the vulnerable tribal population through mobile vans in places with very negligible healthcare facilities. It provided services like immunization, antenatal care to pregnant women (All India Women's Conference, n.d.). Later the fund Skippo helped to provide family planning programs also along with medical services in the innermost rural areas of India (Ghate, 1982). In the vehicle based mobile clinic, there were altogether five health care workers including a female doctor, nurse, trained health worker and a driver. After working for strengthening the program in 1952, the AIWC was able to attract funds from different countries like Canada, the United Kingdom, and New Zealand and extended its services by adding number of mobile vans. But later on, there are various ups and down in the interest of the implementation of the mobile health clinic over the period due to its limitations of extending health care (Venkatesh, 2018). During the late 1990s, the MHC was found to deliver primary care in various hard-to-reach areas across the country but in a very limited manner. For example, under the Southern Health Improvement Sanity the boat is delivering services in the Sundarban delta of West Bengal since 1997 (Ahuja, 2022). In Gwalior and Bhopal, the mobile health clinics were established in 1992 which served the poor population of urban areas. Through provisioning of the family planning services, child and maternal health care it was able to increase the use of family planning services, and decline in infant mortality (Morrison, 1996). In Tamil Nadu, mobile health clinics were used for the first time in 1977 under the Primary Health Centers. But in the mid-1980s, the mobile health clinics did not culminate as fixed health care centers were found to be acknowledged more.

But when it came to notice that though health infrastructure was improved but had not reached the remote areas in 2002 the Government of Tamil Nadu again introduced mobile health clinics and distribute them to different districts to provide health care services in the remote inaccessible areas (Dash et al., 2008). In the same year in Orissa also mobile health clinics were introduced in different areas of the state. In 2005 a mobile health clinic (*Sehat ki Sawari*) was launched in two districts of Uttarakhand i.e., Tehri and Chamoli to serve the hard-to-reach disadvantaged population of the area who have to travel long distances for reaching the health centers. This program is functioning in collaboration with the Uttarakhand Health and Family Welfare Society and Hindustan Latex Family Planning Promotion Trust (Department of Medical Help and Family Welfare). The initiative is being carried out with the help of the European Commission's Sector Investment Program in cooperation with Uttarakhand Health and Family Welfare Society (SCOVA) and Hindustan Latex Family Planning Promotion Trust (HLFPPT).

The launch of the National Rural Health Mission in 2005 is the turning point to increase the demand for mobile health clinics in India. After the commencement of the National Health Mission (NHM), the use of MHC has boomed because NHM tries to increase access to health care, particularly to people living in remote, difficult, under-served, and unreached areas (National Health Mission, 2018). Thus, MHCs are used as a strategy to take healthcare to the doorstep of the underserved population. Public–private partnership model is adopted to expand the outreach program of the mobile health clinics (Ministry of Health & Family Welfare, 2015). In the 6th

Common Review Mission, it was stated that in India 1307 mobile medical units were functioning in 349 districts of India (National Health Mission, 2015).

Different states have adopted this healthcare model to provide healthcare services in remote areas. For example, an outreach program known as *Jeewan Jyoti Yojana* served the tribal areas of Madhya Pradesh with a high concentration of Scheduled Caste and Scheduled Tribe since 1988 (National Health Mission Madhya Pradesh, n.d.). But after the launch of NHM, the scheme was renamed as Deen Dayal Mobile Health Clinic and expanded its services in the year 2006. It provided basic health care services, awareness of sanitation and hygiene, health prevention on different communicable and non-communicable diseases to improve the health indicators of the population. Similarly, in Rajasthan also the tribal population living in the desert areas faces difficulties to access health care facilities as it is far away from the villages and most importantly the poor socio-economic condition makes them unable to afford it. To reach this population, the government of Rajasthan implemented the program Rajiv Gandhi Rural Mobile Medical Unit in 2008–09. Under this program, monthly health camps were planned to provide free medical checkups and medicines (National Health Mission Rajasthan, n.d.). Similarly, to serve the hard-to-reach underserved population where people have no health care facilities in villages of North and Dhalai districts of Tripura helicopters were used. The health teams visit the designated villages to provide health care services like immunization, antenatal, and postnatal care, awareness campaign on hygiene and other health related issues (National Health Mission Tripura, n.d.). In Assam, about three million people are living on the riverine islands. Being situated in the vulnerable riverine areas the people of Assam hardly got an opportunity to avail the benefits of any health programs as they are beyond the reach of any doctor or health workers. Considering the plight of this population, in 2004–2005 the Centre for North East Studies and Policy (C-NES) came up with a major intervention called Boat Clinic to overcome the geographic accessibility barriers and fill the gap in health services. At first, the boat named "Ship of Hope in a Valley of Flood" was introduced in the Dibrugarh district of Assam and was able to receive an award from the World Bank for its innovative concept. After that UNICEF also helped C-NES to gradually extend its services in other districts. Later, in 2008, the National Rural Health Mission, Government of Assam collaborated with C-NES to reach the far-flung riverine islands of the Brahmaputra (Centre for North East Studies and Policy Research, n.d.). On one hand, the National Rural Health Mission incur the operational costs as well as payment of the human resource of the boat clinic and on the other hand, the C-NES is responsible to take care of the boats such as their construction, insurance (Ministry of Health & Family Welfare, 2015). At present, through the public–private partnership between the C-NES and the National Health Mission the boat clinic has been functioning in thirteen districts of Assam to provide primary health care to the *char-chapori*. It provides basic health care services such as routine immunization, family planning, screening of both communicable (HIV, tuberculosis) as well as non-communicable diseases (diabetics, cataracts), vector-borne diseases to the inhabitants of the Brahmaputra islands through a boat equipped with OPD, laboratories, and pharmacies.

There are several organizations offering primary healthcare through mobile health clinics. A not-for-profit organization known as HelpAge which is widely known as Asia's largest mobile healthcare network for elders currently provides healthcare services to 2000 community locations across 24 states of India. Similarly, Wockhardt Foundation initiated the Mobile 1000 program provides primary health care free of cost in the slums of Mumbai (Wockhardt Foundation, n.d). And now it has been successful to reach more than 4000 villages in 20 states of India. The objective of these vans is to fill the gap in primary healthcare in India through the ADCR formula i.e., awareness, diagnosis, cure, and referral. It is creating awareness in the villages regarding sanitation, hygiene practices, safe drinking water, maternal and child healthcare, diseases like HIV, tuberculosis, and diabetes (Mobile 1000, n.d.; Wockhardt Foundation, 2019). At present in India total 200 mobile vans are operating in different states of India under Wockhardt Limited.

5.7 Role of Mobile Health Clinics During Disaster and Pandemic

Disasters have a significant impact on healthcare facilities, making it difficult for patients to get timely and adequate medical care. In a situation like that a mobile health clinic is an alternative for providing medical service to disaster victims who face challenges in accessing healthcare facilities due to the disruption of infrastructure (Ahmad et al., 2008). A study found that along with making provision of emergency medical services it ensures that routine services such as immunization should not be disrupted in the post-disaster period (Maghfiroh et al., 2022). In the year 2004, a massive tsunami hit the Northern coast of Indonesia's Sumatra Island so as a relief effort MHC was arranged through converting buses and small vehicles with the help of great support from foreign relief organizations. Even at that time helicopter mobile clinics were also introduced to provide immediate healthcare services for the disaster victims who did not have access to any healthcare (Rassekh et al., 2014). The MHC proves to be a viable option to treat the ill and help the disabled flood victims who are unable to obtain medical care because of logistical issues and destroyed medical facilities due to the flood in Malaysia in the year 2006 (Ahmad et al., 2008). In India, when Gujarat was affected by a devastating earthquake in 2001 immediate curative healthcare services were provided through mobile health clinics (ReliefWeb, 2017). Within a very short period, small buses were converted to mobile clinics to reach the underserved population. In Assam, boat clinics reach to render health care services in the flood-hit inaccessible riverine islands (Government of Assam, n.d.). Similarly, the World Health Organization deployed a medical emergency Mobile Medical Team during the massive flood in South Sudan to provide health care to the affected populations with special attention to children and women (World Health Organization, 2020). Thus MHC takes an active part in emergency rescue efforts and steps in to substitute nearby health facilities that are devastated by disasters.

The COVID-19 pandemic has severely impacted the healthcare system, causing routine vaccination to be disrupted and non-communicable diseases to be ignored. Due to the travel restrictions, suspension of transportation facilities and fear of coming in contact with the virus of COVID-19, there is a huge decline in in-person preventive care and regular healthcare visits in the health facilities. To address the health needs of the population and reduce barriers this unique and innovative mobile health clinic was used extensively as an alternative strategy to deliver health care to the vulnerable population after the outbreak of the pandemic. It has been observed that in many slums of India, MHCs are used to screen patients having common illnesses such as cough, colds, and body aches. It is deployed with doctors in high-risk zone areas wherever the numbers of positive cases are on the rise to maximize immediate identification, isolating potential spreaders and treating the people who test positive (Corburn et al., 2020). In Assam, door-to-door screenings and swab collection to test COVID-19 were conducted through mobile health clinics (Government of Assam, n.d.). To battle against COVID-19, the Chhattisgarh government also organized 60 mobile medical units to provide door-to-door testing and treatment facilities along with COVID-19 vaccine doses in the municipal corporations and slum areas of the state (The Indian Express, 2021). It can be said that along with reaching the underserved areas MHC has served enormously at the time of disaster and pandemics to the affected population over the period.

5.8 Conclusion

Mobile Health Clinics have the potential to deliver primary care not only in underserved areas but also at a time when static healthcare facilities are undergoing crisis due to the unexpected emergence of a pandemic. It can be used as an alternative to deliver health care at the doorsteps of the vulnerable population in both rural and urban areas. This paper underlines the pressing need to prepare for future to handle any public health emergencies by expanding the use of the MHCs and their services through integration into the health care delivery system as it has the potential to address the primary health care needs of the population at the time of public health emergencies. It can be concluded that while fixed health care delivery gets disrupted during disasters or impaired during the time of pandemics, mobile health clinics can be deployed to reach those affected people to provide primary care.

References

Ahmad, R., Mohamad, Z., Noh, A. Y., Mohamad, N., Hamzah, M. S., Mohammed, N. A., Baharudin, K. A., & Kamauzaman, T. H. (2008). Health major incident: The experiences of mobile medical team during major flood. *The Malaysian Journal of Medical Sciences: MJMS, 15*(2), 47–51.

Ahmed, J. U., Rahanaz, M., & Siddique, R. (2019). Friendship floating hospitals: Healthcare for the riverine people of Bangladesh. *Journal of Developing Societies.* https://doi.org/10.1177/0169796X19826763

Ahuja, A. (2022). *Boat clinics are taking healthcare to the remote and inaccessible islands of sundarbans.* https://swachhindia.ndtv.com/boat-clinics-are-taking-healthcare-to-the-remote-and-inaccessible-islands-of-sundarbans-68908/

All India Women's Conference. (n.d.). Retrieved from https://www.aiwcmumbai.com/index566b.html?option=com_content&task=view&id=70&Itemid=96

Beks, H., Ewing, G., Muir, R., Charles, J., Paradies, Y., Clark, R., & Versace, V. L. (2020). Mobile primary health care clinics for Indigenous populations in Australia, Canada, New Zealand and the United States: A scoping review protocol. *JBI Evidence Synthesis, 18*(5), 1077–1090. https://doi.org/10.11124/JBISRIR-D-19-00057

Caires, A. L. (2017). Mobile health care for people who are homeless. *Creative Nursing, 23*(3), 151–157. https://doi.org/10.1891/1078-4535.23.3.152

Centre for North East Studies and Policy Research (C-NES). https://www.c-nes.org/programmes/boat-clinics/

Corburn, J., Vlahov, D., Mberu, B., Riley, L., Caiaffa, W. T., Rashid, S. F., Ko, A., Patel, S., Jukur, S., Martínez-Herrera, E., Jayasinghe, S., Agarwal, S., Nguendo-Yongsi, B., Weru, J., Ouma, S., Edmundo, K., Oni, T., & Ayad, H. (2020). Slum health: Arresting COVID-19 and improving well-being in urban informal settlements. *Journal of Urban Health: Bulletin of the New York Academy of Medicine, 97*(3), 348–357. https://doi.org/10.1007/s11524-020-00438-6

CSRBOX Desk. (2017, April 15). *A list of 10 mobile medical units in India-reaching the unreached through CSR projects.* https://csrbox.org/India_CSR_news_A-list-of-10-Mobile-Medical-Units-In-India-Reaching-the-Unreached-through-CSR-Projects_15

Dash, U., Muraleedharan, V. R., Prasad, B. M., Dash, S. D., & Acharya, L. S. (2008). *Access to health services in under privileged areas. A case study of mobile health units in Tamil Nadu and Orissa.*

Dhanvantari Raths to Also test for Dengue, Malaria (2020, July 5). *Times of India.* Retrieved from https://timesofindia.indiatimes.com/city/ahmedabad/dhanvantari-raths-to-also-test-for-dengue-malaria/articleshow/76791272.cms

Fils-Aimé, J. R., Grelotti, D. J., Thérosmé, T., Kaiser, B. N., Raviola, G., Alcindor, Y., Severe, J., Affricot, E., Boyd, K., Legha, R., Daimyo, S., Engel, S., & Eustache, E. (2018). A mobile clinic approach to the delivery of community-based mental health services in rural Haiti. *PLoS ONE, 13*(6), Article e0199313. https://doi.org/10.1371/journal.pone.0199313

Geoffroy, E., Harries, A. D., Bissell, K., Schell, E., Bvumbwe, A., Tayler-Smith, K., & Kizito, W. (2014). Bringing care to the community: Expanding access to health care in rural Malawi through mobile health clinics. *Public Health Action, 4*(4), 252–258. https://doi.org/10.5588/pha.14.0064

Ghate, A. (1982). Family planning and voluntary organizations. *Yojana, 26*(9), 15–18.

Government of Assam. Health & Family Welfare (n.d.). https://nhm.assam.gov.in/schemes/mobile-medical-unit-

Government of Assam. Health & Family Welfare (n.d.). Retrieved from https://nhm.assam.gov.in/schemes/mobile-medicalunitmmu#:~:text=MMU%20at%20a%20glance%3A&text=MMU%20in%20Tea%20Gardens%20(TG)%3A%20Initially%2080%20numbers%20of,three%20years%20since%20its%20inception

Guruge, S., Hunter, J., Barker, K., McNally, M. J., & Magalhães, L. (2010). Immigrant women's experiences of receiving care in a mobile health clinic. *Journal of Advanced Nursing, 66*(2), 350–359. https://doi.org/10.1111/j.1365-2648.2009.05182.x

Hill, C., Zurakowski, D., Bennet, J., Walker-White, R., Osman, J. L., Quarles, A., & Oriol, N. (2012). Knowledgeable Neighbors: A mobile clinic model for disease prevention and screening in underserved communities. *American Journal of Public Health, 102*(3), 406–410. https://doi.org/10.2105/AJPH.2011.300472

How Do Mobile Health Clinics Improve Access to Healthcare? (n.d.). Tulane University. https://publichealth.tulane.edu/blog/mobile-health-clinics/

HelpAge India. Mobile Healthcare. (n.d.). Retrieved from https://www.helpageindia.org/our-work/welfare-development/mobile-healthcare/

Khanna, A., & Narula, S. (2016). Mobile health units: Mobilizing healthcare to reach unreachable. *International Journal of Healthcare Management, 9*, 160108025751002. https://doi.org/10.1080/20479700.2015.1101915

Kojima, N., Krupp, K., Ravi, K., Gowda, S., Jaykrishna, P., Leonardson-Placek, C., Siddhaiah, A., Bristow, C. C., Arun, A., Klausner, J. D., & Madhivanan, P. (2017). Implementing and sustaining a mobile medical clinic for prenatal care and sexually transmitted infection prevention in rural Mysore, India. *BMC Infectious Diseases, 17*(1), 189. https://doi.org/10.1186/s12879-017-2282-3

Kumar, M. M., Pathak, V. K., & Ruikar, M. (2020). Tribal population in India: A public health challenge and road to future. *Journal of Family Medicine and Primary Care, 9*(2), 508–512. https://doi.org/10.4103/jfmpc.jfmpc_992_19

Maghfiroh, M. F. N., & Hanaoka, S. (2022). Mobile clinics: Medical service strategy for disaster healthcare response operation. *Journal of Industrial Engineering and Management, 15*(3), 470–483. https://doi.org/10.3926/jiem.3941

Malone, N. C., Williams, M. M., Smith Fawzi, M. C., Bennet, J., Hill, C., Katz, J. N., & Oriol, N. E. (2020). Mobile health clinics in the United States. *International Journal for Equity in Health, 19*(1), 40. https://doi.org/10.1186/s12939-020-1135-7

Ministry of Health and Family Welfare. (2015). *Operational guidelines for mobile medical units*. Available at: https://nhm.gov.in/New_Updates_2018/NHM_Components/Health_System_Stregthening/MMU/Mobile_Medical_Units.pdf

Ministry of Health and Family Welfare Government of India. (n.d.). *National health policy, 2017*. Retrieved September 19, 2022, from https://www.nhp.gov.in/nhpfiles/national_health_policy_2017.pdf

Mobile 1000. https://www.mobile1000.org/

Mobile Van Service Launched to Diagnose TB Cases in the District. (2021, June 16). The Hindu. https://www.thehindu.com/news/national/tamil-nadu/mobile-van-service-launched-to-diagnose-tb-cases-in-the-district/article30189783.ece

Morrison, C. (1996). India's mobile health teams set pace for progress in urban communities. *Population Concern News, 11*, 3.

Nandi, S., Joshi, D., Prasad, V., & Murugan, G. (2017). *Outsourcing of mobile medical units in Chhattisgarh: A case study*. Study on the impact of privatization of public health services. https://www.researchgate.net/publication/319480991_Outsourcing_Of_Mobile_Medical_Units_in_Chhattisgarh_A_Case_Study

National Health Mission. (2015). 9th common review mission report 2015. Ministry of Health and Family Welfare, Government of India. Available at: https://nhm.gov.in/images/pdf/monitoring/crm/9th-crm/Report/9th_CRM_Main_Report.pdf

National Health Mission. (2018). 12th common review mission report 2018. Ministry of Health and Family Welfare, Government of India. Available at: https://nhm.gov.in/New_Updates_2018/Monitoring/CRM/12th/12th-CRM_Report.pdf

National Health Mission Madhya Pradesh. (n.d.). https://www.nhp.gov.in/madhya-pradesh_pg

National Health Mission Rajasthan. (n.d.). http://nrhmrajasthan.nic.in/MMU%20Status%201.htm#:~:text=To%20take%20care%20the%20problem,in%20the%20year%202008%2D2009

National Health Mission Tripura. (n.d.). http://www.nhsrcindia.org/sites/default/files/Health%20Camp%20through%20Helicopter%20Service%20in%20Tripura%281%29.pdf

Ndayizigamiye, P., & Maharaj, M. (2016). *Mobile health adoption in Burundi: A UTAUT perspective*. https://doi.org/10.1109/GHTC.2016.7857342

Neke, N. M., Gadau, G., & Wasem, J. (2018). Policy makers' perspective on the provision of maternal health services via mobile health clinics in Tanzania—Findings from key informant interviews. *PLoS ONE, 13*(9), Article e0203588. https://doi.org/10.1371/journal.pone.0203588

Oriol, N. E., Cote, P. J., Vavasis, A. P., Bennet, J., Delorenzo, D., Blanc, P., & Kohane, I. (2009). Calculating the return on investment of mobile healthcare. *BMC Medicine, 7*, 27. https://doi.org/10.1186/1741-7015-7-27

Our Mobile Clinics Reach Children in Kasai, DRC. (2017, October 20). https://reliefweb.int/report/democratic-republic-congo/our-mobile-clinics-reach-children-kasai-drc

Patient Engagement Hit. How Mobile Health Clinics Drive Care to Vulnerable Patients. (n.d.). https://patientengagementhit.com/features/how-mobile-health-clinics-drive-care-to-vulnerable-patients

Peters, G., Doctor, H., Afenyadu, G., Findley, S., & Ager, A. (2014). Mobile clinic services to serve rural populations in Katsina State, Nigeria: Perceptions of services and patterns of utilization. *Health Policy and Planning, 29*(5), 642–649. https://doi.org/10.1093/heapol/czt052

Post, P. A. (2017). *Mobile health care for homeless people: Using vehicles to extend care*. National Health Care for the Homeless Council. 2007. https://www.nhchc.org/wpcontent/uploads/2012/02/mobilehealth.pdf

Rassekh, B. M., Shu, W., Santosham, M., Burnham, G., & Doocy, S. (2014). An evaluation of public, private, and mobile health clinic usage for children under age 5 in Aceh after the tsunami: Implications for future disasters. *Health Psychology and Behavioral Medicine, 2*(1), 359–378. https://doi.org/10.1080/21642850.2014.896744

Rousseau, E., Bekker, L. G., Julies, R. F., Celum, C., Morton, J., Johnson, R., Baeten, J. M., & O'Malley, G. (2021). A community-based mobile clinic model delivering PrEP for HIV prevention to adolescent girls and young women in Cape Town, South Africa. *BMC Health Services Research, 21*(1), 888. https://doi.org/10.1186/s12913-021-06920-4

Specchio Dei Tempi. (n.d.). *Mobile clinics to bring care to the poorest villages.* Retrieved from https://www.specchiodeitempi.org/en/progetto/for-myanmar/

Spoth, T. (2008). *Choppers for doctors: Motorcycles help health workers traverse Lesotho's mountains.* https://www.pih.org/article/choppers-for-doctors-motorcycles-help-health-workers-traverse-lesothos-moun

"The Mobile Clinic—Time for review of a Community Health Project in India." (2004, November 11). https://reliefweb.int/report/india/mobile-clinic-time-review-community-health-project-india

The Indian Express. (2021, June 13). *Chhattisgarh govt: In 7 months, mobile medical units benefitted over 5 lakh slum dwellers.* https://indianexpress.com/article/india/chhattisgarh-mobile-medical-units-for-slum-dwellers-benefitted-5-lakh-7357264/

The Hans Foundation (n.d.). *Hans medical mobile units—Primary health care.* https://thehansfoundation.org/health/

Trivedi, U., Omofoye, T. S., Marquez, C., Sullivan, C. R., Benson, D. M., & Whitman, G. J. (2022). Mobile mammography services and underserved women. *Diagnostics (Basel, Switzerland), 12*(4), 902. https://doi.org/10.3390/diagnostics12040902

United Nations Office for the Coordination of Humanitarian Affairs. (2010). KENYA: Camel clinics bring condoms to nomads. *PlusNews.* https://reliefweb.int/report/kenya/kenya-camel-clinics-bring-condoms-nomads

Venkatesh, A. (2018). *Mobile medical units: In history and beyond.* Foundation for Rural Recovery and Development. https://forrad.org/mobile-medical-units-in-history-and-beyond/

Whelan, C., Chambers, C., Chan, M., Thomas, S., Ramos, G., & Hwang, S. W. (2010). Why do homeless people use a mobile health unit in a country with universal health care? *Journal of Primary Care and Community Health, 1*(2), 78–82. https://doi.org/10.1177/2150131910372233

Williams, A. M., Botsford, B., Mortensen, P., Park, D., & Waxman, E. L. (2019). Delivering mobile eye care to underserved communities while providing training in ophthalmology to medical students: Experience of the Guerrilla Eye Service. *Clinical Ophthalmology (Auckland, NZ), 13*, 337–346. https://doi.org/10.2147/OPTH.S185692

Wockhardt Foundation: 200th Healthcare Van Launched Under 'Mobile 1000' Program'. (2019). *India CSR network.* https://indiacsr.in/wockhardt-foundation-200th-healthcare-van-launched-mobile-1000-program/

Wockhardt Foundation. (n.d). *Annual report, 2015–16.* http://www.wockhardt.com/files/report-on-csr-activities-wockhardt-foundation.pdf

World Health Organization. (1978). *Declaration of Alma-Ata, International Conference on Primary Health Care, Alma-Ata, USSR, September 6–12, 1978.* Geneva, Switzerland.

World Health Organization. (2019, December 26). *Delivering health in some of the worlds' worst crises through mobile clinics and medical teams.* https://www.who.int/news-room/feature-stories/detail/delivering-health-in-some-of-the-worlds-worst-crises-through-mobile-clinics-and-medical-teams

World Health Organization. (2020). *Increasing access to life-saving primary healthcare services in South Sudan's flood-affected areas.* https://www.afro.who.int/news/increasing-access-life-saving-primary-healthcare-services-south-sudans-flood-affected-areas

Yu, S., Hill, C., Ricks, M. L., Bennet, J., & Oriol, N. E. (2017). The scope and impact of mobile health clinics in the United States: A literature review. *International Journal for Equity in Health, 16*(1), 178. https://doi.org/10.1186/s12939-017-0671-2

Health Digitalization and Its Impact on Frontline Workers: A Study of Anganwadi Workers from Poshan Abhiyan

6

Vaishnavi Mangal

Abstract

This chapter explores digital tools and technologies used by community health care workers, Anganwadi workers in India for health service delivery. Anganwadi Workers are the primary workforce of the Integrated Child Development Scheme (ICDS). The Anganwadi Workers are a community-level workforce responsible for implementing various programs under the ICDS scheme, which covers programs related to prenatal and post-natal care, maternal nutrition, and children's health. Recently, to digitize health service delivery, the Indian Government introduced a digital application called Poshan Tracker for these Anganwadi Workers to keep records and track their activities. Besides this, informally, Anganwadi Workers have started using other texting apps like WhatsApp to connect to their clients because of increasing digital connectivity among people. This chapter is based on the primary, qualitative study on the feasibility of this technology-mediated medium in India and how Anganwadi Workers use these digital mediums for their work. The research explores the use of digital applications has helped this ground-level workforce in their service delivery and what other digital platforms, like (WhatsApp and Facebook) they are using to connect to their clients; what change the introduction of mobile phone-based digital apps has brought to their work regarding efficiency and service delivery; and what are the advantages and problems they have been facing in this sudden digitization of their work. The chapter covers socio-technical issues around usage, practices and the feasibility of use of digital applications among healthcare workers, and the enabling systematic support health care anganwadi workers need in their work. The chapter, hence, will be able to provide insight on enabling environment needed by anganwadi workers to use the apps and device, and how informal use of apps like Whatsapp can contribute to better health-tech application for these workers.

V. Mangal (✉)
Doctoral Fellow, Faculty of Medicine and Health, Norwegian University of Science and Technology, Trondheim, Norway
e-mail: vaishnavi.mangal@ntnu.no; vaishnavimangal6896@gmail.com

6.1 Background

Every sector is leveraging the power of digital technology and public health, and public health service delivery is one of them. There are a wide

S. S. Acharya et al. (eds.), *Paradigm Shifts in Population and Health in India*, Sustainable Development Goals Series, https://doi.org/10.1007/978-981-95-1719-0_6

range of digital public health technologies available—from social media to wearables to mobile apps to big data and artificial intelligence. All this has been promising speed, affordability and effectiveness of public health services in India and abroad. Various institutions like WHO and governments across the world have developed frameworks and guidelines to use digital technologies to improve public health outcomes (WHO). The term "digital public health" is being used more frequently in public health discourse, which emphasizes the significance of digital technologies in public health services. This phrase became widely used after the release of Public Health England's digital-first policy in 2017. It is now used to define a variety of public health initiatives that take into account and make use of digital technologies.

The literature continues to use a variety of definitions and conceptualizations of digital public health as interest in the topic grows among academics and professionals. Regarding how they conceptualize the functions of digitalization and digital transformation in digital public health, the definitions that are now available vary. Which definition would help public health practises and results the most is still up for debate. By encapsulating the intent of their practice and offering a clear road map for ongoing development, public health researchers and practitioners can better advance the field by achieving greater consensus on the definition of digital public health and the role of digitalization and digital transformation in this definition (Iyamu et al., 2021). According to review by Iyamu et al. (2021) the purpose of digitalization is to increase efficiency and provide value to patients, and it has been defined in the literature as a sociotechnical process that entails integrating digital technology into current operations and duties. Data generation that is automated and more efficient may be made possible by the integration of digital technology into current operations. The use of computer systems and electronic health records at primary health care clinic is an illustration of digitalization because it enables the generation of health data throughout the service delivery process, ensuring that such data may be used to inform disease prevention, surveillance, and health care quality improvement.

In India, public health programs are adding digital components like dashboards, mobile applications to make service delivery easier for the workers as well as the people. Poshan Abhiyaan or National Nutrition Mission uses technology for real time monitoring of the program. The Common Application System (CAS), also known to as the monitoring system or app, is a centralized, real-time monitoring system that is used to more effectively track the community services provided by Anganwadi Workers (AWWs). This is for the aim to achieve functional goal of "bringing operational efficiency". In order for this program to operate effectively, a surveillance infrastructure that is based on monitoring frontline staff members and their activities in accordance with the widely held belief in "data-driven governance" is required, where they report to the government in India.

This chapter examines the role of digitization on the frontline worker and their work. The Anganwadi workers have been asked to use the Poshan Tracker app for data entry and Real-time Monitoring of their work. The app is necessary for their work and is monitored based on the data entered in them. Yet, there is a lack of research on how workers feel about using technology interventions, how it has changed their work, how they go about their daily lives, and what function these systems have. This research addresses some of these concerns by examining how a digital intervention like ICDS-CAS and Poshan Tracker affects AWWs' interactions with community members and their own work. It contributes to a critical analysis of India's digital technology-driven public health program delivery. Anganwadi services are one of the largest public health service delivery program in the world. There are 20 lakh (2 Million) employees which are part of program (PTI, 2019). This research was done using the qualitative method of enquiry to look at the burden of anganwadi workers and how introduction of digital tool have changed that. It also looks at socio-technical issues that have arisen with the introduction of the technology and the infrastructural and programmatic issues that workers face. It also looks at role of the mobile applications and how it has transformed the very nature of job and care work of the workers- and how these workers are dealing with it.

6.2 Indian Healthcare System and Digitalization

India's healthcare system has historically been underfunded, with no government since independence having spent more than 4% of GDP on health. The regulatory mechanism to control the private sector has been weak and has not been prioritized historically by any ruling governments. Historically, most of the budget allocation for health have been spent on the training and practice of medical graduates in India, which leaves less money for health system building and strengthening. Access to doctors, medicines, and diagnostic facilities is primary concern for most people in India. Government health facilities continue to have limited access to medications and medical supplies due to underfunding, shoddy logistics, and procurement procedures. Only a select few Indian states have established enough funding, procurement, and distribution systems for medical supplies and diagnostics. Most health services are concentrated in cities and urban areas, cutting off large population which lives in rural and tribal parts of the country. The reach of Primary Health Care is very low, despite programs like the National Rural Health Mission, whose primary aim was to provide basic primary services in rural areas (Inequality Report, 2021, n.d.).

Both at the Central and state levels, underfunding of government health programs has been a major source of contention. Given their limited resources, state governments, who are required by the Constitution to pay for public health and hospitals, are constrained in what they can offer. From around 32% of total tax funds during the 13th Finance Commission (2010–2014) to 42% during the 14th Finance Commission, there have been initiatives to increase tax devolution from the federal government to state governments for health (2015–2019). However, state governments in India have challenged this. Tax financing has been directed to Central Government-sponsored nationwide schemes on health, which often does not fit the epidemiological needs of that specific state. There are many health programs being run concomitantly by Central and State governments, which leads to confusion about accountability.

To introduce more patient-centric solutions and bridge gaps in health service delivery as stated above, the Indian government, under the umbrella of Digital India, aims to revolutionize the health system in India by launching several programs and missions, introducing mobile applications for health services and creating a long term vision for digital health services in India. Part of it was the launch of National Digital Health Mission. Along with this, mobile applications and several web-based portals have been launched to track the health service delivery and ease the experience of health service providers as well as users. Some recent examples of such application are (a) Launch of the Co-Win app for COVID vaccinations (2021) (b) the Application for *Ayushman Bharat* scheme, which provides health insurance to eligible beneficiaries and also connect people to primary health care (c) web based portal called NI-KSHAY (Ni-end, Kshay-Tuberculosis) which is a patient management system under National Tuberculosis Elimination Program (NTEP) (d) Poshan Tracker (Poshan-Nutrition) (Wadhwa, n.d.). Digital Technology in public health in India is being proposed as next big thing which can transform Indian Healthcare. India has emerged as a one of the leading countries using digital technology for healthcare and public health services. India has been taking active steps in this direction-under the umbrella campaign of "Digital India" which was launched in 2014 to promote use of digital goods social needs. India was one of the countries in 2016 to propose a resolution on Digital Health at WHO General Body Meeting. India's 2017 National Health Policy also proposes Telemedicine service as integral part of Health Service delivery centers in India.

6.3 National Nutrition Mission (Poshan Abhiyaan)

Poshan Abhiyaan or National Nutrition Mission (NNM) was launched by the current Government of India in 2017. It aims to provide a convergence mechanism for the country's response to malnutrition, improve nutrition among children, pregnant women, and lactating mothers. The NNM takes stock of all the nutrition related programs/schemes in the country on the target population. This is a grand scheme with one of its goal being convergence of all nutrition related programs/scheme running for different target groups in our population. India has a population of 1.37 billion according to the National Family Health Survey 5, severe wasting has increased in children aged under 5, which was 7.5% in 2015–16 (4th round of NFHS), has increased to 7.7% in this round. For treating malnutrition, multiple interventions such as timely breastfeeding, age-appropriate complementary feeding, full immunization, and vitamin A supplementation are essential. Anaemia is a cause of worry in children as well as in women in the reproductive age group (14–45). Many programs, like Integrated Child Development Services, Nutrition Rehabilitation Centers, the Right to Food Act etc. exist already but they function in silos and have no convergence because of fragmented health system, which NNM aims to do (Aggarwal & Kakkar, 2019).

There have been various schemes to provide adequate nutrition and education to children in the age group 0–6 years, constituting a population of 158 million in our country (Census, 2011). The first step in this direction was the Integrated Child Development Services (ICDS), launched in 1975. It was one of the world's largest schemes to cater to women and children and was formed to improve the nutritional and health status of children 0–6 years of age, pregnant women, and lactating mothers. Its objectives also included laying the foundation for proper physical, social, and psychological development of children to reduce child mortality, morbidity, malnutrition, and school dropouts among children. It also focused on enhancing the mother's capacity to care for children's needs. It worked in coordination between various departments and covers preschool, basic healthcare tips, and non-formal education. This scheme integrates all the services which children need for their development. This "package of service" provides integrated care from one single source. Convergence of all services has been a vital feature of the ICDS scheme. The Anganwadi center acts as a point to provide these services (Aggarwal & Kakkar, 2019).

In 2017, NITI Ayog, India's apex decision-making body, launched National Nutrition Strategy (NNS) formed to effectively focus on nutrition and more effective action to achieve nutritional objectives, which will help fulfil Niti Ayog's National Development Agenda (Aggarwal & Kakkar, 2019).

National Nutrition Mission addresses the problem of lack of real-time measurement of nutritional determinants, which affects the target action for most vulnerable mothers and children. NNS also promotes measures like community mobilization, which can help effect behavioral change. NNS envisions a malnutrition-free India, aligning it with other government missions like *Swacchh Bharat* and *Swasth Bharat*. The action taken by the government for this is to ensure a convergence of effort and a continuum of care by innovating service delivery measures (Aggarwal & Kakkar, 2019).

Convergence is one of the goals under NNM, which aims to converge all the schemes addressing malnutrition and real-time monitoring of the work being done. Technological applications have been introduced for this monitoring, and Anganwadi workers are incentivized to use these applications. These mobile-based applications like ICDS-CAS and Poshan Tracker also are part of this. The Nutrition Mission includes other activities like Social Audits and Jan Andolan to create awareness on various health and nutrition-related subjects. Hence in the long term, NNM aims to bring the necessary social and behavioral change in the community (Aggarwal & Kakkar, 2019).

6.4 Use of ICT in Nutrition Delivery in India

Anganwadi workers and female supervisors can access smartphones and tablets that come pre-configured with the Poshan Abhiyaan Common Application Software. The implementation of the NNM is hinged on the pillars of supporting the development of services for the vulnerable populations, which mainly includes:

- Technology (Integrated Child Development Scheme (ICDS)—computer application software);
- Convergence Action Planning;
- Behavioral Change Communication; and
- Capacity building.

To monitor activities under National Nutrition Mission, an ICT based real-time monitoring system (ICT-RTM) has been proposed. The ICT-RTM driven by ICDS Common Application Software (CAS) has two components. One component is Mobile application for field functionaries and Supervisors. The mobile application, named as *Poshan Tracker* app, with modules which corresponds to each of the 10 out of 11 registers (except stock register) used by Anganwadi Workers (AWWs). The lady supervisors use the mobile application on tablet to monitor the work of Anganwadi workers and review performance of Anganwadi Centers. It also has a web-based application with dashboard which is used by the upper level officers to review the performance of the health workers and the program on a regular basis.

The Integrated Child Development Scheme-Common Application Software (ICDS-CAS) (Ministry of Women and Child Development) aims to:

- improve the efficiency and effectiveness of Anganwadi workers as a job aid;
- track each children's nutrition status;
- automate growth chart generation;
- automate ICDS registers;
- monitor timeliness and quality of services delivered;
- Provide real-time reports, alerts, and dashboards to all the six tiers of nutrition governance and enable prompt action for decision supports.[1]

There were eight modules in the ICDS-CAS known as Common Care or ComCare. Inside each module, the anganwadi worker fills different forms as before, but now in a digital mode. These modules tells workers things they need to do, from household management to how to maintain records.

The ICDS-CAS (2018–2021) was replaced by POSHAN 2.0, which was introduced in 2021. The primary differences between the two are (a) the direct replacement of ICDS-CAS with Poshan Tracker, (b) the addition of budgetary provisions for ungraded Anganwadis (Saksham Anganwadis), and (c) the ranking of all subnational governments on a national scale based on six key performance indicators (KPIs). It is possible to generalize the results in POSHAN 2.0 because the data is carefully collected at the point of transition from ICDS-CAS to POSHAN 2.0 (SP et al., 2022).

6.5 Workers Problems and Issues

The recently introduced changes do not take into account the burden of work on AWW. Time use analysis of workers by Jain et al. (2020) shows that though a smartphone-based application is available and they have been given the option to skip using the paper registers, AWWs spend a large portion of their working hours filling out their paper registers. It might hinder them from spending the necessary amount of time conducting house visits and assisting adolescent girls, pregnant women, and nursing mothers, this

[1] (i) Anganwadi worker, (ii) Supervisor, (iii) Block, (iv) District, (v) State/Union Territory, (vi) Central Project Management Unit.

is a problem that the government can fix. The predicted time spent on important tasks needs to be adjusted in order to better reflect the work realities of AWWs.

While most AWWs were aware of the notion of convergence, there is little actual convergence between "health" and "nutrition" operations. AWWs attributed this lack of convergence to immediate linkage problems between the two sectors, including divergent agendas across the sectors, technological unfamiliarity with the other sector, worries about data sharing, and a lack of incentives. However, AWWs shared more general organizational problems (infrastructure limitations and a mismatch in job expectations) and urban contextual difficulties (migrant population, unmapped areas, and cultural barriers) that constrained their sector-specific and cross-sector responsibilities. Also, AWWs voiced many worries about their evolving duties and weren't always open to adjustments to their traditional positions and working styles. Additionally, there is not enough training and supervision provided to them (Ramani et al., 2021).

Many studies done on ICDS have found that the quality of food is subpar and is not enough to provide the desired nutrition to children. There is no doubt that it is difficult and discouraging for AWWs to work in such circumstances, as these gaps have also been noted in this study too (Ramani et al., 2021).

The study by Ramani et al. further states that for the evolving duties AWWs are now required to do, AWWs need to be better prepared. Some AWWs in their research claimed that the "digital conversion" of data was a technical issue. Most people didn't like being closely watched and thought that it wasn't appropriate for the informal work duties they had first agreed to. Also AWWs do not have enough technical support to overcome daily difficulties. Another recent study from rural Bihar and Madhya Pradesh has identified similar difficulties. The study had also noted that AWWs felt more prepared to engage in community service after using the new software, but social barriers like mistrust and doubt affect their use (Gopalkrishnan et al., 2020).

Also, starting in 2021, mobile phones and Poshan Tracker is to be required for use by all Anganwadi staff. There have been delays in the procurement and delivery of the mobile phones, despite government plans to provide them. They are unable to download the app on their own personal smartphones, which jeopardizes the entire project. Because they are contract employees, anganwadi staff frequently lack the funds for a recharge because their compensation is based on the amount of data they upload to their mobile devices for Poshan Abhiyaan. They need to receive more training, and moving totally to a tech-based platform without fixing the bugs makes it difficult for them to operate efficiently.

Programs in the social sector have recently seen a top-down drive towards techno-solutionism. Sanitation workers in Pune and Accredited Social Health professionals in Haryana are only two examples of low-income workers who have been frequently forced to adopt technology by the Center and numerous State governments. As previously mentioned in this literature review, even the required use of Aadhaar has created a number of real-world issues in rural areas, making it occasionally impossible for individuals to receive government benefits. By changing them from carers to compliant data collectors, the deployment of such gadgets by health professionals, such as anganwadi workers, is bound to drastically alter their operations. Employees at anganwadis are already perceived as doing "menial" data collection jobs and needing supervision (Bansal, 2021).

The accessibility and availability of cell phones and 4G networks is also a foundational element of the technology-centered strategy. There are further ways to use technology to aid healthcare workers in their work. In order to push back against these top-down illusions at the policy level, this can be done by working with the workforce and their unions to develop, test, and demonstrate technologies that assist caring chores and propose technology alternatives from scratch.

The study explored the impact of the digital app Poshan Tracker on the work of Anganwadi workers in Delhi. It is a qualitative exploratory study with purposive sampling. The secondary data and research has been reviewed and further corroborated with primary data collected and analyzed in this smaller study undertaken by the researcher. Data provides maximum insights into the phenomenon under examination.

Based on the literature review, the gaps which have been found are as follows:

- There is a dearth of literature on the impact of the mHealth app on healthcare workers in India. In this case, Poshan Tracker was introduced for AWWs in August 2020 and was made mandatory for AWWs in March 2021. It is a recent introduction, and there is a dearth of standards and tools as digital health solutions are fast evolving. This results in a lack of evidence to form normative guidelines on using the app.
- There is a lack of research on implementing ICDS in urban areas (Ramani et al., 2021), and this study intends to shed light on the working of the Poshan Scheme (previously ICDS) in urban slums of Delhi.

6.6 Rationale of Study

Digital health and digital health intervention are being introduced as solutions to gaps in health system functioning, especially in public health service delivery in India. This study focuses on National Nutrition Mission and Nutrition Delivery schemes in this study. This is because these schemes are crucial to health of marginalized, i.e., women and children.

6.7 Research Methodology

This research was conducted using a qualitative methodology that incorporates primary data collection. In this study, the researcher assesses the effectiveness of a digital mobile application intervention. The study examines the benefits and drawbacks of using mobile applications to deliver health services by Anganwadi workers. It investigates the intervention's effectiveness. The exploratory technique was chosen as the type of methodology since the research is exploratory and the pertinent questions or answers are unknown, necessitating in-depth interviews and analysis by looking at the issue from several angles. The research topic is current, with limited secondary literature, and the impact of mobile applications on the Anganwadi workers is a new and unexplored area. The participants for the research, Anganwadi workers, are drawn through a snowball sample accrued via original informants' interviews to optimize sample diversity. Approval and consent were taken from anganwadi workers before interviewing them, and proper privacy is maintained.

6.8 Sampling Design

The research explored how the POSHAN Abhiyaan's introduction of mHealth technology and applications have affected the work done by anganwadi workers, and how it has shaped, altered, and affected the work done by anganwadi workers. In this research, the bottom up approach has been used, i.e., at anganwadi worker's level.

A through interview research was done with Anganwadi workers to get their viewpoints. First, the researcher spoke with the Anganwadi Union representatives, who have represented the Anganwadi workers for a long time. After this, the researcher connected to the 18 Anganwadi workers for the interview through union representatives. The workers were recruited through referrals by the Anganwadi Union Members. The initial contacts were made in January 2022, but the data was collected in June 2022 when the anganwadi centers opened after COVID induced lockdown. The researcher was initially introduced to 3 workers, one in Inderlok, one in Bhalswa, and one in Jahangirpuri, and the researcher recruited 15 other workers through snowball sampling in June 2022. The name of workers has been changed to preserve anonymity.

The sampling used is purposive sampling, based on the criteria that the respondent should be:

(a) Anganwadi worker
(b) Should be working in Delhi
(c) Have been in service for more than 4 years, so the information from Anganwadi workers on how they used to work pre-Poshan Tracker and CommCare and what changes the introduction of Poshan Tracker has brought can be covered.

The principle of saturation was followed in this research. This allowed the researcher to conduct an additional interview if needed to reach clear conclusions.

6.9 Area of Study

The interviews were conducted with Anganwadi workers in 3 urban slum settlements in North West district of Delhi-

- Jahangirpuri
- Bhalswa
- Inderlok

6.10 Analysis

With the introduction of POSHAN Abhiyaan and its real-time monitoring system in 2018, pregnant women, nursing moms, and children at risk are seen as body politic that can be detected, followed, and managed by digital technology. It divides the concept of dietary well-being and health into digestible categories and statistics that can be recorded, researched, and streamlined to meet goals. The digital aspect and digitization of the nutrition mission serve this goal (SP et al., 2022). However, workers remain confused and their changing job description and lack of adequate training confuses them about their work. In research by Ramani et al. (2021), it says that AWWs feel confused as outreach and campaign organizers when they seem to be pre-school teachers. Even though the AWW's major responsibility is to care for pregnant and lactating women, they are now spending a lot more time on gathering, collating, and uploading government data than they did in only ICDS time. The AWWs work and their priorities have radically changed as a result Poshan Abhiyaan's decision to change community healthcare as something that can be traced, recorded, and monitored through digital applications and dashboards. Along with this, rapid transformation without enough preparation put AWWs in a state of tension, confused between the differences between previous program and new schemes (Ramani et al., 2021; SP et al., 2022) POSHAN 2.0 was launched in 2022, and four schemes were merged as part of it. The four schemes are Anganwadi services, Poshan Abhiyaan, the Scheme for Adolescent Girls, and the National Crèche Scheme (Kaskar, 2022). The rapid changes in schemes, along with merger and introduction of new ones have left anganwadi workers in a constant state of confusion as well as uncertainty about their job roles.

6.11 Worker's View on Transition from ICDS to Poshan Abhiyaan

In this study, when asked about the Poshan Abhiyaan scheme, AWWs reported that while they know about it, they see it as ICDS only, but now with increased responsibility and technology component. The workers were not aware of details of POSHAN 2.0 as a program or its larger goals. No worker was aware about different aspects of Poshan Abhiyaan and why it has been introduced and the purpose for it. One worker said that the scheme was to keep a check if AWWs are doing their work, and if they are distributing food to the beneficiaries, which was irregular and hard to track before the mobile application. The worker said their work is being monitored because of everyday data entry. Another worker from Inderlok, said that in Poshan Abhiyaan, the number of beneficiaries has increased, and it now includes teenage girls too. Workers conflated National Nutrition Month with the whole program. NNM is the month of September every year is celebrated as the *Rashtriya Poshan Maah* or the National Nutrition Month across the country, as one activity in Poshan Abhiyaan.

6.12 Change in Nature of Work

The anganwadi workers in various studies (SP et al., 2022; Ramani et al., 2021) have said that the nature of work has changed, and the paperwork and documentation has increased with the change in program. Workers says that for activities they do in center, they have to take photos which have to be sent to their supervisors, parents of the children and in the mobile application. Workers all over the country has been opposing the introduction of mobile app and digitization of work. In Maharashtra, workers protested by returning 80,000 phones back to the government (Swaddle & Kalia, 2021). The workers said that they will return to manual data and record keeping, as earlier. Similar protest has been seen in Haryana, Tamil Nadu, and Delhi too against the introduction of phone by the government.

Anganwadi workers under Poshan Mission have to celebrate two community based events every month, and they do anything from Mahila Mandal meeting, meeting of teenage girls, celebrating the birthday of children, and *godhbharai* of pregnant women (baby shower of women where they are given nutritious food).

Workers in this research in Delhi expressed same frustration with community based events and "*Jan Andolan*" they have to organize as part of Poshan Abhiyaan. Workers from Jahangirpuri area said that since their centers are close by, for *Jan Andolan* they coordinate with each other and often organize a rally in community on important topics of public awareness like sanitation, COVID-19, pollution etc. Worker M from Bhalswa reported that she was asked to organize a plantation drive *(poshan vatika)* by the supervisor and since she did not have money. No nursery nearby was ready to give plants sampling at a lower, affordable cost with GST bills, she has to ask children to bring pots from their home and they did activities in that only and sent those photos to supervisor (Worker M, Bhalswa, 19/06/22).

Workers are struggling under constant demand of data which is being asked from them. The app, workers report, is like a toy or an alarm that constantly keeps ringing and asking them for data. The data entry requirements and the constant app updates come without adequate training support.

However, some workers in this research said that there are some advantages to this shift in digital mode, in which they can just enter weight and height and app lets them know in which quantile the child is in, which then they inform parents about. The determination of malnutrition status has become easier through the app. If a child is in red zone in Poshan Tracker app (severely malnourished) they inform the parents and local health center, and the program supervisor can also immediately see and take action on it because it is updated in the app. Worker R2 (17/06/2022) and P (21/06/2022) from Inderlok block in Delhi said that due to this constant attention children's health status has improved in their centers. The growth monitoring aspect of the whole Poshan Mission provides corrective measures needed for the children immediately, workers reported. Another worker said that the regular tracking of the activities has made it difficult for the workers and supervisors to siphon off food or funds, which used to happen in pre 2018 (Worker R, Bhalswa, 14/06/22). She said that the food supply to the beneficiaries is regular because it is tracked.

As evident in this chapter, there has been four major changes in the job description of anganwadi workers from ICDS to Poshan Abhiyaan:

- The worker's roles and responsibilities under Poshan Abhiyaan has expanded drastically, and now they are community mobilizer too, along with pre-school teachers and sitters of the community children.
- The AWWs did not receive any orientation and training for these new responsibilities, which has resulted in confusion between the new programs (Poshan Abhiyaan) and old one (ICDS).
- Workers are facing problems in conducting activities for community based events because

of lack of funds provided by the government and tedious reimbursement process.
- However, workers have reported that the benefit they see is it is easier to quantify children in different malnutrition category SAM, malnourished, and healthy through the app.

The workers now play the role of pre-school teachers, community mobilization managers, and data collectors, but with meager salaries. The top-down way expectations are put on AWWs indicate that government and administration do not respect them as professionals. The way POSHAN Abhiyaan was introduced without any consultation with AWWs says there is a lack of space for AWWs' consent and agency. The workers lack the funds to organize these events, and there are harsh reimbursement documentation requirements, including producing GST bills and documentation proof (in the form of photos). This leads to workers spending their own money and incurring financial losses for doing work for which the government is supposed to give them money.

AWWs do not physically share space with their co-workers despite the existence of unions because each individual lives and works in their own centers. The requirement for employment, even at the risk of exploitation, limits their ability to bargain, and whenever they do, like they did protest in Delhi in 2022, it was brutally crushed with suspension of 900 workers (Newslive Staff, 2022). In this research too, workers from Inderlok reported that researcher 2 workers from their projects were also suspended because of protesting, and all they are afraid to say anything against government as government has been brutal towards them ("*We are now all fearful to say anything against government. They should not have been suspended, they were long time workers but government these days show no mercy (Worker R, Inderlok, 17/06/2022)*".

The introduction of Community Based Events has changed the nature of work and now they are indulging in a lot of work which is not beneficial for the community, (like taking out cycle rally for the *jan andolan.* They also lack resources for it but have to do because of the government mandate.

In POSHAN Abhiyaan, AWWs also have to do community based events, as part of outreach in the community. Previously (as part of ICDS program), they were only pre-school teachers for the community, but now roles have been expanded. Research by Ramani et al. (2021) shows that AWWs feel confused and agitated about these new roles as they considered themselves are pre-school teacher, not program organizer as well as managers. In the auto-ethnographic work done on AWWs in Tamil Nadu by P et al. (2022), the workers reported same issue there.

The government is required to send the necessary monies to the AWWs in advance for planning and carrying out community based special events. Participants in study by SP et al. (2022) also noted that workers frequently put up their own money to organize these expensive events because funding did not move on time. However, there is a constant demand of photos. The evaluation process, which evaluates the nationwide districts based on defined measures like the total number of submitted images from the events, is quite competitive. In the end, the AWWs struggle to meet demands imposed by the datafication of development goals due to the pressure supervisors feel to portray the quantitative success of their region. The end result of this is that workers are being pressurized for the increased work, but with no support and training on the new additional work.

Workers reported that they had to work long hours to feed data on the app, along with internet issues. The slow server made it more difficult to enter data. The workers reported that supervisors ask them for data anytime, at any moment. This becomes difficult to respond to due to non-functionality of app because of internet and other data upload issues.

According to the research, SP et al. (2022) the AWWs in Tamil Nadu shared experiences vis. a. vis. cost of the mobile phone. The research states that the workers themselves were responsible for paying for the damages. Despite the fact that the policy mandates that 5% of the procurement cost be set aside for phone repair, this nonetheless occurred. Once someone receives a phone for business use, they keep it, and regardless of who actually owns the phone, people start using it for their own needs, this creates a personal dependency, as was intended by the officials. They can't risk losing control of this tool. Due to the way the ICDS application was created and the incentives associated with collecting data for AWWs, it would be difficult to function without a phone for longer than a few days.

Similar experiences have been reported by workers in this study. The AWWs were provided phones and they have been using the same devices. Many of the mobile devices has stopped working, or malfunction frequently, which has forced workers to use their personal phone for the work. 18 out of 21 workers in this study reported that they have been using their personal devices for running the app.

There is huge internet bill which workers often struggle with. The workers are paying for the internet out of their own pockets and have not received any compensation for it. There was 200 rupees compensation for the recharge but many workers have not got it yet also, the government-mandated sim is from telecom company Vodafone, whose internet connection does not work in many anganwadis. The internet is prepaid, and 200 rupees recharge did not last the whole month.

Hence, for the workers, their work has increased with the introduction of the mobile app. Previously they just had to maintain all the data records in the register, but now they have to do it in both register and phone. Documentation has become more rigorous, maintaining the same data in two modes. The research by Jain et al. (2020) on time use patterns by AWWs in Madhya Pradesh states that even though a smartphone-based application is available and they have the choice to forego using paper registers, it is discovered that AWWs spend a significant portion of their working hours filling out their paper registers. This is a problem that the government can solve because it could prevent them from spending the required amount of time making house visits and helping adolescent girls, pregnant women, and nursing mothers (Jain et al., 2020). The same is the situation in the urban slums of Delhi, where workers spend a lot more time doing the documentation work than engaging in the care workers as they are supposed to by their job roles.

6.13 Data Requirements and Resultant Socio-technical Issues

The app has fundamentally changed how the AWW interacts with different stakeholders in both their personal and professional life, which have an influence on their productivity and jeopardizes the standard of care provided to the community. Workers had control over the type of conversation they wanted to have with the community prior to the launch of the app. They chose the direction the conversation would take based on their knowledge of the community and the rapport they built with them over time. For the app to increase the quality of the data, a precise set of questions must be answered in a particular order. The employees said the previous method, which allowed them to fill out forms, was easier (SP et al., 2022). The same can be seen here. AWWs, previously trusted community health workers, have now turned into data collection agent from the community, and the constant demand for data from the community make the community suspicious about AWWs.

Anganwadi worker held the view that the home visit alert of the app is not new, as they used to do home visits previously too on their own estimates, a worker said that: *"for example, if a child is not coming to the centre, we will go to his house and ask why he's not coming. We used to do home visits for immunisation, asking if the mother has got all the injections and everything. It is not new, we used to do it before also, it is just app tells us when to go now. We used to do it previously too, so it is nothing new" (Worker B. Jahangir Puri, 13.06.22).*

The home visit introduction schedule remains one of the biggest problems for AWWs. Previous to the introduction of the app, AWWs used to do home visits on their own estimates, making sure they did it when the clients were at home and when they had wrapped up their center work. However, now the app tells them to do visits on a specific day and post photos of same on app as proof. The software regularly issues reminders to the workers and controls the deliverables as mentioned earlier. The system for collecting data via apps requires some visual proof of house visits. In the study by SP et al. (2022) in rural Nilgiris of the Tamil Nadu region, geographically dispersed home made it very difficult for AWWs to travel to each home on given date and collect data. This also resulted in the AWWs incurring the financial cost and their work hours increasing as they travel far to collect data.

The low level of digital literacy and trust in the community often stops beneficiaries from sharing information with workers. To verify phone numbers, an OTP would be sent to the beneficiaries' phone numbers and work has to ask them and fill that OTP in app to verify it. However, many beneficiaries refused to share those OTPs with the workers.

Due to the digitization of daily tasks, there is an implied, unstated requirement that employees must possess a foundational understanding of computers and phones. While the remuneration for the Anganwadi job is fixed, there is also a discretionary portion that is dependent on doing extra responsibilities. They also receive a standard monthly bonus of Rs. 500, which is determined by the community's nutrition-related data that the AWWs input to the monitoring app. For each month, AWWs must upload at least 60% of the data to qualify for the incentive. Also, helpers receive Rs. 250 per month for starting the Anganwadi. The older workers who have been working for a long time reported that they have faced difficulties in getting used to mobile phones (SP et al., 2022; Ramani et al., 2021).

So from the above narratives, we can see how strict the data requirements from AWWs are. They have been working at night, they have been spending their own money and resources for this. The workers have to enter the data of everything they do in the app. The workers face issues such as interacting with the community for digital requirements, and in a digitally low-literate society, it hampers their reputation in the community the work. Firstly, their work has increased and the strict data-keeping requirements force them to take data on physical registers as well as the app. Anganwadi staff members continue to record data on their physical registers and upload it to their phones as they had in the past. But, there is much pressure to get it right when they switch from paper to app because it is challenging to fix a mistake once data is posted to the app, making the process stressful and subject to criticism. Also, there are stricter deadlines for uploading data, and Anganwadi employees' performance is immediately timestamped, which led to some respondents reporting fraudulent entries rather than deadline violations.

The workers add data of the distribution of food and take home ration, supplementary nutrition programs, and immunization status of children and pregnant mother. Recently from December 2021, Aadhaar is necessary for new beneficiaries to register. July 10, 2022 was the deadline provided to seed aadhaar for every beneficiary receiving care from Anganwadi. The linking was made compulsory for beneficiaries to access supplementary nutrition and food provided at the centers. While conducting this field work too, all the anganwadi workers told that they have been busy in linking aadhaar card of every child and mother and verifying it (*Anganwadi Centres Rush to Verify Children Beneficiaries' Aadhaar*, 2022).

6.14 Discussion

The only pre-implementation research before introducing this scheme and ICT method was on usability, not how the project will affect AWWs' job in general. As a result, the app has caused AWWs to incur financial, cognitive, and emotional expenses that are mostly going unreported to management. They pay for their internet bills, CBE bills, have to work long hours, and leave them with no time for the actual care work. The app also negatively impacts the workers' interactions with the community, their supervisors, assistants, Anganwadi children, and their families, which in most cases impacts their professional and personal lives. The app and its requirement like OTP has turned the workers relationship with community bitter. The worker have no agency over their own work, they cannot delete the clients and they cannot access the data they enter, which makes their work more difficult and impacts their performance indicator for fault of their own.

Real-time data entry is largely viewed with scepticism due to rural areas' poor internet accessibility. In addition to maintaining eleven registers, an Anganwadi employee who makes much less than the minimum wage must now log data on the program. The employees have been particularly told not to get rid with the actual registers. There are also differences between states in the distribution of smartphones and the regularization of funding for data recharges. Additionally, employees are paying out of pocket extra money for data recharge.

Workers also mention how work hours have increased to the point where some of them stay up until the wee hours of the morning entering data into the application. In order to receive support at home, older workers' families occasionally need to be taught how to utilize the program, according to ICDS managers.

The data that is gathered by the program is still another undefined part of the overall procedure. Monitoring changes in the nutrition situation-this has been claimed to make easier with the availability of consistent data on child nutrition. The information has not been made accessible, though. Recently, on April 1, 2022, the administration informed the parliament that, in contrast to the 19% reported in the NFHS statistics, the country's rate of severe acute malnutrition according to data gathered from Poshan Tracker is 2%. However, the dashboard for Poshan Tracker currently available on the internet only provides information about the application's coverage; therefore no direct conclusions regarding the state of nutrition can be made from it. In order to protect the privacy of women and children who get services through the Anganwadi programs, it is stated that the data should not be made public. However, it needs to be made more obvious how a system of accountability or openness may be upheld throughout the entire data management process. There needs to be public access to aggregated data, in a way that maintain privacy and confidentiality for the sake of tracking nutrition goals.

The role of workers have fundamentally changed. AWWs collect maternal and child health data at pre-natal, post-natal and infant stages. The huge amount of data asked from them can be described as "avalanche of numbers" (Hacking, 1982) where "record keeping is an end in itself" (Gupta, 2012). AWWs are collecting data in their registers, as well as those in the mobile application too. The constant demand of evidence in the form of photos of everything creates a tyranny of transparency on the workers.

The launch of the mobile app has blindly *datafied* several facets of AWW's operations and has disregarded their worries and requirements. Due to invisible labour, unheard-of levels of smartphone surveillance, and the gap between the app's supposed technical subject and the real experiences of AWWs, relationships have become strained and workers endure misery (SP et al., 2022).

6.15 Impact of Digitization of Work on the Job Roles of Anganwadi Workers

The digitization of the work has changed goals for Anganwadi workers by focusing on numerical targets and statistical data, which is now used to measure their performances. In this research, one of the key themes that emerged is that the ICT and digital interventions are forced upon the workers from the top, and this top-down approach of policy implementation with no adequate time for training has left them confused about their nature of work. The focus is on data entry, and numbers are required-this demand for numbers and data has changed the notion of care work that is done by workers.

Workers were used to the process of and collection of data, which they used to maintain in their registers. They used to collect, maintain, and manage data in their physical registers, hence the presence of data was always there in the system, even before the introduction of technology. However, the data collection was secondary to the work they did, and the data collection was an administrative record requirement.

The introduction of the app has changed the motive of data collection-it is now for real-time monitoring so immediate action can be taken. However, this has made Anganwadi workers data collectors first and care workers for the community as second. The app acts as a tool to monitor and control the workers, where workers are constantly asked to update data-so that it can go on the dashboard. The salaries and compensation for all the work remain unchanged.

Workers in this research reported that while the ICDS program has been expanded into Poshan Abhiyaan and now Poshan 2.0 it has come with additional charges like community based events and *Jan Andolan*-for holistic nutritional awareness. However, this has increased the job responsibility for workers in the community, and the compensation system-which is reimbursement based-remains slow. The additional requirement of paperwork like GST bills to claim makes it difficult to file for compensation. Moreover, workers are expected to put up a façade that they are organizing a community by conducting these events as asked by apps. Workers in this research reported that they have been doing community outreach on their own based on the needs and assessment of the particular people in the community, but now those interactions are dictated by apps-when and how should they happen-what should be asked-which is contingent on the data which is needed by the apps and dashboard.

The informal and volunteer nature of the job of workers makes it impossible for the workers and the top-down nature of decision-making excludes them from the decision-making process. The workers in this research reported that they were not made to be part of the consulting and feedback process.

Since the workers are the lowest in the hierarchy, they have no bargaining power and are excluded from any program and policy consultations, with new changes forced on them. This has turned their focus away from their relationships with the children and the community, toward the state's expectations of statistical performance in terms of care and health. This moves their primary responsibility of caring for the community to taking care of the state's needs. They face numerous obligations and limitations. Care work is inherently tricky under a system of bureaucratic apathy. The workers are left completing the data requirements and achieving the milestones set by the government (like organizing two community based events per month) instead of doing work that will benefit the people in the community. The only difference between Anganwadi workers and census takers is that Anganwadi workers are aware of the social and cultural context of the community they serve because they are from the same community and know people from communities because their job is to care for them.

The argument of the government for real-time monitoring has been to plug the gaps in data flow and use the incoming coming data for immediate action. While real-time monitoring has brought some glaring gaps in health system delivery into focus, this insistence on data is not just for plugging these gaps. This also serves as an example of data-driven governance in this age of neoliberalism, where the success of a program is totally dependent on the one who is lowest in the hierarchy, i.e., Anganwadi workers in this case.

The new data gathering regime then acts as a window into governments' way of functioning, where the AWW is the sole representative of the state dealing with the populace. It seems that AWWs are under more pressure to pay more attention to the data work as there is more emphasis on the data performance and data audits. This has complete redesigned of workflow architecture as well as the definition of work in the fields of nutrition, health, and care. The ICDS-CAS project's emphasis on data collecting demonstrates how nutrition or health are treated as data process and end in themselves. Those in positions of authority in the government can promote technology-aided data gathering and its utilization as a scientific process by focusing on the capacity to monitor, aggregate, and centrally evaluate this data. The transition from the whims and rigidity of paper to the modernity of a digital, quickly updated, complete data system is portrayed as a reasonable process. As a result, in this perspective, the data intermediary is equipped with technology and goes through their own "modernization" process (Gupta, 2001). For AWWs, challenging this data-regime has costs, not the least of which is the moral obligation that has been placed on them to uphold the fiction of effective public services and increase the accuracy of the statistical modelling of health. Together with regular pressures, the relationship with supervisors has broken down; supervisors themselves work in a hierarchy that is not designed for feedback. Each level of authority depends on the next as a result of creating zero sum competitions across districts, which forces supervisors to increase their reliance on AWWs in an effort to meet the demands of the new regime (SP et al., 2022).

This has changed their relationship with their supervisors too, as in this study workers in interviews said that their supervisors are aware of the unreasonable amount of work and expectations put on the workers but they do not have any power to do anything. The focus on data-based reporting and surveillance have centralized the whole process and even supervisors are not left with any power to resolve workers' issue or help workers in any way. This has reduced the flexibility for workers to negotiate their terms of work-when their work is measured by the data they enter. The goal of state here, hence is not "to care for citizen" but "to show" that they care for the citizens by showing the data. Workers now believe that the only thing that matters is the data they feed- and the only thing they have to do is to maintain the dashboard, since their incentives are tied to it.

The standard that govern anganwadi care work hence have changed. Previously workers have autonomy to decide when they wanted to enter the data, and data entry was a secondary thing to their main work of taking care of children. They had autonomy over the process, but now that agency has been lost.

References

Aggarwal, P., & Kakkar, R. (2019). National nutrition strategy: The needed timely modification to make integrated child development scheme more effective. *The Indian Journal of Pediatrics, 86*(7), 628–632. https://doi.org/10.1007/s12098-019-02869-9

Bansal, V. (2021, August 12). How healthcare workers in India fought a surveillance regime and won. *Coda Story*. https://www.codastory.com/authoritarian-tech/indian-health-workers/

2011 Census of India | Office of the Registrar General & Census Commissioner, India. India. [Web Archive] Retrieved from the Library of Congress. https://www.loc.gov/item/lcwaN0017959/

Gopalakrishnan, L., Buback, L., Fernald, L., Walker, D., Diamond-Smith, N., In Addition to the CAS Evaluation Consortium. (2020). Using mHealth to improve health care delivery in India: A qualitative examination of the perspectives of community health workers and beneficiaries. *PLoS ONE, 15*(1), e0227451.

Gupta, A. (2001). Governing population: The integrated child development services program in India. *States of Imagination: Ethnographic Explorations of the Postcolonial State,* 65–96.

Gupta, A. (2012). *Red tape: Bureaucracy, structural violence, and poverty in India.* Duke University Press.

Hacking, I. (1982). Biopower and the avalanche of printed numbers. *Humanity in Society, 5*, 279–295.

Iyamu, I., Xu, A. X. T., Gómez-Ramírez, O., Ablona, A., Chang, H. J., Mckee, G., & Gilbert, M. (2021). Defining digital public health and the role of digitization, digitalization, and digital transformation: Scoping review. *JMIR Public Health and Surveillance, 7*(11), Article e30399. https://doi.org/10.2196/30399.PMID: 34842555;PMCID:PMC8665390

Jain, A., Walker, D. M., Avula, R., Diamond-Smith, N., Gopalakrishnan, L., Menon, P., Nimmagadda, S., Patil, S. R., & Fernald, L. C. H. (2020). Anganwadi worker time use in Madhya Pradesh, India: A cross-sectional study. *BMC Health Services Research, 20*(1), 1130. https://doi.org/10.1186/s12913-020-05857-4

Kaskar, Z. (2022, September 22). *Watch | Pressured to downplay malnourishment numbers: Ex-anganwadi workers speak.* The Wire. https://thewire.in/video/watch-pressure-downplay-malnourishment-numbers-ex-anganwadi-workers

Ministry of Health and Family Welfare. (2022). *More than 50 digital health services/applications integrated with Ayushman Bharat Digital Mission (ABDM).* Press Information Bureau (PIB) Delhi (Release ID: 1845845). https://pib.gov.in/PressReleasePage.aspx?PRID=1845845

Ministry of Science and Technology, 2022, 28th October, Union Minister Dr Jitendra Singh Union Minister Dr Jitendra Singh says, India has emerged as a leading country in the world in delivery of Digital Health services, Press Release. https://pib.gov.in/PressReleaseIframePage.aspx?PRID=1871545

National Family Health Survey (NFHS-5). (n.d.). *Rchiips.org*. http://rchiips.org/nfhs/factsheet_NFHS-5.shtml

Newslive Staff. (2022, March 16). Big blow: Delhi HC denies petition of protesting Anganwadi workers and helpers. *NEWS9LIVE*. https://www.news9live.com/india/big-blow-delhi-hc-denies-petition-of-protestinganganwadi-workers-and-helpers-159361

Poshan Tracker. (n.d.). Retrieved 06 June 2022, from https://www.poshantracker.in/

PTI. (2019). Government plans to upgrade 2.5 lakh anganwadi centres in next 5 years: Women and Child Development Ministry official. https://economictimes.indiatimes.com/news/politics-and-nation/governmentplans-to-upgrade-2-5-lakh-anganwadi-centres-in-next-5-years-women-and-child-development-ministryofficial/articleshow/72828637.cms

Ramani, S., Sridhar, R., Shende, S., Manjarekar, S., Patil, S., Pantvaidya, S., Fernandez, A., & Jayaraman, A. (2021). Implementing a 'convergent' framework of action against childhood malnutrition in urban informal settlements of Mumbai: Frontline perspectives. *Journal of Family Medicine and Primary Care, 10*(10), 3600–3605. https://doi.org/10.4103/jfmpc.jfmpc_2526_20

SP, A. M., Vaghela, P., & Pal, J. (2022). Counting to be counted: Anganwadi workers and digital infrastructures of ambivalent care. *Proceedings of the ACM on Human–computer Interaction, 6*(CSCW2), 1–36. https://doi.org/10.1145/3555177

Swaddle, T., & Kalia, S. (2021, September 1). Anganwadi workers return 80,000 faulty smartphones given for data collection. *The Swaddle*. https://theswaddle.com/anganwadi-workers-return-80000-faulty-phonesgiven-for-data-collection/

Part III
Emerging challenges in Health

Trend and Correlates of Unmet Need for Healthcare in India

7

Sandhya R. Mahapatro

Abstract

While India has made significant strides in health indices under the initiative of universal healthcare access, the unmet medical need is still substantial. As per the 75th National Sample Survey round, around 12% of ailed people were not accessing healthcare services from facilities despite reported illness. To ensure universal access to healthcare access, the identification of factors impedes healthcare access is crucial for appropriate policy intervention. The present paper attempts to fill this gap through analysing the trend and correlates of unmet need for healthcare. Various rounds of National Sample Survey data are used for analysis. The findings suggest despite the rhetoric of universalisation of healthcare, a substantial share of ailed persons could not access care from health facilities. Although the unmet need declined over time, the socioeconomic differentials in unmet needs are widening and acceptability related unmet need was more than the health system barriers. The findings from the regression analysis show that ailed persons belong to low economic class and from underdeveloped regions have higher unmet need. Community level interventions to create health awareness prioritising the marginalised and younger age group is important for reducing the acceptability related barriers. A multisectoral policy approach with strategies to address geographical heterogeneity is required for reducing overall unmet medical needs.

S. R. Mahapatro (✉)
Nabakrushna Choudhary Centre for Development Studies, Bhubaneswar, India
e-mail: sandhyamahapatro@gmail.com

7.1 Introduction

With the stated goal of reducing inequalities in health outcomes and equity in healthcare access, health system reforms were widespread across the globe, especially in developing countries (Subirats et al., 2014). Health equity is of particular concern in the Indian context in the light of widening economic inequality as health inequality escalates with income inequality (Joe et al., 2008). Studies have shown that in India individuals with the greatest need for healthcare had the least likely to meet their healthcare needs (Sen et al., 2002). In India, the parallel transition in demographic and epidemiological profiles poses major challenges to the healthcare system such as rising demand for services & cost of care, the inadequacy of infrastructure etc. To overcome such challenges, reforms in the health sector have been witnessed since the last decade through the emphasis on universal access to healthcare.

S. S. Acharya et al. (eds.), *Paradigm Shifts in Population and Health in India*, Sustainable Development Goals Series, https://doi.org/10.1007/978-981-95-1719-0_7

Equity in healthcare access is reiterated in various policy documents from the Bhore committee report to National Health Policy 2017. The paradigm shifts in the health sector appeared through innovative health policies and programmes in the past few years exemplified by the National Rural Health Mission, the National Health Mission, Rashtriya Swasth Bima Yojna, National Health Policy, and National Health Protection Scheme have attempted to provide adequate & quality healthcare to the poor and vulnerable. With the introduction of various policy interventions under universal health coverage, health indices show an improvement. Nevertheless, the discourses on equity in healthcare continue as still a group of ailed people were not able to meet the need for medical care. As evident from National Sample Survey data self-reported approximately 12% could not access health care resulting in unmet needs during the period 2017–18 although the share is declining over time.

Examining the access barriers assumed special significance recently in the context of structural reforms, income inequality and the poverty level of the county where more than 1/5th of the population is still below the poverty line, a major contributor to health inequality which is further accompanied by gaps in social differentiation of caste, religion and gender. Unless the mechanisms that constraints access to healthcare are addressed explicitly, the mandate of universal health coverage will unlikely to occur and equity in healthcare access will remain a noble aspiration. An assessment of the key factors that contribute to unmet medical needs is important as forgone healthcare is associated with prolonged illness and higher treatment costs (Tidikis & Strasen, 1994) and widens health inequality.

While identifying the factors that act as barriers, often the access to health care was evaluated based on the actual utilisation with little consensus on analysing the reasons for unmet medical need and doing so, excluded a population group whose need for medical care could not turn into demand. Unmet medical need is the widely accepted indicator of exploring the barriers to healthcare access (Alin et al., 2010; Hwang et al., 2017; Cylus & Papanicolas, 2015). Studies on health-seeking behaviour show that health system challenges such as unavailability of services, poor quality, skewed allocation of resources, high cost of care affected the use of healthcare, especially for the poor and vulnerable (Gumber et al., 2012; Hwang, 2018; Kiwanuka et al., 2008). The widening income inequalities accompanied by the increasing cost of care perhaps push many families to forgo care and perpetuate inequalities in healthcare. Findings from studies in this line reveal that in India health spending among the lower income class was relatively higher and in backward regions poor pay more for utilisation of inpatient care services from public health centres (Mahapatro et al., 2018; Das & Mohanty, 2019). Despite the provision of financial support, poor were not motivated to access services from a health facility (Kuuire et al., 2015; Fjaer et al., 2017) also found in studies. The unmet medical need thus is not only the failure of the health system in providing care but also arises out of personal choice, preference, norms etc. The factors associated with the unmet need for healthcare thus would not be same (Hwang, 2018) and reason for experiencing unmet medical need require a different policy approach (Allin, 2010; Sibley, 2011).

Research studies to date in India, often engaged in investigating the determinants of health outcomes in terms of healthcare utilisation (Roy & Chaudhuri, 2008; Prinja et al., 2012; Borooah, 2010, Balarajan et al., 2011; Scaria, 2017; Baru et al., 2010; Mukherjee et al., 2011). Undoubtedly, the findings of these studies provide guidance for policy action, however, not sufficient to address the barriers as the patients who were not able to access care were overlooked. These studies thus, failed to include the perspective of non-users of healthcare that act as a barrier to use healthcare. Literature on unmet medical need in India mainly examined the prevalence and measurement of inequities (Ghosh, 2014; Pandey et al., 2017) with little emphasis on the barriers mostly supply side (Banerjee et al., 2004) or limited to certain diseases (Kanungo et al., 2015). The reason being with the implementation of universal healthcare coverage and decline in cost-based barriers unmet medical need is assumed to decline significantly.

Understanding the factors contributing to unmet medical need is a matter of concern for the health care system and individual wellbeing and hence, call for a detailed investigation. This study intends to fill the gap in the literature on unmet medical need for healthcare in India.

Given this, the objective of the paper is (1) to compare the trend in the type of unmet need. 2) To understand the factors associated with unmet need for health care.

7.2 Conceptual Framework on Correlates of Unmet Need

'Unmet need' for healthcare is the widely used indicator that measures barriers to access healthcare. Unmet need broadly assessed through clinically assessed need where the respondent was not satisfied with the services received and subjective assessment of the need for care that does not turn into a demand for care. This study has followed the latter approach as used in many studies as the patient is the best judge of his/her health status (Cavelieri, 2013). Further, the study followed the classification used in literature to understand the factors that are related to different types of unmet need arising out of availability, accessibility and acceptability of health care (Chen & Houm, 2002).

Unmet medical need is defined in this study as those individuals' reported illness during last 15 days from the date of the survey but could not sought care due to various reasons. This measure identifies the individuals who have encountered barriers that prevent access (Allin et al., 2010; Garcia et al., 2014). Studies have shown that the unmet need for healthcare arises due to the barriers of health system which depends on the availability of healthcare resources, cost of care (Sibley & Glazier, 2009; Allin & Masaria, 2009; Nelson & Park, 2006) and also the acceptability of healthcare that influenced by users capabilities such as wage or income loss, personal circumstances, attitudes etc. These are the perceived barriers or the expressed demand that defines unmet need. There are other unobserved demand-side barriers that were unexpressed. This includes people who have no demand (untreated) or lack of seriousness of ailment (Low perceived need) when there is an objective need for it. 'Untreated' cases include those ailed people who have no demand for healthcare services. Besides, people's perception of illness which is not a tangible barrier but a disincentive to seek healthcare and hence creates inequity. It is defined as 'low perceived need' in the study. This category differs from 'untreated' cases because people were aware of their health issues, and they were using other alternative sources of healthcare which has not happened with untreated cases.

The conceptual model of unmet need for healthcare access is presented in Fig. 7.1. It is believed that the mechanisms that influence access to healthcare through these indicators were not mutually exclusive rather the interaction of these creates barriers to access healthcare services. Understanding the socioeconomic differentials in these indicators and the factors associated with them will enable us to draw inferences about the underlying barriers that cause inequities in healthcare access.

7.3 Data, Measures, and Method

The study used cross-sectional data from the various rounds of the National Sample Survey such as the 60th, 71st and 75th rounds. This survey aimed at generating basic quantitative information on the behaviour of the sample households seeking treatment (for ailments) during the last 15 days and during the last 365 days. Information about inpatients was collected during the last 365 days while the outpatient information was collected during the last 15 days to avoid recall lapses. In the present analysis, we have used individual-level data on outpatients during in last 15 days to explore the underlying reasons for the unmet need for healthcare.

7.4 Measurement Indicators

Unmet need is analysed using the question 'whether the ailed persons seek medical advice during the last 15 days which s/he did not receive'

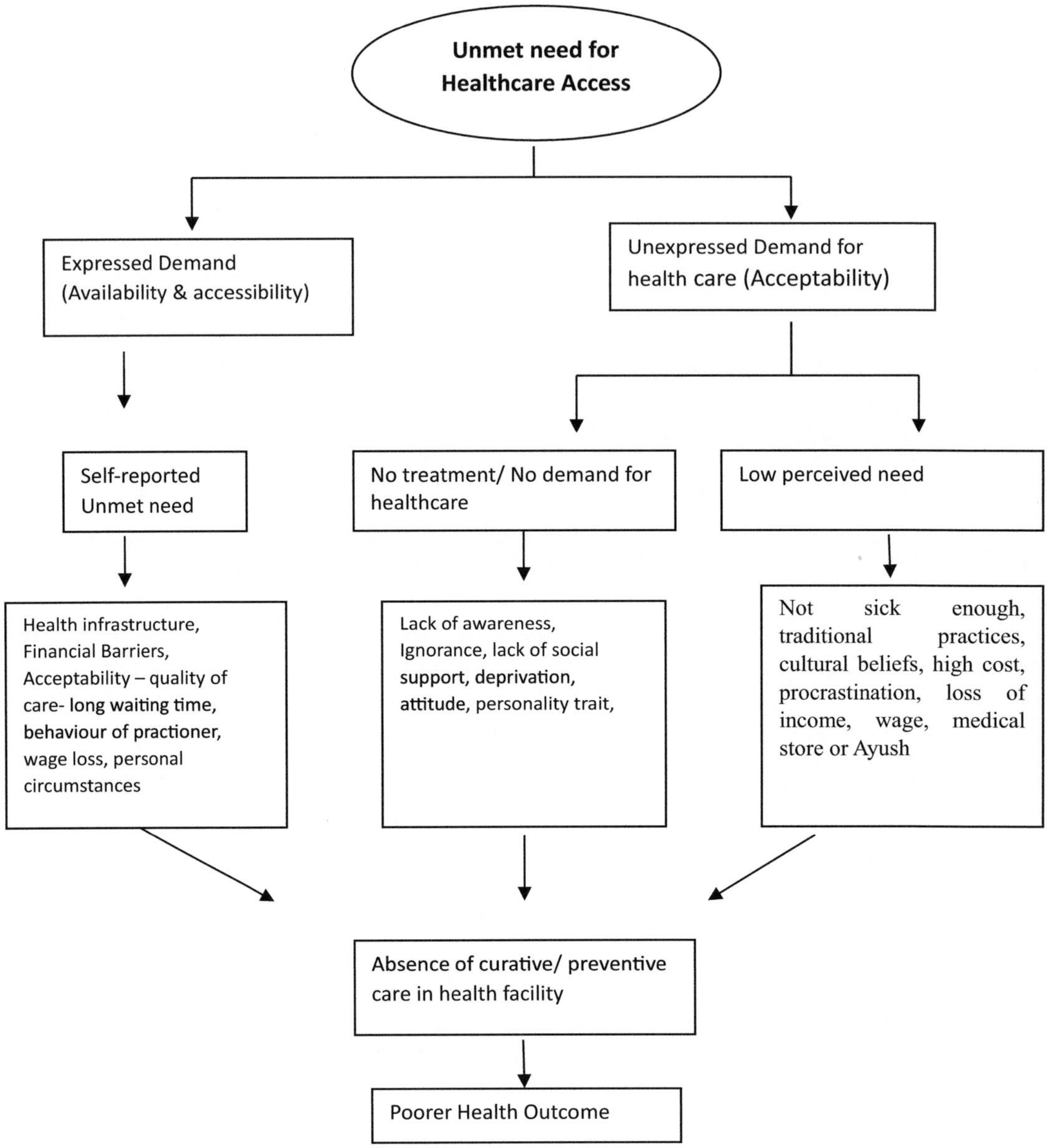

Fig. 7.1 Conceptual framework on unmet need for healthcare

and 'the reasons for not taking medical advice'. The responses for not accessing healthcare from health facilities were divided broadly into two categories: acceptability issues that include cases related to untreated, and low perceived need (illness not serious). The other category includes access barriers that include health system challenges and other reasons.

7.4.1 Health System Barrier (Availability/Accessibility)

This category includes those ailed people who sought medical care but could not access it. It is based on the single question asked in the data set to those who reported ailment during the last 15 days 'Reason for not seeking medical advice'. The response to the question is multiple and related to the non-availability of health facilities, poor quality of care, long waiting times, and higher costs. Besides, 'Other' reasons are also included in this category which may include arising due to social stigma, wage loss or other personal circumstances.

7.5 Acceptability Barrier

7.5.1 Low Perceived Needs

This category relates to those who considered their ailment not serious enough to warrant accessing healthcare from the facility. In the data, set it is stated as a reason for not seeking medical advice, but what influences their perception of their own health needs to be explored. Dependency on traditional practitioners, quacks, use of the medical store, Ayush, cultural beliefs, attitudes etc. perhaps influences it.

7.5.2 Untreated

This category relates to those who had not taken any treatment despite they have reported having an ailment that would warrant treatment. In the data set the question that was asked to ailed people 'nature of treatment'. Those who have reported no treatment were considered untreated. In the data set, the reason for having no demand for healthcare was not explicitly mentioned. It is believed that lack of health knowledge, lack of social support, ignorance and attitudes are expected to be the reason for not seeking any treatment.

In the data set, while asking the reason for not accessing healthcare, information was collected on health system issues and financial barriers which are clubbed as 'unmet need'. While for the other two indicators the barriers arise mainly from the user perspective and the reasons were not specified. The socioeconomic characteristics of the ailed person for each response were examined to understand the pattern of inequality in each of the responses and explore the barriers.

For the regression analysis, the socioeconomic and demographic variables such as social group, economic status, educational level, gender, age and place of residence were used as explanatory variables in our analysis.

7.6 Trends in Unmet Need for Health Care

Figure 7.2 presents the trends in unmet need for health care from 2004 to 2018. The overall unmet need for care that was reported as 15.7% in 2004–05 declined to 11.7% in 2017–18. (Fig. 7.2). The rural–urban differential in unmet needs suggests that it was higher in rural than urban in all the rounds of NSS although the gap declines over time. The unmet need for healthcare in the rural area remains almost stagnant between 2004–05 and 2014–15.

Moreover, the results depict unmet medical need remains high in rural area and the percentage share remains almost stagnant over the years. However, the latest NSS shows a decline for both rural and urban areas.

7.7 Unmet Need for Health Care by Underlying Reported Reasons

Distribution of unmet needs by the reasons show long waiting as a reason for non-utilisation of healthcare increased from 1% in 2004–05 to 4.5% in 2017–18. Non-utilisation of healthcare due to financial reasons, however, shows a huge dip. However, the non-utilisation of health care due to the low perceived need that illness is not serious increased from 35.5% in 2004–05 to 62% in 2017–18 (Table 7.1).

Moreover, the demand-side barriers contributing to the unmet need for healthcare access increased whereas access barriers related to healthcare services provided by the government are declining. For instance, the non-utilisation of services due to the non-availability of medical facilities declined from 9.5% in 2004–05 to 5.7% in 2017–18.

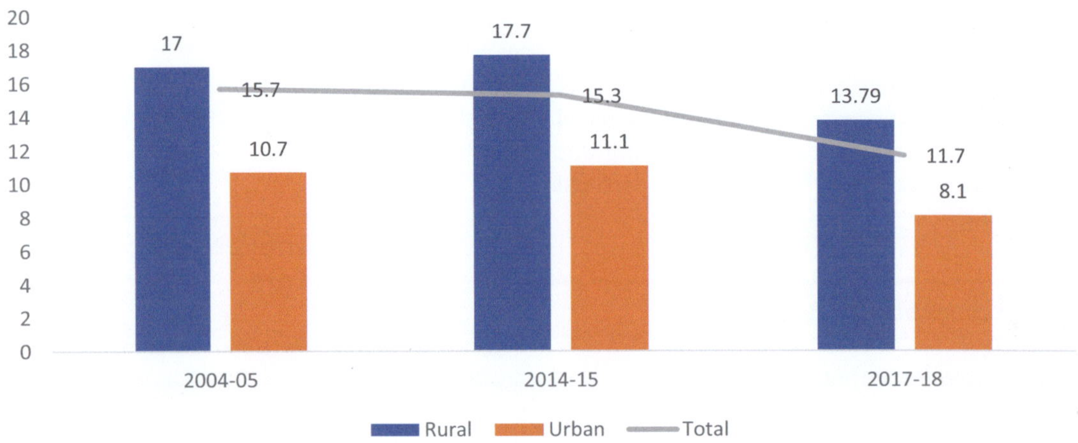

Fig. 7.2 Trends in unmet need for health care, 2004–2018

Table 7.1 Trend in Unmet need for medical care by reasons for unmet need, 2004–05 to 2017–18

Unmet need	2004–05	2014–15	2017–18
Accessibility/ availability	37.13	16.31	12.18
No medical facility	9.49	9.16	5.69
Financial reasons	26.62	4.65	2.04
Long waiting	1.02	2.5	4.45
Acceptability	62.88	83.69	87.82
Lack of faith	2.79	2.66	1.16
Illness not serious	35.55	47.47	62.46
No demand	10.15	23.32	15.03
Others	14.39	10.24	9.17

Source National sample survey rounds

7.8 Socioeconomic Differentials in Unmet Need

Table 7.2 presents the characteristics of an ailed person by the type of unmet medical need for 2004–05 and 2017–18. Irrespective of type, the unmet medical need was higher in the lower economic class. For instance, in 2017–18 while 2.3% of ailed people from low economic class reported no treatment, it declines to 1.3% for the higher economic class. A similar pattern was observed for other healthcare barriers as well. A variation in unmet medical need according to economic status among individuals reporting illness was not serious was observed. Individuals reporting illness not serious was much higher in the lower economic class (9.5%) than the richer class (4.6%) in 2017–18 while class differential was not observed in 2004–05. Acceptability-related unmet medical need due to no treatment and availability barriers was higher among SC/ST than general caste, low educated and those living in the rural area. From the table it was observed that while 3% of SC/ST in 2017–18 reported unmet medical need due to no treatment, it was 1.4% for others, whereas no caste differentials were observed in 2004–05. This reveals while there was no significant difference observed among the socioeconomic group by various types of unmet needs during 2004–05, the differentials widened over time and were observed in all the socioeconomic indicators for 2014–15 and 2017–18.

The trend in the type of unmet need by socioeconomic differentials reveals, while untreated cases among low economic class were 1.7%, it increases to 5% in 2014–15 and further declined to 2.3% in 2017–18. Likewise, illness not serious was a major reason and was higher in 2017–18 compared to 2004–5 among the low economic class.

The educational differentials in unmet need suggest a higher non-utilisation among illiterates

Table 7.2 Socioeconomic and geographic differential in unmet need for care by type of unmet need, 2004–05 to 2017–18

Background characteristics	Unperceived unmet need		Self-reported unmet need		Total	Unperceived unmet need		Self-reported unmet need		Total	Unperceived unmet need		Self-reported unmet need		Total
	Untreated	Illness not serious	Health service barriers	Other		Untreated	Illness not serious	Health service barriers	Other		Untreated	Illness not serious	Health service barriers	Other	
	2004–05					2014–15					2017–18				
Economic class															
Low (Q1)	1.7	6.0	9.9	2.8	20.4	5.0	10.6	5.3	1.7	22.2	2.3	9.5	2.3	1.3	15.3
Middle (Q2)	1.4	5.5	5.8	2.5	15.2	4.4	7.5	3.4	1.5	16.8	1.2	6.0	0.7	0.9	8.9
Higher (Q3)	1.4	5.2	2.0	1.3	9.8	2.1	4.8	1.0	1.6	9.4	1.3	4.6	0.3	0.9	7.0
Sex															
Male	1.7	5.5	6.2	2.2	15.5	3.6	7.4	3.2	1.3	15.5	1.7	7.4	1.6	1.3	12.0
Female	1.4	5.7	6.4	2.4	15.8	3.5	7.2	2.7	1.8	15.1	1.8	7.5	1.5	0.9	11.5
Caste group															
Scheduled Caste/tribe (SC/T)	1.4	5.5	10.0	2.7	19.6	6.4	7.4	4.4	2.2	20.2	3.0	9.1	1.9	0.9	14.9
Others	1.6	5.6	5.1	2.2	14.4	2.7	7.2	2.5	1.4	13.7	1.4	7.0	1.3	1.1	10.7
Education															
Illiterate	1.5	5.7	8.5	2.8	18.4	4.2	7.0	3.9	1.5	16.6	2.6	8.1	1.5	1.3	13.5
Primary/secondary	1.6	5.6	5.5	2.1	14.7	3.6	8.1	2.9	1.6	16.1	1.4	7.5	1.6	1.0	11.5
Higher secondary	1.5	5.6	2.9	1.5	11.5	2.9	6.8	1.9	1.5	13.2	1.0	5.2	1.0	0.8	7.9
Graduate and above	2.1	4.4	0.5	0.7	7.7	2.1	7.1	1.0	2.4	12.2	0.9	6.4	0.0	0.8	8.1
Geography															
Rural	1.7	5.7	7.7	2.6	17.7	4.1	8.0	4.0	1.6	17.6	2.2	8.3	2.0	1.2	13.8
Urban	1.3	5.4	2.7	1.4	10.7	2.7	5.9	1.0	1.6	11.1	0.9	5.9	0.5	0.8	8.1
Total	1.6	5.6	6.3	2.3	15.7	3.6	7.3	2.9	1.6	15.3	1.8	7.5	1.4	1.1	11.7

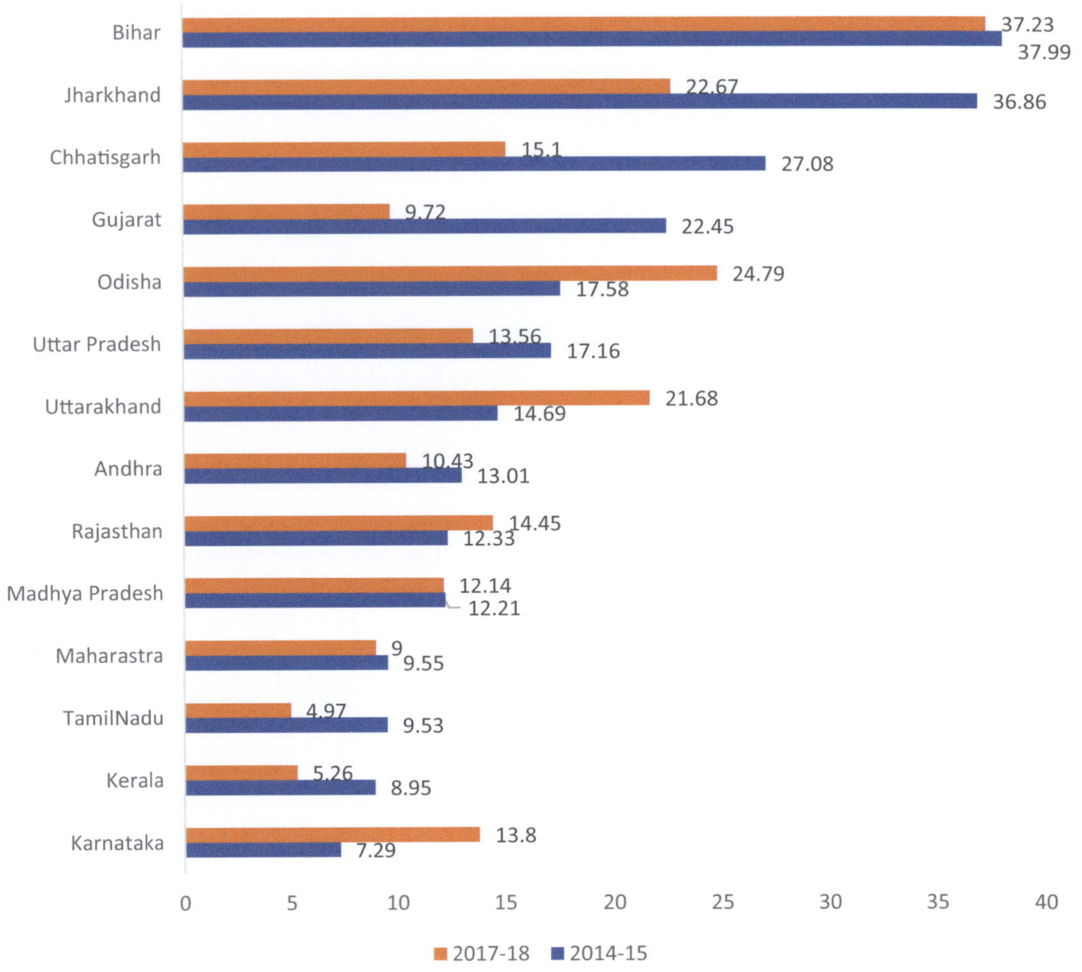

Fig. 7.3 Trends in unmet need for health care across the states, 2014–15 and 2017–18

for both 2014–15 and 2017–18 and it declines with an increase in education level. Except for the 'other reason' a notable rural–urban difference irrespective of the type of unmet need was observed for all subcategories.

A regional pattern of unmet need for care further show the regional level health system functioning and the contextual factors have significant influence to the health-seeking behaviour. The unmet medical need is found higher in many of the poor states of India (Fig. 7.3).

For the year 2017–18, unmet need for medical care is highest in Bihar (38%) followed by Chhattisgarh (27%), Odisha(24.8%), Jharkhand (15%) and whereas individuals not availing service from health institution is lower in developed regions. For instance, non-utilisation of healthcare was 7.2% and 5.2% in Karnataka and Kerala respectively. These facts signify a direct association of poverty, backwardness, poor functioning of health care, and low level of health literacy with the use of health care in states of India.

The change in the prevalence of unmet needs between 2014–15 and 2017–18 reveals Odisha, Uttarakhand, Karnataka show a significant decline in the utilisation of health care from health care centres both public/private. On the other hand, Gujarat, Jharkhand, Chhattisgarh, Uttar Pradesh etc., shows the percentage of ailed person reporting non-access to health care from healthcare facility has declined.

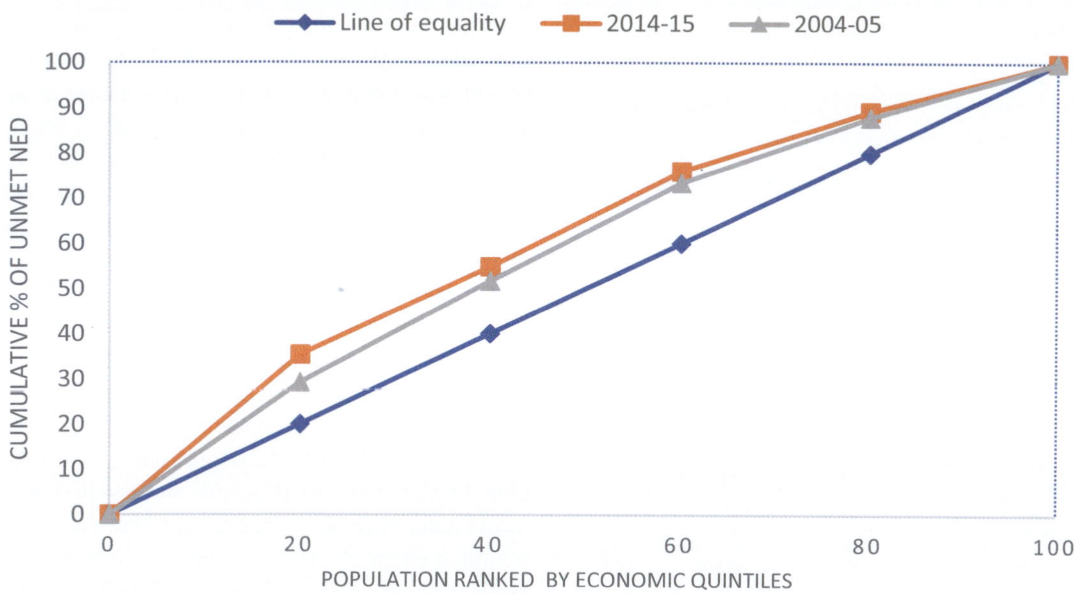

Fig. 7.4 Concentration curve for the ailed person with unmet need, 2004–05 and 2014–15

Moreover, the pattern of non-utilisation varies over the period by socioeconomic characteristics. The concentration of unmet need is higher among the lower socioeconomic class than their counterpart in recent as compared to earlier rounds The concentration curve (Fig. 7.4) that measures the inequality in healthcare access lies below the line of equality indicating health care access are pro-poor.

The CI value was (-0.17) and (-0.19) for 2004–05 and 2014–15 respectively indicating the economic inequality among the non-users of health services increases marginally in 2014–15. The increase could be perhaps associated with the widening of income inequality in the country which is linked with healthcare utilisation apparent through increased CI value for unmet need.

7.9 Analysis of the Association of Unmet Need with Socioeconomic Factors

The results of multivariate logistic regression on correlates of unmet needs are shown in Table 7.3. The odds of not accessing health care were higher among the low educated, those living in rural area, and the low caste and low economic group. For instance, the odds of having an unmet need for health care were lower among the literate as compared to the illiterates. The odds of unmet need for care were 10%, 21% and 23% lower among those who attained primary, secondary and higher education than the illiterates. Likewise, ailed people belonging to the middle and rich economic groups were 21% and 31% less likely to have unmet needs than the poor economic class.

The probability of unmet needs was higher among the ailed person living in the rural area than those are in urban. Ailed people having the chronic disease were less likely to report unmet needs and younger and middle age group people have more unmet needs than the older people.

7.10 Discussion

The present study has examined the socioeconomic differentials and correlates of unmet medical need in India. The findings suggest that the unmet need for healthcare has declined over the time, however the socioeconomic differential has widened. The study finds reasons for unmet

Table 7.3 Association of socioeconomic and geographic factors with unmet need for healthcare, 2017–18

Background variables	Odds ratio	Std error	$p > [z]$
Current age			
60+®			
0–14	0.83***	0.05	0.002
15–34	1.29***	0.08	0
35–44	1.23***	0.08	0.002
45–59	1.04	0.06	0.517
Sex			
Male®	1	1	1
Female	0.92**	0.03	0.014
Household size	1.02***	0.01	0.006
Economic status			
Lower®			
Middle	0.79***	0.03	0
Upper	0.69***	0.04	0
Caste			
SC/ST®			
Others	0.84***	0.03	0
Level of education			
Illiterates®			
Primary	0.90**	0.04	0.023
Secondary	0.79***	0.04	0
Graduate and above	0.77***	0.05	0
Sector			
Rural®			
Urban	0.88***	0.03	0.001
Ailment			
Acute®			
Chronic	0.30***	0.01	0
Regions			
South®			
North	0.99	0.06	0.793
Central	1.14**	0.06	0.025
East	1.56***	0.08	0
West	0.89*	0.06	0.082
North east	2.28***	0.18	0
Pseudo R^2	0.0757		
N	43,218		

Source Estimated from National Sample Survey data, 2017–18

need are complex and influenced both by demand side and supply side factors. Of all the reasons, acceptability barriers constitute significant share and it increases over time with a decline in accessibility barriers. Despite the stronger commitment of the government for providing affordable and accessible healthcare to all, ailed people belonging to low socioeconomic groups have a higher unmet medical need.

With the rise of neo-liberalism which is adhered to a market-oriented society and accordingly with reforms in the health system, the role of non-state actors become prominent in India and consequently, healthcare becomes unaffordable to the poor. In this line studies find that individuals with less income are less likely to obtain medical services despite having serious health issues (van Doorslaer et al., 2004; Mohammadbeigi, 2013) owing to relatively higher out of expenditure than those rich (Mahapatro et al., 2018; Das & Mohanty, 2019). The cost of care as a reason for unmet need has declined substantially with time, however, economic status is the key determinant and the probability of non-access to health care in low-income families is significant. Financial constraints accompanied by a lack of health knowledge, the belief of low risk of developing the disease, indirect costs such as informal charges, and transport (Haomiao et al., 2004; Israel, 2016; Waters et al., 2013) in low-income families resulted in higher unmet need for medical care. Apart from such vulnerabilities, the expansion of community resources such as retail drug stores may likely to reduce healthcare utilisation from the facility (Petkova, 2008) though the association does not find true in other studies (Gao et al., 2012). A cross-tabulation of those reporting illness not serious seeking an alternative source of treatment suggests more than 3/4th of them depend on pharmaceutical stores (NSS). This may be attributed to many reasons such as poverty, poor transportation, time constraint or poor quality of services. In this line studies have shown that the higher acceptability barrier among the poor arises if health services are substandard in terms of quality, effectiveness, and appropriateness or if the patient lack trust in health facility (Cook-Craig et al., 2012; Aline et al., 2010) and hence, they rely on advice from friends and family, drug stores and other informal sources of treatment.

The rural–urban differential in unmet need for medical care suggests that not seeking any treatment and health system barriers account for higher unmet need in rural areas and is patterned by caste differential. The urban biases in health care services in terms of allocation of resources and expenditure create constraints in utilising health care services (Dillip & Duggal, 2004; Garg & Karan, 2009; Baru et al., 2010; Mondal et al., 2014) in the rural area. This is further reflected through higher unmet medical need among the marginalised group. Analysing higher unmet need among SC and ST, studies show lack of treatment owing to inherent discriminative practices resulted in poor health outcomes among the lower social group (Balarajan et al., 2011; Baru et al., 2010; Borooah, 2010; Mukherjee et al., 2011; Scaria, 2017) along with unavailability services in remote rural areas. Travel cost, waiting time also opportunity cost force poor people to forgo care along with limited health knowledge (Penchansky & Thomas, 1981). The regional pattern of unmet medical need reveals that the unmet need was higher in backward states compared to developed ones. Low level infrastructure, cultural norms along with financial burden restrict individuals specifically the lower class as they had to spend more on hospitalisation (Dash & Mohanty, 2019).

A non-linear association of unmet need with age suggests younger have higher unmet need than older. Although the seriousness of illness was lower among younger, substituting the work time to seek care may discourage them not to visit the hospital (Mukherjee & Karmakar, 2008; Cavelieri, 2013) as that might affect their wage. It is needless to mention that such untreated morbidity in the long run affects their productivity, health status and poses challenges to the healthcare system as the country is moving toward an ageing society. Unmarried Individuals or those living alone have lower demand for health care. This is also evident from the association of family size with unmet need that individuals in large families are more likely to seek treatment. Having a chronic illness is also positively correlated with the probability of experiencing an unmet medical need, as the fact of being hampered in daily activities because of health problems (Cavelieri, 2013). These results reveal the fact that recurrent care needs might force to forgo treatments due to the increasing economic burden. The socioeconomic status of ailed person intersecting with the quality of care resultant a higher likelihood of reporting difficulties in meeting their health care needs.

There are some limitations observed in this study. As the ailed person has not reported what type of care was required, it was unable to know the unmet need arose from which level of medical care. Further, responses were self-reported morbidity based on subjective assessment of the ailed person and were not clinically verified. Thirdly, the study has not analysed unmet need according to disease pattern, hence limited in analysing the severity of illness. This study was based on cross-section data, however, the collection of information about an individual over time will provide how the pathways contributing unmet need, especially among the poor will explore in more detail whether recurrent illness may discourage them not to access care.

7.11 Conclusion

Despite the rhetoric of universal healthcare coverage, a certain section of the population in India is deprived of accessing medical care. This study aims to uncover the association of socioeconomic factors with unmet medical need. The key findings of the study are: First, the socioeconomic differentials in unmet need are widening although the overall unmet medical need is declining. Secondly, the barriers related to the acceptability of healthcare services consist of a major proportion and unmet need for health care was pro-poor. Unmet need for healthcare was mainly concentrated in rural areas, younger age, and backward regions and among the socioeconomically marginalised group.

With the implementation of NRHM, investment in health infrastructure has been increased extensively, however in rural areas, the marginalised are yet deprived of health care. This is more apparent from the unavailability of the facility that poses major challenges to the health-care system in achieving universal health care access. Unmet need due to acceptability barriers contributes substantially to overall unmet need which is mainly based on perceptions. Health promotion efforts that are not targeted at the poor are likely to increase socioeconomic disparities. Increasing health literacy and prioritising the younger age group is important to reduce acceptability related unmet need. State-specific policies to improve the efficiency of health care delivery system and trained community workers who were key to facilitating to use healthcare, especially in poor resource settings are desirable. Further research is required to address the acceptability barriers for appropriate strategies and interventions. Policies and programmes thus should be designed and implemented to remove socioeconomic and regional inequalities and ensure equity in healthcare access. A multisectoral policy approach with strategies to address geographical heterogeneity is required for reducing unmet need.

References

Allin, S., Grignon, M., & Le Grand, J. (2010). Subjective unmet need and utilization of health care services in Canada: What are the equity implications? *Social Science and Medicine, 70*(3), 465–472.

Balarajan, Y., Selvaraj, S., & Subramanian, S. V. (2011). Health care and equity in India. *The Lancet, 377*(9764), 505–515.

Banerjee, A., Deaton, A., & Duflo, E. (2004). Wealth, health, and health services in rural Rajasthan. *American Economic Review, 94*(2), 326–330.

Baru, R., Acharya, A., Acharya, S., Kumar, A. S., & Nagaraj, K. (2010). Inequities in access to health services in India: Caste, class and region. *Economic and Political Weekly, 49–58*, 38.

Borooah, V. (2010). *Inequality in health outcomes in India: The role of caste and religion* (pp. 179–207).

Cavalieri, M. (2013). Geographical variation of unmet medical needs in Italy: A multivariate logistic regression analysis. *International Journal of Health Geographics, 12*(1), 27.

Chen, J., & Hou, F. (2002). Unmet needs for health care. *Health Reports, 13*(2), 23–34.

Cook-Craig, P., Ely, G., Flaherty, C., Dignan, M., & White, C. R. (2012). Seeking health advice from social networks in low-income urban neighbourhoods. *American Journal of Health Behaviour, 36*(6), 723–735. https://doi.org/10.5993/ajhb.36.6.1

Cylus, J., & Papanicolas, I. (2015). An analysis of perceived access to health care in Europe: How universal is universal coverage? *Health Policy, 119*(9), 1133–1144.

Dash, A., & Mohanty, S. K. (2019). Do poor people in the poorer states pay more for healthcare in India? *BMC Public Health, 19*(1), 1020.

Dilip, T. R., & Duggal, R. (2004). Unmet need for public health-care services in Mumbai, India. *Asia-Pacific Population Journal, 19*(2), 27–40.

Ebid, A., & Abdel-Wahab, E. (2006). Bronchial asthma and COPD: Impact of pharmaceutical care on outcomes and quality of life in Egyptian patients. *Bulletin of Pharmaceutical Sciences-Assiut University, 29*(1), 167.

Fjær, E. L., Stornes, P., Borisova, L. V., McNamara, C. L., & Eikemo, T. A. (2017). Subjective perceptions of unmet need for health care in Europe among social groups: Findings from the European social survey (2014) special module on the social determinants of health. *The European Journal of Public Health, 27*(suppl_1), 82–89.

Gao, W., Dang, S., Yan, H., & Wang, D. (2012). Care-seeking pattern for diarrhea among children under 36 months old in rural western China. *PLoS ONE, 7*(8), 43103.

Garcia-Subirats, I., Vargas, I., Mogollón-Pérez, A. S., De Paepe, P., Da Silva, M. R. F., Unger, J. P., & Vázquez, M. L. (2014). Inequities in access to health care in different health systems: A study in municipalities of central Colombia and north-eastern Brazil. *International Journal for Equity in Health, 13*(1), 10.

Garg, C. C., & Karan, A. K. (2009). Reducing out-of-pocket expenditures to reduce poverty: A disaggregated analysis at rural–urban and state level in India. *Health Policy and Planning, 24*, 116–128.

Ghosh, S. (2014). Health sector reforms and changes in prevalence of untreated morbidity, choice of health-care providers among the poor and rural population in India. *International Journal of Health Policy and Management, 2*(3), 125.

Gumber, A., Dhak, B., & Lalitha, N. (2012). Declining free health care and rising treatment costs in India: An analysis of national sample surveys 1986–2004. *Journal of Health Management, 14*(2), 97–116.

Haomiao, J., Santana, A., & Lubetkin, E. I. (2004). Measuring risk perception among low-income minority primary care patients. *The Journal of Ambulatory Care Management, 27*(4), 314–327.

Hwang, J. (2018). Understanding reasons for unmet health care needs in Korea: What are health policy implications? *BMC Health Services Research, 18*(1), 557.

Hwang, J., Guilcher, S. J., McIsaac, K. E., Matheson, F. I., Glazier, R., & O'Campo, P. (2017). An examination of perceived health care availability and unmet health care need in the city of Toronto, Ontario, Canada. *Canadian Journal of Public Health, 108*(1), 7–13.

Israel, S. (2016). How social policies can improve financial accessibility of healthcare: A multi-level analysis of unmet medical need in European countries. *International Journal for Equity in Health, 15*(1), 41.

Kanungo, S., Bhowmik, K., Mahapatra, T., Mahapatra, S., Bhadra, U. K., & Sarkar, K. (2015). Perceived morbidity, healthcare-seeking behaviour and their determinants in a poor-resource setting: Observation from India. *PLoS ONE, 10*(5), Article e0125865.

Kiwanuka, S. N., Ekirapa, E. K., Peterson, S., Okui, O., Rahman, M. H., Peters, D., & Pariyo, G. W. (2008). Access to and utilisation of health services for the poor in Uganda: A systematic review of available evidence. *Transactions of the Royal Society of Tropical Medicine and Hygiene, 102*(11), 1067–1074.

Kuuire, V. Z., Bisung, E., Rishworth, A., Dixon, J., & Luginaah, I. (2015). Health-seeking behaviour during times of illness: A study among adults in a resource poor setting in Ghana. *Journal of Public Health, 38*(4), 545–553.

Mahapatro, S. R., Singh, P., & Singh, Y. (2018). How effective health insurance schemes are in tackling economic burden of healthcare in India. *Clinical Epidemiology and Global Health, 6*(2), 75–82.

Mohammadbeigi, A., Hassanzadeh, J., Eshrati, B., & Rezaianzadeh, A. (2013). Decomposition of inequity determinants of healthcare utilization, Iran. *Public Health, 127*(7), 661–667.

Mondal, S., Lucas, H., Peters, D., & Kanjilal, B. (2014). Catastrophic out-of-pocket payment for healthcare and implications for household coping strategies: Evidence from West Bengal, India. *Economics Bulletin, 34*(2), 1303–1316.

Mukherjee, A. N., & Karmakar, K. (2008). Untreated morbidity and demand for healthcare in India: An analysis of national sample survey data. *Economic and Political Weekly, 2008*, 71–77.

Mukherjee, S., Haddad, S., & Narayana, D. (2011). Social class related inequalities in household health expenditure and economic burden: Evidence from Kerala, south India. *International Journal for Equity in Health, 10*(1), 1.

Nelson, C. H., & Park, J. (2006). The nature and correlates of unmet health care needs in Ontario, Canada. *Social Science and Medicine, 62*(9), 2291–2300.

Pandey, A., Ploubidis, G. B., Clarke, L., & Dandona, L. (2017). Horizontal inequity in outpatient care use and untreated morbidity: Evidence from nationwide surveys in India between 1995 and 2014. *Health Policy and Planning, 32*(7), 969–979.

Penchansky, R., & Thomas, J. W. (1981). The concept of access: Definition and relationship to consumer satisfaction. *Medical Care, 1981*, 127–140.

Petkova, V. B. (2008). Pharmaceutical care for asthma patients: A community pharmacy-based pilot project. *Allergy and Asthma Proceedings, 29*(1), 55.

Pitkin Derose, K., & Varda, D. M. (2009). Social capital and health care access: A systematic review. *Medical Care Research and Review, 66*(3), 272–306.

Prinja, S., Kanavos, P., & Kumar, R. (2012). Health care inequities in north India: Role of public sector in universalizing health care. *The Indian Journal of Medical Research, 136*(3), 421.

Roy, K., & Chaudhuri, A. (2008). Influence of socioeconomic status, wealth and financial empowerment on gender differences in health and healthcare utilization in later life: Evidence from India. *Social Science and Medicine, 66*(9), 1951–1962.

Scaria, S. (2017). Caste and gender in relation to health inequality: A village study from Kerala. *South Asia Research, 37*(1), 1–18.

Sibley, L. M., & Glazier, R. H. (2009). Reasons for self-reported unmet healthcare needs in Canada: A population-based provincial comparison. *Healthcare Policy, 5*(1), 87–101.

Tidikis, F., & Strasen, L. (1994). Patient-focused care units improve service and financial outcomes. *Healthcare Financial Management: Journal of the Healthcare Financial Management Association, 48*(9), 38–40.

van Doorslaer, E., & Masseria, C. (2004). *Income-related inequality in the use of medical care in 21 OECD countries.*

Waters, E. A., Hay, J. L., Orom, H., Kiviniemi, M. T., & Drake, B. F. (2013). "Don't know" responses to risk perception measures: Implications for underserved populations. *Medical Decision Making: An International Journal of the Society for Medical Decision Making, 33*(2), 271–281.

8 A Comprehensive Assessment of Nutritional Anemia Among Adolescent in India: An Evidence from CNNS (2016–2018)

Sampurna Kundu, Subhojit Shaw, Madhushree Banerjee, and Balram Paswan

Abstract

Nutritional anemia is a condition caused by iron deficiency that affects both boys and girls throughout the lifecycle. The present study evaluates nutritional anemia in association with various anthropometric, biochemical, dietary, and sociodemographic behaviors among the adolescents of India. The study utilizes the first-ever nationally representative Comprehensive National Nutrition Survey (CNNS) data (2016–2018). The statistical tools used include bivariate analysis and multivariate ordered logit model to achieve the study objectives. In India, micronutrient deficiencies have a significant association with anemia except for vitamin B12 deficiency. Iron deficit people are likely to have a significantly higher prevalence of anemia at all severity levels (Mild: 26%; Moderate: 33%; Severe: 5.2%). The proportional odds ratio is higher among stunted individuals, showing more likely to develop anemia than non-stunted individuals. Dietary diversity depicts the proportional odds ratio is significantly lesser for those intaking the food groups, dairy products, (AOR: 0.62; *p*-value: 0.000) and flesh foods like meat and fish (AOR: 0.68; *p*-value: 0.039). The study showed that a good diet in adolescent girls could protect against anemia in women in the reproductive age-group. Food diversification among high-risk populations should focus on context-specific and integrated nutrition intervention programs to reduce anemia among adolescents.

S. Kundu (✉)
Postdoctoral Research Fellow in Epidemiology, Faculty of Health and Life Sciences, University of Exeter, UK, Exeter, United Kingdom
e-mail: sampurna34@gmail.com

S. Shaw
Department of Development Studies, International Institute for Population Sciences, Deonar, Mumbai, India

M. Banerjee
Public Health Nutrition, The Maharaja Sayajirao University of Baroda, Vadodara, India

B. Paswan
International Institute for Population Sciences, Mumbai, India

8.1 Introduction

According to WHO, adolescence is the age period between 10 and 19 years for both sexes. It is the formative stage of life when the maximum physical, psychological, and behavioral changes occur (Verma et al., 2013). Increased nutritional needs at this phase of life relate to the fact that they gain up to 50% of adult weight, more than 20%

S. S. Acharya et al. (eds.), *Paradigm Shifts in Population and Health in India*, Sustainable Development Goals Series, https://doi.org/10.1007/978-981-95-1719-0_8

of adult height, and 50% of adult skeletal mass during this period (Gebreyohannes et al., 2014). Required micronutrients for adolescent growth and development are calcium, iodine, vitamin A, zinc and folic acid, and iron (Mittal et al., 2011). Among various micronutrients, iron needs are high in adolescent girls than adolescent boys due to the expansion of blood volume associated with the adolescent growth spurt and the onset of menstruation (Dallman, 1992; Kumar et al., 2018; Meier et al., 2003). Nutritional anemia in iron deficiency is the most widespread form of malnutrition among women and children and adolescents (Kotecha & Medicine, 2011). The adolescent stage is a window of opportunity in the life cycle to address malnutrition problems. During the adolescent growth spurt, the risk of nutritional anemia, specifically iron deficiency anemia, reappears for both boys and girls (Soliman et al., 2014). Inadequate dietary intake, defective iron absorption, increased iron requirements due to repeated pregnancies and lactation, insufficient iron reserves at birth, the timing of umbilical cord clamping, frequency of infections in children, and excessive physiological blood loss during adolescence and pregnancy are some of the causes responsible for the high prevalence of anemia in India.

Nutritional anemia can be an isolated condition caused by a nutritional deficiency (e.g., iron, folate, vitamin B12), or it may develop secondary to another disease or its treatment. Low serum ferritin among children and adolescents with normal C-reactive protein levels is considered as a biomarker for iron deficiency [Ministry of Health and Family Welfare (MoHFW), 2019]. Folic acid, B vitamin, is needed to form heme, the pigmented, iron-containing portion of the hemoglobin in red blood cells (erythrocytes). A deficient intake of folic acid impairs young red blood cells' maturation, which results in anemia (Chen et al., 2019). Zinc is a catalyst for many enzymes needed for red blood cell production; thus, anemia is associated with zinc deficiency (Badham et al., 2007). A hand full of the study suggests adjuvant zinc therapy's effects for improving anemia with significant improvement of hemoglobin levels within 3 weeks (Fukushima et al., 2009). Vitamin B12 and folate are necessary for forming healthy red blood cells, which repair body cells and tissues, and DNA synthesis. Both folic acid and Vitamin B12 are involved in the synthesis of nucleic acids and amino acids. Folate can lead to macrocytic (enlarged red blood cell) anemia. Vitamin B12 is found primarily in animal-origin foods, and risks for deficiency are therefore higher where access to these foods is limited (Simpson et al., 2010). There is ample research on iron deficiency anemia and its effect on adolescent girls, but there is a need to focus on adolescent boys at the same time [Chalise et al., 2018; Kumar et al., 2018; Ministry of Health and Family Welfare (MoHFW), 2019; Mittal et al., 2011]. Several factors associated with iron deficiency anemia (IDA), like dietary diversity, reflect the concept that increasing the variety of foods and food groups in the diet helps ensure adequate intake of essential nutrients and promotes good health to reduce IDA (Tolentino et al., 2007).

The prevalence of IDA is 6–8 times higher in countries where there is little dietary intake of meat. The majority is 70% in Southeast Asia and 44% in sub-Saharan Africa. In developing countries, the prevalence of IDA is 42% in women (Olumakaiye et al., 2010). India has the highest prevalence of iron deficiency anemia among women, including adolescents, worldwide (Rai et al., 2018). Low iron status may be caused by inadequate dietary intake, low absorption, parasitic infection, and medical conditions that cause internal bleeding (Anand et al., 2014; Olumakaiye et al., 2013). Maintaining iron status in the body, a balanced diet is essential for the healthy growth and development of children and adolescents [Ministry of Health and Family Welfare (MoHFW), 2019]. In India, a study suggests that inadequate intake of dietary iron, poor bioavailability, and inadequate concurrent intake of dietary micronutrients appear to be the primary factors responsible for the high prevalence of anemia and iron deficiency among young women (Thankachan et al., 2007). Another study suggested that young rural women had low serum ferritin and folate levels, possibly due to inadequate food and iron and folic acid intake (Pathak et al., 2004). Similarly, a study in Bangladesh on adolescent girls attending schools in 14 Dhaka city reveals that 31% of these girls consumed less than 50% RDA for iron and 10% less than 50% energy (Ahmed et al., 1998). It is estimated that nearly 300–400 million in India are vegetarian, ranging from abstinence of poultry products, meat, fish, roots, and tubers (Borude, 2019). Other than vegetarian and non-vegetarians, vegan, Lacto, or Lacto-Ovo vegetarian constitute (1.6%) in India (Agrawal et al., 2014). Previous studies in India are sporadic and are mostly based on cross-sectional case studies. In India, a program like (WIFS, National Iron Plus Initiative Program) *Anemia Mukt Bharat,* 2018 aims to reduce the prevalence of anemia among women in the reproductive age-group to achieve Global Nutrition Target-2 by 2025.

There has not been much work to examine the nutritional anemia attributable to micronutrient deficiency. There is a need to focus on their dietary pattern because they will soon enter the maternal phase. The present study aims at evaluating factors affecting nutritional anemia among adolescents in India. This is achieved through the characterization of the various anthropometric, biochemical, sociodemographic, and dietary behaviors. We hypothesized that exclusively vegetarian diets typically in the absence of fish, meats and poultry are less likely to be related to nutritional anemia than the non-vegetarian diet.

8.2 Materials and Methods

8.2.1 Data Source and Population

The present study has used Comprehensive National Nutrition Survey (CNNS) 2016–2018, the first-ever nationally representative nutrition survey of children and adolescents in India. This survey is based on multi-stage sampling covering both rural and urban households. The national representative sample survey includes children and adolescents (0–19) years across 30 states comprising 112,316 samples with anthropometric measures and 51,029 samples for blood, urine, and stool test.

The study sample for this specific study comprises 35,830 adolescents (10–19) years. The information collected includes (a) household characteristics-household member roster; and socio-economic status (b) environmental condition-access to and use of safe drinking water; access to and use of sanitation facilities; and hygiene practices, (c) health status-morbidity, (d) dietary intake-dietary diversity. Unlike other nationally representative surveys (NFHS, DHS, AHS, and NNMB), CNNS had collected information on direct and indirect nutrition assessment data on anthropometry, biochemical, and dietary.

8.2.2 Measures

8.2.2.1 Outcome Variable

The outcome variable, iron deficiency anemia level, has been marked by low hemoglobin (Hb) concentration in the blood samples. The phlebotomists collected the blood sample after taking the consent from the adolescents' parents/caregivers. In the present study, the 'anemia' variable has been categorized into 4-categories as being suggested by (WHO, 2015) when Hb is <12 'non-anemic'; Hb $\leq$ 11 and >12 'mild anemia'; Hb > 11 'moderate anemia'; and Hb < 8 as 'severe anemia'.

8.2.2.2 Explanatory Variables

The study has used direct nutrition assessment components, namely, anthropometry, biochemical, and dietary variables with various indirect sociodemographic covariates to assess anemia among the adolescents. The sociodemographic background variables include the age of the adolescent, gender, residence, religion, caste, mother's education, and wealth index; anthropometry variables include stunting, underweight and BMI; biochemical variables include iron deficiency, vitamin-D deficiency, zinc deficiency, vitamin-A deficiency, vitamin B-12 deficiency, folate deficiency, consumption of IFA tablets, consumption of deworming tablets; and finally the dietary variables has been classified as minimum dietary diversity—(a) grains, roots and tubers; (b) legumes and nuts; (c) dairy products (milk, yogurt, cheese); (d) flesh foods (meats, fish poultry, and liver/organ meats); (e) eggs; (f) vitamin-A rich fruits and vegetables and (g) other fruits and vegetables. The aforesaid covariates were controlled to estimate the effect (β coefficient) on adolescents' anemia.

The unit-level explanatory variables of CNNS data have been coded into sub-categories, where gender is coded as 1 'males' and 2 'females. Residence type is a dichotomous variable with the where 1 'rural' and 2 'urban' respectively. The religion variable has been coded as, 1 'Hindu', 2 'Muslim', and 3 'others'. In Indian society is distinguished by different social groups: 1 'Scheduled Caste' (SC); 2 'Scheduled Tribe' (ST); 3 'other backward class (OBC); 4 'others', where the SC/ST population are the most deprived class of people. Mother's level of education has been classified into six categories: 0 'no schooling'; 1 '<5 Completed Years'; 2 '5–7 Completed Years'; 3 '8–9 Completed Years'; 4 '10–11 Completed Years'; and 5 '≥12 Completed Years'. While measuring the economic status, wealth index variable with the quintile categories as: 1 'poorest'; 2 'poor'; 3 'middle'; 4 'rich'; and 5 'richest' has been used from the dataset.

The anthropometric measurement of adolescent children whose height-for-age *Z*-score is below minus two standard deviations (−2 SD) and whose weight-for-age *Z*-score is below minus two standard deviations (−2 SD) from the median of the reference population are classified as stunting and underweight. Similarly, using the WHO Child Growth Standards BMI-for-age below minus two standard deviations (−2 SD) has been marked as low BMI for the adolescents. All the aforesaid anthropometric variables have been coded as dichotomous measures.

The biochemical measures like deficiency of iron have been marked by serum ferritin <15 μg/l; vitamin-D deficiency as serum 25(OH)D concentration < 12 ng/mL (30 nmol/L); zinc deficiency as serum zinc concentration < 65 μg/dl; Vitamin-A deficiency as serum retinol concentration < 20 μg/dL; Vitamin B-12 serum vitamin B12 < 203 μg/ml; and folate deficiency as serum erythrocyte folate < 151 ng/ml. In addition, various food items have been grouped into seven broad categories following minimum dietary diversity (WHO, 2015). Furthermore, the consumption of deworming tablets, micronutrient deficiencies, and dietary variables was made dichotomous for the analysis.

8.2.3 Statistical Analysis

To examine the association between adolescent' anemia and different explanatory variables, bivariate analysis with an array of χ^2 has been used. In the present study, the outcome variable category is in the form of an ordinal scale-non-anemia, mild anemia, moderate anemia, and severe anemia. We have used multivariate ordered logistic regression model to examine the effect of anthropometric, biochemical, dietary, and other sociodemographic variables on anemia. Additionally, using the adjusted prevalence, we have estimated the projected number of adolescents' anemia (Table S1). Let Y be the ordinal outcome variable, in this case it is the anemia levels, and p_1, p_2, p_3 and p_4 be the proportions in each level, such as, 'non-anemic', 'mild', 'moderate' and 'severe', respectively. The logarithm of odds are as follows:

$$\text{Non-anemic, } \log\left(\frac{p_1}{p_2 + p_3 + p_4}\right), \tag{8.1}$$

$$\text{Non-anemic or Mild, } \log\left(\frac{p_1 + p_2}{p_3 + p_4}\right), \tag{8.2}$$

$$\text{Non-anemic or Mild or Moderate, } \log\left(\frac{p_1 + p_2 + p_3}{p_4}\right), \tag{8.3}$$

The assumption of proportional odds, which means that all the independent variables have an identical effect at each category of the outcome variable, has been tested using the likelihood ratio test of proportionality. Test for the existence of multicollinearity was done with the help of variance inflation factor (VIF).

Suppose Y^* is the unobserved dependent variable

$$Y^* = x^T \beta + \varepsilon$$

where x is the vector of predictor variables, β is the vector of regression coefficients, and ε is the error term. Since, Y^* is unobserved, we observe the categories of responses

$$Y = \begin{cases} 0 \text{ if } & Y^* \leq \mu_1 \\ 1 \text{ if } & \mu_1 < Y^* \leq \mu_2 \\ 2 \text{ if } & \mu_2 < Y^* \leq \mu_3 \\ 3 \text{ if } & \mu_3 < Y^* \end{cases}$$

where μ_i's are externally imposed endpoints of the observable categories of the outcome variable. Then the ordered logistic regression model uses the observations on Y, which are a form of censored data on Y^*, to fit the parameter vector β.

8.3 Results

8.3.1 Prevalence of Anemia

The spatial variation in anemia among adolescents can be seen across India. The distribution of anemia among adolescents has been sporadic (Fig. 8.1).

Overall, in India across the age-group of 10–19 years, the prevalence of anemia is 28.34%, and is maximum in the state West Bengal (44.01%), followed by Tripura (38.73%) and Assam (37.98%). Across different regions, Telangana in the Southern-region has the highest severe anemic condition (3.01%), while the lowest can be found in Tripura (0.27%) in the Northeastern region. Moderate and mild anemia was highest in the eastern region of West Bengal (17.43%) and (26.29%) respectively (Fig. 8.1). The lowest moderate anemia can be found in Manipur (2.3%) in the Northeastern region, and Kerala in Southern India has the lowest mils anemia (5.17%). On the contrary, Kerala, Manipur, and Nagaland have least anemic adolescents.

From the bivariate results, as shown in Table 8.1, it can be observed that with increasing age, there is a significant decrease in the prevalence of mild level of anemia, with the maximum being in the age 10 (25%). In contrast, for moderate anemia, the highest is in the age 17 (14%) and severe in age 18 (2%). Gender wise it can be found that females have a significantly higher prevalence of anemia at all severity levels (Females: Mild 25%, Moderate 16.3%, Severe 1.5%). Religion is also shown to have a significant association with anemia, with maximum mild anemia being among Muslims (21%), moderate (11%) and severe (2%) anemia being among other religions. The caste factor depicts a significant role to play with the maximum prevalence of anemia at all levels of severity among the scheduled tribes (Mild: 21%; Moderate: 15%; Severe: 1.5%). The wealth index shows that the prevalence of anemia is significantly more among the poor wealth quintile.

Among indicators measuring malnutrition, stunting is significantly associated with anemia, and at all levels, if anemia, the prevalence is higher among stunted youths (Mild: 20%; Moderate: 11.5%; Severe: 1.6%). Micronutrient deficiencies have quite a significant association with anemia except for vitamin B12 deficiency. Iron deficit people are observed to have a significantly higher prevalence of anemia at all severity levels (Mild: 26%; Moderate: 33%; Severe: 5.2%). Similarly, prevalence of anemia at all severity levels is higher among youths with vitamin D deficiency (Mild: 21%; Moderate: 11%; Severe: 0.8%), vitamin A deficiency (Mild: 23%; Moderate: 11%; Severe: 1.6%), folate deficiency (Mild: 14%; Moderate: 8%; Severe: 0.5%). Prevalence of anemia is significantly higher among youths who do not consume deworming tablets (Mild: 17%; Moderate: 10%; Severe: 1.3%). Dietary behavior plays a significant role in the prevalence of anemia among youths. The consumption of the following food groups-grains, roots and tubers; legumes and nuts; milk products; fish and meat; and eggs, have shown significant association with prevalence of anemia, that is, the prevalence, as well as the severity, is less among those who consume these food groups.

8.3.2 Regression Analysis

Table 8.2 shows the multivariate ordered logistic regression model depicting the effects of biochemical and sociodemographic factors on anemia

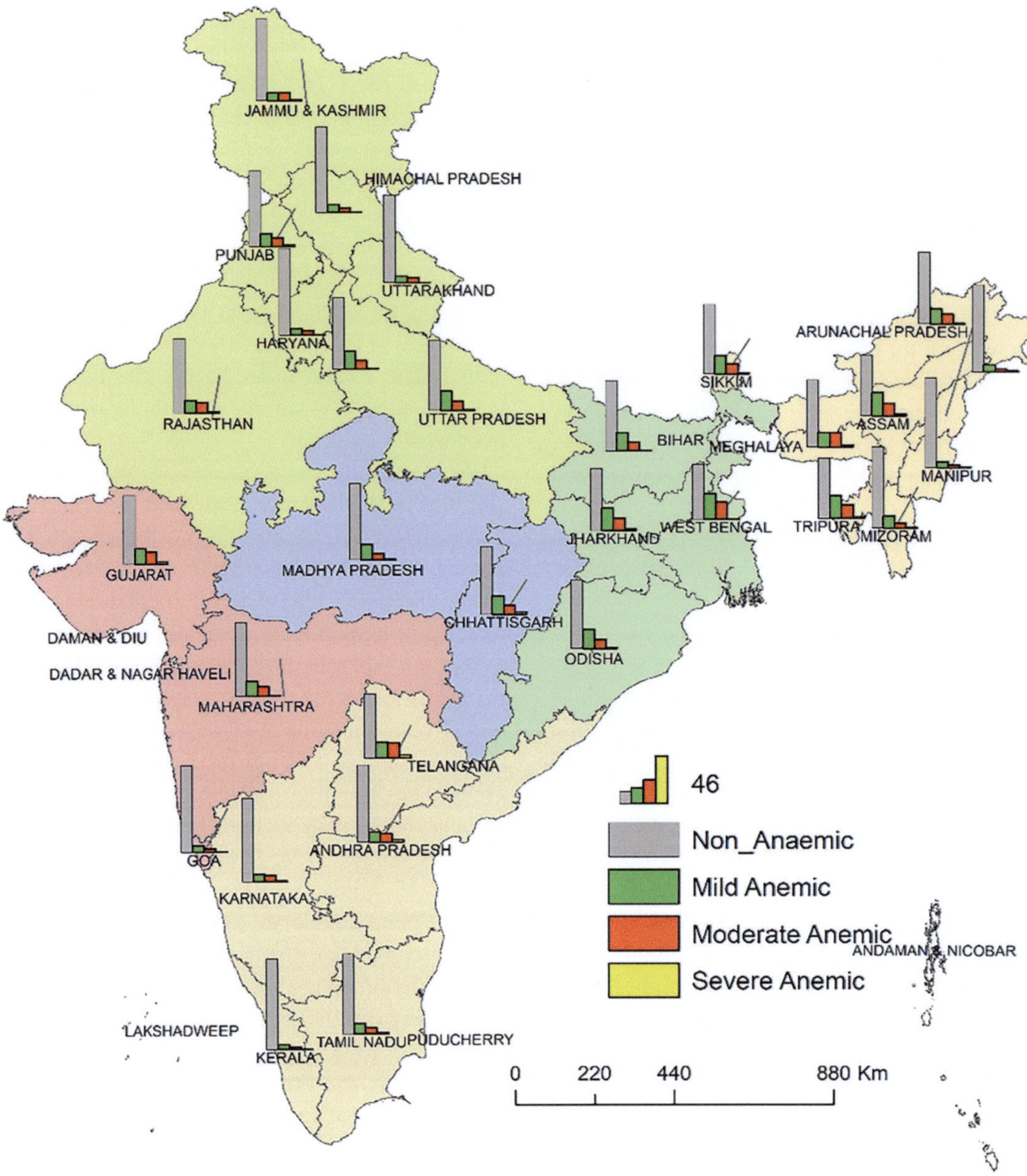

Fig. 8.1 Spatial distribution of non-anemia; mild anemia; moderate anemia; and severe anemia across India's different states

levels among adolescents aged 10–19. The findings show the covariates' proportional odds ratio is significant across the ordered outcome variable of anemia. With the respondents' increasing age, the chances of developing anemia decrease and change proportionally across the levels of the outcome variable (AOR: 0.94; *p*-value: 0.000). The results show that females are more likely to develop anemia across the severity levels of anemia than men (AOR: 3.34; *p*-value: 0.000). Education was found to have no significant impact on the regression model. The proportional odds ratio is observed to decrease with the increasing wealth quintiles significantly compared to the poorest quintile.

Table 8.1 Anthropometric, biochemical, dietary behavior and socio-demographic characteristics-wise prevalence of elevated anemia among adolescents age (10–19) years (India, 2016–18)

	Non-anaemic	Mild	Moderate	Severe	χ^2 (*p*-value)
Age of the respondent					
10	66.51	24.76	8.43	0.3	0.000
11	70.1	19.64	9.85	0.41	
12	72.41	19.76	6.98	0.84	
13	70.6	19.19	9.87	0.33	
14	72.52	15.94	10.14	1.4	
15	70.61	17.38	11.08	0.93	
16	70.8	16.32	11.69	1.19	
17	72.71	12.19	13.96	1.14	
18	75.63	10.97	11.52	1.88	
19	77.78	12.74	8.69	0.79	
Gender					
Male	85.7	9.8	4.16	0.35	0.000
Female	57.29	24.89	16.32	1.49	
Religion					
Hindu	72.13	16.85	10.13	0.89	0.000
Muslim	68.6	20.72	9.93	0.75	
Others	74.13	13.36	10.75	1.75	
Caste					
SC	68.71	18.49	11.55	1.25	0.000
ST	63.28	20.59	14.64	1.49	
OBC	75.47	14.85	9.03	0.65	
Others	72.26	18.32	8.64	0.78	
Mothers' education					
No schooling	75.7	18.2	4.82	1.29	0.000
<5 completed years	71.73	18.72	8.11	1.44	
5–7 completed years	72.66	17.69	8.91	0.73	
8–9 completed years	75.33	15.34	8.86	0.47	
10–11 completed years	79.26	13.74	6.06	0.94	
≥12 completed years	75.39	16.66	7.43	0.52	
Wealth index					
Poorest	65.4	21.71	12.06	0.83	0.000
Poor	70.68	18.05	10.23	1.04	
Middle	71.62	17.03	10.27	1.08	
Rich	73.49	15.59	10.31	0.61	
Richest	77.39	13.85	7.76	1	
Stunting					
No	72.98	16.59	9.74	0.69	0.000
Yes	66.86	20.03	11.48	1.62	
Underweight					
No	59.08	31.95	8.72	0.25	0.669
Yes	58.2	20.11	21.69	0	
BMI					

(continued)

Table 8.1 (continued)

	Non-anaemic	Mild	Moderate	Severe	χ^2 (*p*-value)
No	70.72	17.81	10.45	1.02	0.146
Yes	73.36	16.46	9.57	0.62	
Iron deficiency					
No	77.2	16.59	6.09	0.12	0.000
Yes	36.33	25.76	32.71	5.2	
Vitamin-D deficiency					
No	72.3	16.89	9.82	0.99	0.011
Yes	66.54	21.43	11.24	0.79	
Zinc deficiency					
No	72.26	17.5	9.6	0.63	0.000
Yes	64.49	19.19	13.79	2.53	
Vitamin-A deficiency					
No	71.75	17.32	10.2	0.72	0.000
Yes	64.21	23.4	10.79	1.6	
Vitamin-B12 deficiency					
No	69.13	19.2	10.79	0.88	0.059
Yes	73.84	16.48	8.34	1.35	
Folate deficiency					
No	68.11	19.29	11.39	1.21	0.000
Yes	77.54	14	7.95	0.52	
Consumption of IFA tablets					
No	72.38	16.73	9.95	0.93	0.053
Yes	66.14	21.39	11.73	0.75	
Consumption of deworming tablets					
No	71.37	17.26	10.41	0.96	0.001
Yes	72.74	17.07	9.41	0.78	
Grains, roots and tubers					
No	73.61	14.56	10.49	1.35	0.044
Yes	71.47	17.61	10.08	0.85	
Legumes and nuts					
No	72.22	16.63	10.17	0.98	0.006
Yes	70.43	18.83	10.03	0.71	
Dairy products					
No	70.08	18.64	10.32	0.96	0.000
Yes	73.72	15.52	9.91	0.86	
Flesh foods					
No	71.5	17.23	10.33	0.94	0.000
Yes	80.76	16.39	2.85	0	
Eggs					
No	71.53	17.32	10.23	0.92	0.000
Yes	79.56	13.06	6.67	0.71	
Vitamin A rich fruits and vegetables					
No	69.38	11.47	17.67	1.48	0.830

(continued)

Table 8.1 (continued)

	Non-anaemic	Mild	Moderate	Severe	χ^2 (*p*-value)
Yes	71.79	17.3	10	0.9	
Other fruits and vegetables					
No	70.18	13.22	15.6	1.01	0.637
Yes	71.78	17.27	10.04	0.91	

The proportional odds ratio is higher among stunted individuals, thus showing them to be more likely to develop anemia than non-stunted individuals (AOR: 1.60; *p*-value: 0.000). Among the various micronutrient deficiencies, iron deficit (AOR: 7.25; *p*-value: 0.000), zinc deficit (AOR: 1.31; *p*-value: 0.000), vitamin A deficit (AOR: 1.50; *p*-value: 0.000) individuals, has more chances of developing anemia, whereas, vitamin D deficit (AOR: 0.85; *p*-value: 0.037) and folate deficit (AOR: 0.73; *p*-value: 0.000) individuals has lesser chances. The dietary diversity covariates depict that the proportional odds ratio is significantly lesser for those intaking the food groups, dairy products (AOR: 0.62; *p*-value: 0.000) and flesh foods like meat and fish (AOR: 0.68; *p*-value: 0.039).

8.4 Discussion

The present study has shown the significant sociodemographic, biochemical, anthropometric, and dietary factors affecting anemia among youths in the age-group of 10–19. The age shows a significant decrease in the prevalence of mild-level of anemia, with the maximum being at the age 10, whereas for moderate anemia, the highest is 17 and severe at age 18. A similar study in Nepal has shown the prevalence of anemia was exceptionally high among 15–19-year-olds and female adolescents compared to young (10–14 years) and male adolescents (Chalise et al., 2018). Gender wise it can be found that females have a significantly higher prevalence of anemia at all severity. Another study revealed that anemia was more prevalent in girls who were more than 14 years of age compared to girls who were less than 14 years of age (Rati et al., 2014). Religion has also shown a significant association with anemia. Interestingly, respite of predominantly non-vegetarian diet Muslim adolescents have higher anemia level than others. A study revealed that tea drinking is a popular custom across Muslim countries, including Saudi Arabia. It is usually consumed both before and after all meals; tea is a beverage that harmfully affects an individual's iron levels due to its high polyphenol content, which inhibits nonheme iron absorption; thus, Muslim population could have a high level of prevalence of anemia (Alzaheb & Al-Amer, 2017). The caste factor depicts a significant role to play with the maximum prevalence of anemia at all levels of severity among the scheduled tribes. Being socially deprived class, the ST adolescent population might have the inaccessibility of sufficient nutritional food. A study revealed that 89.1% of scheduled tribes were affected by anemia. The wealth index shows that the prevalence of anemia is significantly more among the poor indices.

Among indicators measuring malnutrition, stunting is significantly associated with anemia, and at all levels of anemia, the prevalence is higher among stunted youths. A study in Bangladesh identified that malnutrition (BMI-for-age *Z*-score $\leftarrow$ 2SD) is a significant risk factor of anemia among adolescent girls. Studies conducted in similar settings also found that lower BMI is associated with a higher rate of anemia among adolescent girls (Mistry et al., 2017). However, contradictory to this, BMI had not significantly been associated with anemia among adolescent girls from rural India (Schulze et al., 2019). Micronutrient deficiencies have quite a significant association with anemia except for vitamin B12 deficiency. Iron deficit people are likely to have a significantly higher prevalence of anemia at all severity levels (Wirth et al., 2018). A study

Table 8.2 Multivariable ordered logistic regression model output showing the anthropometric, biochemical, dietary behavior, and socio-demographic characteristics on anemia among adolescents age (10–19) years (India, 2016–18)

	AOR	SE	*p*-value
Age of the respondent	0.940	0.014	0.00
Gender			
Male	1.000		
Female	3.342	14.97	0.00
Religion			
Hindu	1.000		
Muslim	1.154	0.144	0.25
Others	0.617	0.077	0.00
Caste			
SC	1.000		
ST	1.192	0.164	0.201
OBC	0.721	0.078	0.002
Others	0.896	0.096	0.305
Mothers' education			
No schooling	1.000		
<5 completed years	1.331	0.379	0.315
5–7 completed years	1.309	0.364	0.333
8–9 completed years	1.332	0.370	0.303
10–11 completed years	0.891	0.255	0.686
≥12 completed years	0.967	0.278	0.906
Wealth index			
Poorest	1.000		
Poor	0.745	0.177	0.215
Middle	0.559	0.126	0.01
Rich	0.493	0.109	0.001
Richest	0.439	0.099	0.00
Stunting			
No	1.000		
Yes	1.596	0.140	0.000
Iron deficiency			
No	1.000		
Yes	7.252	0.631	0.000
Vitamin-D deficiency			
No	1.000		
Yes	0.845	0.068	0.037
Zinc deficiency			
No	1.000		
Yes	1.315	0.113	0.001
Vitamin-A deficiency			
No	1.000		
Yes	1.500	0.154	0.00
Folate deficiency			
No	1.000		
Yes	0.726	0.058	0.00
Consumption of deworming tablets			
No	1.000		
Yes	0.761	0.058	0.00
Grains, roots and tubers			
No	1.000		
Yes	0.965	0.096	0.719
Legumes and nuts			
No	1.000		
Yes	1.187	0.096	0.039
Dairy products			
No	1.000		
Yes	0.777	0.061	0.001
Flesh foods			
No	1.000		
Yes	0.676	0.128	0.039
Eggs			
No	1.000		
Yes	0.957	0.176	0.811
Vitamin A rich fruits and vegetables			
No	1.000		
Yes	0.831	0.188	0.415
Other fruits and vegetables			
No	1.000		
Yes	0.961	0.246	0.877
Cut 1	0.298	0.506	
Cut 2	1.779	0.508	
Cut 3	4.263	0.526	

suggested that the low DDS reflected low iron consumption from dietary sources; thus, the low availability of dietary iron and high iron requirements is closely linked to depleted iron status (Olumakaiye et al., 2010, 2013).

Similarly, the prevalence of anemia at all severity levels is higher among youths with zinc deficiency, vitamin D deficiency, vitamin A deficiency, folate deficiency. A study revealed a significant positive association between serum 25(OH)D concentrations and serum iron among African Americans in a US Cohort study (Smith et al., 2015). The high prevalence of mild and moderate anemia demands due emphasis to bring down the total prevalence of adolescent girls' anemia. In serving soldiers prevalence of macrocytic anemia was more as compared to microcytic (Iron deficiency) anemia (62.5 vs. 27.5) (Kumar et al., 2018). A deficient intake of folic acid impairs young red blood cells' maturation, which results in anemia (Chen et al., 2019). The prevalence of anemia is found to be significantly higher among youths who do not consume deworming tablets. Dietary behavior plays a significant role in the prevalence of anemia among youths.

The consumption of the following food groups-grains, roots and tubers; legumes and nuts; milk products; fish and meat; and eggs, have shown significant association with prevalence of anemia, that is, the prevalence, as well as the severity, is less among those who consume these food groups. Low dietary iron and high iron requirements are closely linked to depleted iron status (Beard & Tobin, 2000). A study suggested that In India, the prevalence of anemia is high because of low dietary intake, low iron (less than 20 mg/day) and folic acid intake (less than 70 μg/day); poor bioavailability of iron (3–4% only) in phytate fiber-rich Indian diet; and chronic blood loss due to infection such as malaria and hookworm infestations. Dietary diversity is the number of foods consumed across and within food groups over a reference period. It is widely recognized as being an essential dimension of diet quality. It reflects the concept that increasing the variety of foods and food groups in the diet helps ensure adequate intake of essential nutrients and promotes good health (Institute of Medicine Standing Committee on the Scientific Evaluation of Dietary Reference Intakes %J Dietary Reference Intakes for Calcium & Fluoride, 1997). Iron deficiency develops gradually and usually begins with negative balance when iron intake does not meet dietary iron's daily needs. This negative balance initially depletes the storage form of iron while the blood hemoglobin level, a marker of iron status, remains normal. Iron-deficiency anemia is an advanced stage of iron depletion (Beard & Tobin, 2000). The low dietary intake of iron and folic acid coupled with poor bioavailability of iron is the primary factor responsible for the very high prevalence of anemia (Kaur, 2014). This is evident from data for India—the prevalence of anemia is higher in Indian adolescents consuming a vegetarian diet (45.8%) as compared to those consuming a mixed diet, which includes animal food (30%) (WHO, 2011).

8.5 Conclusion

In developing countries, anemia is still a major public health concern, particularly among women of reproductive age, especially adolescent girls. The study showed that a good diet in adolescent boys and girls could protect against anemia in women in the reproductive age-group. In India, adolescents belong from 15 to 19 years have the highest prevalence of nutritional anemia. Food diversification among high-risk populations should focus on context-specific and integrated nutrition intervention programs, including nutrition education, mass supplementation with iron and folic acid tablets, treatment of hookworm, and sanitation programs that could reduce the prevalence of IDA among adolescent girls.

Acknowledgements I would like to thank the Population Council of India for providing the CNNS survey data that was used.

References

Agrawal, S., Millett, C. J., Dhillon, P. K., Subramanian, S., & Ebrahim, S. J. N. J. (2014). Type of vegetarian diet, obesity and diabetes in adult Indian population. *Nutrition Journal, 13*(1), 1–18.

Ahmed, F., Zareen, M., Khan, M. R., Banu, C. P., Haq, M. N., & Jackson, A. A. J. P. H. N. (1998). Dietary pattern, nutrient intake and growth of adolescent school girls in urban Bangladesh. *Public Health Nutrition, 1*(2), 83–92.

Alzaheb, R. A., & Al-Amer, O. J. C. M. I. W. S. H. (2017). The prevalence of iron deficiency anemia and its associated risk factors among a sample of female university students in Tabuk, Saudi Arabia. *Clinical Medicine Insights: Women's Health, 10*, 1179562X17745088.

Anand, T., Rahi, M., Sharma, P., & Ingle, G. K. J. N. (2014). Issues in prevention of iron deficiency anemia in India. *Nutrition, 30*(7–8), 764–770.

Badham, J., Zimmermann, M. B., & Kraemer, K. (2007). The guidebook nutritional anemia: Task force sight and life. *The Guidebook Nutritional Anemia, 2007*, 1.

Beard, J., & Tobin, B. J. T. A. J. O. C. N. (2000). Iron status and exercise. *The American Journal of Clinical Nutrition, 72*(2), 594S-597S.

Borude, S. J. O. S. (2019). Which is a good diet—Veg or non-veg? Faith-based vegetarianism for protection from obesity—A myth or actuality? *Obesity Surgery, 29*(4), 1276–1280.

Chalise, B., Aryal, K. K., Mehta, R. K., Dhimal, M., Sapkota, F., Mehata, S., & Sawyer, S. J. P. O. (2018). Prevalence and correlates of anemia among adolescents in Nepal: Findings from a nationally representative cross-sectional survey. *PLoS ONE, 13*(12), e0208878.

Chen, M.-Y., Rose, C. E., Qi, Y. P., Williams, J. L., Yeung, L. F., Berry, R. J., & Crider, K. S. J. T. A. J. O. C. N. (2019). Defining the plasma folate concentration associated with the red blood cell folate concentration threshold for optimal neural tube defects prevention: A population-based, randomized trial of folic acid supplementation. *The American Journal of Clinical Nutrition, 109*(5), 1452–1461.

Dallman, P. (1992). Changing iron needs from birth through adolescence. In *Paper presented at the nestle nutrition workshop series (USA)*.

Fukushima, T., Horike, H., Fujiki, S., Kitada, S., Sasaki, T., Kashihara, N. J. T. A., & Dialysis. (2009). Zinc deficiency anemia and effects of zinc therapy in maintenance hemodialysis patients. *Therapeutic Apheresis and Dialysis, 13*(3), 213–219.

Gebreyohannes, Y., Shiferaw, S., Demtsu, B., & Bugssa, G. J. A. (2014). Nutritional status of adolescents in selected government and private secondary schools of Addis Ababa, Ethiopia. *Adolescence, 10*(11), 11.

Institute of Medicine Standing Committee on the Scientific Evaluation of Dietary Reference Intakes %J Dietary Reference Intakes for Calcium, P., Magnesium, Vitamin D,, & Fluoride. (1997). *Dietary reference intakes*.

Kaur, K. J. E. J. O. Z. R. (2014). Anaemia 'a silent killer'among women in India: Present scenario. *European Journal of Zoological Research, 3*(1), 32–36.

Kotecha, P. V. J. I. J. O. C. M. O. P. O. I. A. O. P., & Medicine, S. (2011). Nutritional anemia in young children with focus on Asia and India. *Indian Journal of Community Medicine, 36*(1), 8.

Kumar, A., Goyal, A., Verma, N., & Mahesh, A. J. I. J. O. A. I. M. (2018). Study of anemia among adolescent school girls and young adults. *International Journal of Advances in Medicine, 5*(4), 877–881.

Meier, P. R., Nickerson, H. J., Olson, K. A., Berg, R. L., Meyer, J. A. J. C. M., & Research. (2003). Prevention of iron deficiency anemia in adolescent and adult pregnancies. *Clinical Medicine and Research, 1*(1), 29–36.

Ministry of Health and Family Welfare (MoHFW), G. O. I., UNICEF and Population Council. (2019). *Comprehensive national nutrition survey (CNNS). National report*. Retrieved from New Delhi.

Mistry, S. K., Jhohura, F. T., Khanam, F., Akter, F., Khan, S., Yunus, F. M., & Rahman, M. J. B. H. (2017). An outline of anemia among adolescent girls in Bangladesh: Findings from a cross-sectional study. *BMC Hematology, 17*(1), 1–8.

Mittal, M., Abhay, R., Yadunath, M., & Vilasrao, J. J. I. J. P. P. S. (2011). An intervention on iron deficiency anemia and change in dietary behavior among adolescent girls. *International Journal of Pharmacy., 3*(1), 40–42.

Olumakaiye, M. F., %J ICAN: Infant, C., & Nutrition, A. (2013). Adolescent girls with low dietary diversity score are predisposed to iron deficiency in southwestern Nigeria. *ICAN: Infant, Child, and Adolescent Nutrition 5*(2), 85–91.

Olumakaiye, M., Atinmo, T., Olubayo-Fatiregun, M. J. J. O. N. E., & Behavior. (2010). Food consumption patterns of Nigerian adolescents and effect on body weight. *Journal of Nutrition Education and Behavior, 42*(3), 144–151.

Pathak, P., Saxena, R., Kapoor, S. K., Dwivedi, S. N., Singh, R., & Kapil, U. J. N. M. C. J. N. (2004). Status of serum ferritin and folate levels amongst young women in a rural community of Haryana. *India. Nepal Medical College Journal: NMCJ, 6*(1), 13–16.

Rai, R. K., Fawzi, W. W., Barik, A., & Chowdhury, A.J.W.S.-E.A.J.O.P.H. (2018). The burden of iron-deficiency anaemia among women in India: How have iron and folic acid interventions fared? *WHO South-East Asia Journal of Public Health, 7*(1), 18–23.

Rati, S. A., Jawadagi, S. J. I. J. O. S., & Researh, D. (2014). Prevalence of anemia among adolescent girls studying in selected schools. *International Journal of Scientific Research, 3*(8), 1237–1242.

Schulze, K. J., Mehra, S., Shaikh, S., Ali, H., Shamim, A. A., Wu, L. S., & Sungpuag, P. J. T. J. O. N. (2019). Antenatal multiple micronutrient supplementation compared to iron–folic acid affects micronutrient status but does not eliminate deficiencies in a randomized controlled trial among pregnant women of rural Bangladesh. *The Journal of Nutrition, 149*(7), 1260–1270.

Simpson, J. L., Bailey, L. B., Pietrzik, K., Shane, B., Holzgreve, W.J.T.J.O.M.-F., & Medicine, N. (2010). Micronutrients and women of reproductive potential: required dietary intake and consequences of dietary deficiency or excess. Part I–folate, vitamin B12, vitamin B6. *The Journal of Maternal-Fetal and Neonatal Medicine, 23*(12), 1323–1343.

Smith, E. M., Alvarez, J. A., Martin, G. S., Zughaier, S. M., Ziegler, T. R., & Tangpricha, V. J. B. J. O. N. (2015). Vitamin D deficiency is associated with anaemia among African Americans in a US cohort. *British Journal of Nutrition, 113*(11), 1732–1740.

Soliman, A., De Sanctis, V., Elalaily, R. J. I. J. O. E., & Metabolism. (2014). Nutrition and pubertal development. *Indian Journal of Endocrinology and Metabolism, 18*(Suppl 1), S39.

Thankachan, P., Muthayya, S., Walczyk, T., Kurpad, A. V., Hurrell, R. F. J. F., & Bulletin, N. (2007). An analysis of the etiology of anemia and iron deficiency in young women of low socioeconomic status in Bangalore, India. *Food and Nutrition Bulletin, 28*(3), 328–336.

Tolentino, K., Friedman, J. F. J. T. A. J. O. T. M., & Hygiene. (2007). An update on anemia in less developed countries. *The American Journal of Tropical Medicine and Hygiene, 77*(1), 44–51.

Verma, R., Kharb, M., & Yadav, S. J. I. J. S. S. I. R. (2013). Prevalence of anemia among adolescents under IBSY in rural block of a district of northern India. *International Journal of Social Sciences and Interdisciplinary Research, 2*(9), 95–106.

WHO. (2011).*Prevention of iron deficiency anaemia in adolescents*. Retrieved from

WHO. (2015).*The global prevalence of anaemia in 2011.*

Wirth, J. P., Rajabov, T., Petry, N., Woodruff, B. A., Shafique, N. B., Mustafa, R., & Rohner, F. J. N. (2018). Micronutrient deficiencies, over-and undernutrition, and their contribution to anemia in Azerbaijani preschool children and non-pregnant women of reproductive age. *Nutrients, 10*(10), 1483.

9 Hysterectomy Practices and Its Associated Factors While Assessing the Rural–Urban Differences

Manali Swargiary, Chandrima Paul, and Sampurna Kundu

Abstract

Hysterectomy is considered one of the most common non-pregnancy-related major surgery performed on women. Studies on hysterectomy in developing countries are limited with many restrictions contributing to it. The developed countries report high prevalence in comparison to the developing countries like India reporting low prevalence. The primary aim of the paper is to examine the national and state-level prevalence of hysterectomy among women aged 40 and above and understand the association of socio-demographic factors, lifestyle habits, and pregnancy history over the individuals undergoing hysterectomy. The Longitudinal Ageing Study in India Wave-1 (2020), a nationally representative survey was used for the study. It is a cross-sectional, national survey of scientific investigation of the health, economics and social determinants of population ageing in India. The survey covered 72,250 older adults, whereas, for the study, females with age 40 or above were considered; thus, we have a sample size of 39,309. Bivariate and multivariate analysis were carried out to achieve the study objectives. Women in the age group 40–50 have mostly undergone hysterectomy (12.7%), which also shows a decreasing prevalence with increasing age. Medical conditions like excessive bleeding (33.6%) be the leading cause of the undergone cases. The odds show that women residing in the urban area are 1.23 times and who belongs to the richest households are 2.16 times more likely to undergo hysterectomy than the rural area and poorer women. The main contributor to the rural–urban differential is the number of pregnancies, wealth, social-group, and lifestyle factors. Undergoing hysterectomy is not mandatory for all cases; unless it is extremely life-threatening which need to made aware of along with other gynaecological morbidities. Measures are needed to ensure suitable and treatment options availed among the respective age groups which are accessible, affordable, and of better quality.

M. Swargiary · C. Paul (✉)
International Institute for Population Sciences, Mumbai, India
e-mail: cpaul250996@gmail.com

S. Kundu
Postdoctoral Research Fellow in Epidemiology, Faculty of Health and Life Sciences, University of Exeter, UK, Exeter, United Kingdom

9.1 Introduction

A hysterectomy is a surgical procedure to remove a woman's uterus. It is the most common non-pregnancy-related major surgery performed on women. This procedure of surgery can be used

S. S. Acharya et al. (eds.), *Paradigm Shifts in Population and Health in India*, Sustainable Development Goals Series, https://doi.org/10.1007/978-981-95-1719-0_9

as a diagnosis for several chronic pain conditions as well as certain types of cancer and infections. After the caesarean section, hysterectomy is the second most frequent surgical procedure for women. This surgical procedure involves removing the uterus and cervix, and in some cases, the fallopian tubes and ovaries. The symptoms leading to the diagnosis of hysterectomy are chronic pelvic pain, continuous vaginal bleeding, uterine cancer, fibroids, pelvic inflammatory disease, uterine prolapse and endometriosis. It is unlikely for women aged 18–35 years to go through hysterectomy unless it is necessary for their well-being.

According to a study conducted on 17,032 women in the UK, 11.1% of them had undergone the process of hysterectomy. Among them, social class plays a moderate degree of influence on hysterectomy rates. Using the lifetable method, it is calculated that 20% of these women have had a hysterectomy by the age of 55 (Vessey et al., 1992). Hysterectomy Surveillance by Centres for Disease Control and Prevention (CDC), 1994–1999, in the US, women aged 40–44 years had a significantly higher hysterectomy rate than any other age group, followed by 45–54 years women. Subsequently, in the 2002–2010 decade, the number of inpatient hysterectomies performed in the United States has declined substantially, with nearly one-fourth of a million fewer procedures in 2010 than in 2002 (Wright et al., 2013). The prevalence of hysterectomy is relatively high in developed countries like the USA, the UK compare to the developing countries. Around the world, the observed rates of hysterectomy ranged from as high as 5.4% in the USA to intermediate rates of 3.4% in Italy to a low of 1.2% in Norway (Domingo & Pellicer, 2009). Fibroids, prolapse, and endometriosis are the dominant causes behind the procedures. The study points out that hysterectomy is a surgical procedure that one in every three women in the United States endures, which makes it one of the most important health issues by its sheer magnitude (Pokras & Hufnagel, 1988). According to the NFHS-4 report [International Institute for Population Sciences (IIPS) and ICF, 2017], 3.2% of hysterectomy cases were recorded in India. States like Andhra Pradesh, Telangana, Bihar, and Gujarat showed high contribution among 15–44 years women. Evidence on the association of hysterectomy with age, less education, and rural residence are consistent with previous community-based research in India (Desai et al., 2019). The dominant reasons behind women undergoing hysterectomy are excessive menstrual bleeding with 56% and fibroids/cysts with 20%. Women in older ages, that is, 45–49 years, belongs to rural areas, with obesity, with no schooling, more parity and low age at marriage is more likely to undergo hysterectomy (Shekhar et al., 2019).

Most of the studies on a hysterectomy in India are carried out based on a small sample size or taking all the women in reproductive age, which doesn't show the nation-wide representation and the risk among the older adults to understand the course of hysterectomy on a large scale. Studies have highly pointed out that hysterectomy over the course of time and across nations can be highly seen among women age 40 and above, which is the main focus in the study to understand the highly risked group of women. Another reason would be most studies in our country are done based on medical or hospital-based without considering the socio-economic and demographic factors influencing the cases which are covered in the study. Our study focuses to assess the national and state prevalence of hysterectomy in India among older adult women, with understanding the influence of some individual and household level associative factors. From the past pieces of literature, it is evident that most women who underwent surgeries of hysterectomy have seen differentials in factors i.e. age, education, etc., that are associated with hysterectomy in India. So, it is very relevant to study the factors associated with hysterectomy in women of ages 40 and above in India. The study follows a particular conceptual framework which is shown in Fig. 9.1.

9.2 Materials and Methods

The present study is based on the Longitudinal Ageing Study in India Wave-1 (2020), a nationally representative survey. The LASI wave-1 is

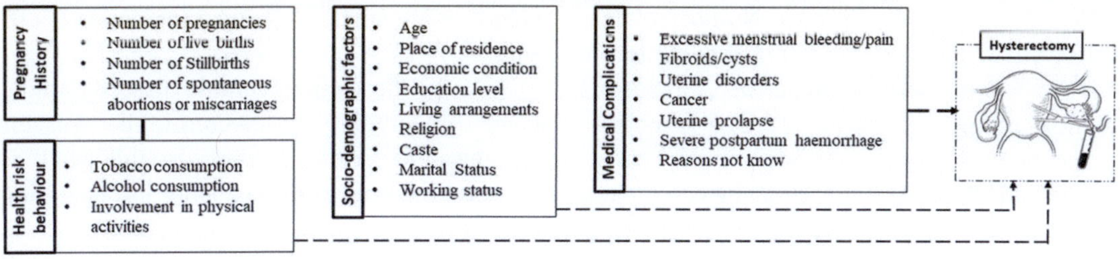

Fig. 9.1 Conceptual framework

a comprehensive study of 72,250 older adults aged 45 and above, including their spouses of less than 45 years. LASI data gives us information about various demographics, economics with retirement and insurance, family and social networks, health and well-being of the elderly in India. It is the world's most extensive longitudinal study on the elderly population [International Institute for Population Sciences (IIPS) et al., 2020]. In the study, the individual file of the LASI Wave 1 survey is utilized for the analysis. Only females with age 40 or above are considered in the sample; thus, we have a sample size of 39,309.

9.2.1 Outcome Variable

The dependent variable of the study is measured by the question asked in the survey, 'Have you undergone an operation to remove your uterus (hysterectomy)?' is used to define our outcome variable and coded as '1' for Yes and '0' No.

9.2.2 Covariates

The independent variables for the study are socio-demographic variables, health risk behaviour, pregnancy history, and the medical reasons for undergoing hysterectomy. Age in this study is taken as 40 and above, thus categorized into 10-year age groups ending with an open group: '40–50', '50–60', '60–70', '70–80', '80+'. The ages below 45 actually involves spouses of the respondents, hence considered in the age group. Place of residence was coded as 'Rural' and 'Urban'. The living arrangements variable had the categories-'living alone', 'living with spouse and others', 'living with spouse and children', 'living with children and others', 'living with others only'. Religion was divided into the categories-'No religion', 'Hindu', 'Muslim', 'Christians', 'Others'. According to the Indian caste system, the various social groups were categorized as-'Scheduled Caste' (SC), 'Scheduled Tribe' (ST), 'Other backward class (OBC)', 'None'. Marital status was divided as 'Currently married', 'Widowed', 'Divorce/Separated', and 'Never married'. Economic condition is measured by monthly per capita consumption expenditure (MPCE) and categorized as: poorest; poor; middle; rich; and richest.

The health risk or lifestyle behaviour were considered as determining factors as well. The smoking behaviour was measured by the variables-Currently smoke tobacco products (No, Yes); Currently consume smokeless tobacco (No, Yes); Ever smoked or consumed tobacco (No, Yes). Drinking patterns were measured by the variables0-Ever consumed any alcoholic beverage (No, Yes); Frequency of consumption of 5 or more drinks on one occasion (No, Less than once a month, 1–3 days per month, 1–4 days per week, Almost daily). The engagement in physical activities was measured by-Involvement in activities like yoga, asanas, meditation etc. (No/Rarely, Yes); Engage in vigorous physical activities (No/Rarely, Yes); Engage in moderate energetic physical activities (No/Rarely, Yes).

Pregnancy history can play a major role too and hence measured by the following variables-Number of pregnancies (0, 1–3, 4–9, 10 or more); Number of Medical Termination of Pregnancy

(MTP) (0, 1, 2, 3, 4 or more); Number of live births (0, 1, 2, 3, 4 or more); Number of stillbirths (0, 1, 2, 3, 4 or more), Number of spontaneous abortions or miscarriages (0, 1, 2, 3, 4 or more).

The medical reasons for undergoing hysterectomy included excessive menstrual bleeding/pain, fibroids/cysts, uterine disorders (rupture)/injury, cancer, uterine prolapse, severe postpartum haemorrhage, and, reasons not know.

9.2.2.1 Statistical Analysis

The state-wise proportion of women who have undergone hysterectomy is depicted through a prevalence map. The bivariate analysis included cross-tabulation, Goodman and Kruskal ɣ, to examine the association between the dependent and independent variables. The ɣ coefficient ranges from −1 to 1, and the formula is represented as

$$\gamma = \frac{N_c - N_d}{N_c - N_d}$$

where N_c and N_d are the number concordant and discordant pairs respectively. The Goodman and Kruskal ɣ, not only tests the association but also the strength of association between the two variables.

Since the medical reasons for undergoing hysterectomy has been asked only to those who have done it, hence these variables have been excluded from the regression model. Also, age, number of pregnancies, MTPs, live births, stillbirths, and spontaneous abortions/miscarriages were taken as continuous variables in the regression analysis. For the multivariate analysis, from the generalized linear model (GLM) framework, the logit link function belonging to the binomial family is used to model the probability of undergoing hysterectomy as a function of the covariates (Murray & Munz, 2015; Prasetyo et al., 2019). Thus, we have the logit regression model as

$$\log\left(\frac{\pi_i}{1 - \pi_i}\right) = x_i^T \beta = \alpha + \beta_i x_i$$

where α is the intercept β_i's are regression coefficients.

To study the socio-economic disparity among women undergoing hysterectomy, the Wagstaff concentration index is used. In this study it has been used measure inequality in undergoing hysterectomy by socio-demographic variables, lifestyle behaviour, and pregnancy history as well. The concentration index (C) is computed as

$$C = \frac{2}{N^2 \mu_h (1 - \mu_h)} \sum_{i=1}^{N} h_i R_i$$

where N is the number of observations, R_i is the deviation of the rank from the mean (or median) rank according to economic condition, h_i is another variable of interest, μ_i is the mean of h, and the minimum and maximum of the variable of interest are the scalar's lower limit and upper limit.

Fairlie (2005) technique of decomposition is used decompose the gap in undergoing hysterectomy by the place of residence of the women (rural/urban). This technique decomposes the gap in undergoing hysterectomy over the place of residence and we observe the percentage contribution of each of the attributable factors.

Thus, a non-linear equation $Y = F(X\beta)$, can be decomposed as:

$$\begin{aligned} Y^r - Y^u = & \left[\sum_{i=1}^{N^r} \frac{F(x_i^r \beta^r)}{N^r} - \sum_{i=1}^{N^u} \frac{F(x_i^u \beta^r)}{N^u} \right] \\ & + \left[\sum_{i=1}^{N^u} \frac{F(x_i^u \beta^r)}{N^u} - \sum_{i=1}^{N^u} \frac{F(x_i^u \beta^u)}{N^u} \right] \end{aligned}$$

where Y^r and Y^u represents undergoing hysterectomy in rural and urban areas with samples N^r and N^u, respectively (Fairlie, 2005). The statistical analysis is carried out in STATA 14.0, map is created using ArcGIS 10.3 and figure using OriginPro.

9.3 Results

The proportion of women who have undergone a hysterectomy in India is 11.45% with the highest being in the state of Andhra Pradesh and Punjab having almost 24% proportion. The lowest practice of hysterectomy is mostly in the North-eastern states including Tripura, Mizoram, Assam, Arunachal Pradesh and Nagaland (Fig. 9.2).

Table 9.1, presents the bivariate results of the proportion of women undergoing hysterectomy according to socio-economic and demographic variables. It can be observed that the percentage of women undergoing hysterectomy decreases significantly with increasing age, that is, starting with 12.7% in the age-group 40–50, it is 4.4% in 80+. The percentage of hysterectomy is significantly higher in urban areas (14.8%) than in rural areas (9.8%). Mostly women living with spouses and others or children have undergone hysterectomy (12%), whereas women living with only others were the lowest proportion to undergo hysterectomy (5.3%). Looking at the marital status of the women, it can be observed that currently, married women are the maximum (12.2%), followed by divorced or separated (10.9%) and unmarried women the lowest (4.6%) to have undergone hysterectomy. With increasing wealth quintile, the proportion of women undergoing hysterectomy also increases, from around 8% in the poorest to 17% in the richest quintile. Women who have done the professional course as part of education, are the maximum who undergoing hysterectomy (53%). The proportion was significantly higher among currently working women (12.12%).

Hysterectomy was also found to be significantly associated with lifestyle behaviours like smoking or consuming tobacco products, drinking alcoholic beverages or being involved in physical activities (Table 9.2). Women who currently smoke tobacco products are strong significantly related to being undergoing hysterectomy (6.6%). Those who have the frequency of consuming five or more drinks on one occasion, like almost 1–3 days per month, have the maximum percentage of undergoing hysterectomy (23.6%).

Among the medical reasons for performing a hysterectomy, excessive bleeding (33.6%), fibroids or cysts (25.6%), uterine prolapse ((16.7%) and disorders (11.2%) are some of the significantly major reasons (Fig. 9.3).

With the increasing number of pregnancies and livebirth the proportion of hysterectomy increased, whereas with an increasing number of stillbirths the proportion decreased (Table 9.3).

The adjusted multivariate regression model shows that women in urban areas have the odds of 1.23 times more of undergoing hysterectomy than women in rural areas. The likelihood of undergoing hysterectomy increases with the wealth quintile of the women (Table 9.4).

The Wagstaff normalized concentration index value for undergoing hysterectomy is 0.16, indicating that it is more concentrated among the well-off section of women (Table 9.5).

The Fairlie decomposition analysis shows that a number of pregnancies around 43%, wealth quintile 13%, caste 10%, tobacco consumption 10% and involvement in yoga, meditation etc. around 6.3% contribution towards the differential in undergoing hysterectomy between rural and urban women (Table 9.6). The number of live births and stillbirths shows a negative percentage contribution indicating the differential is more in the urban direction.

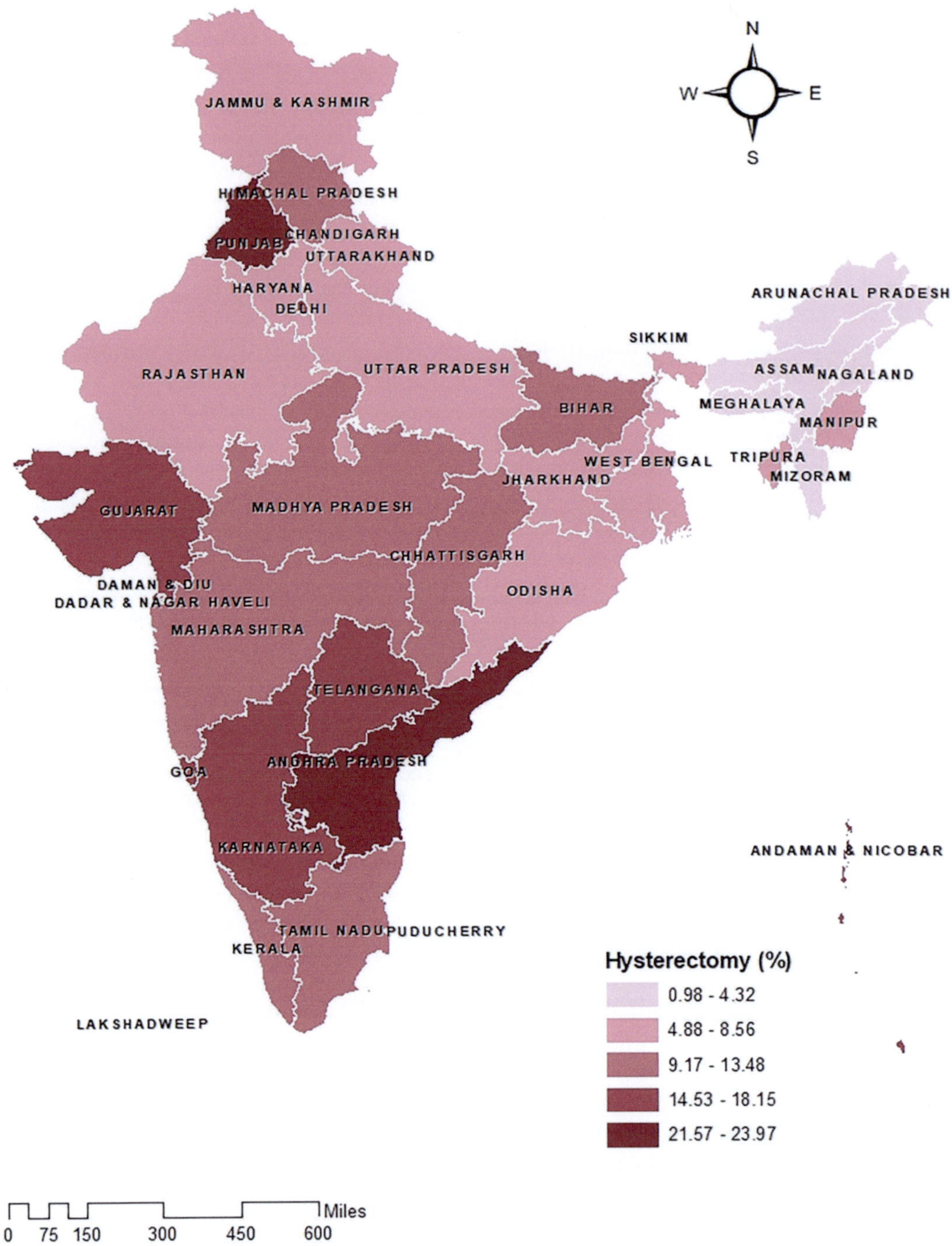

Fig. 9.2 State-wise prevalence of hysterectomy in India

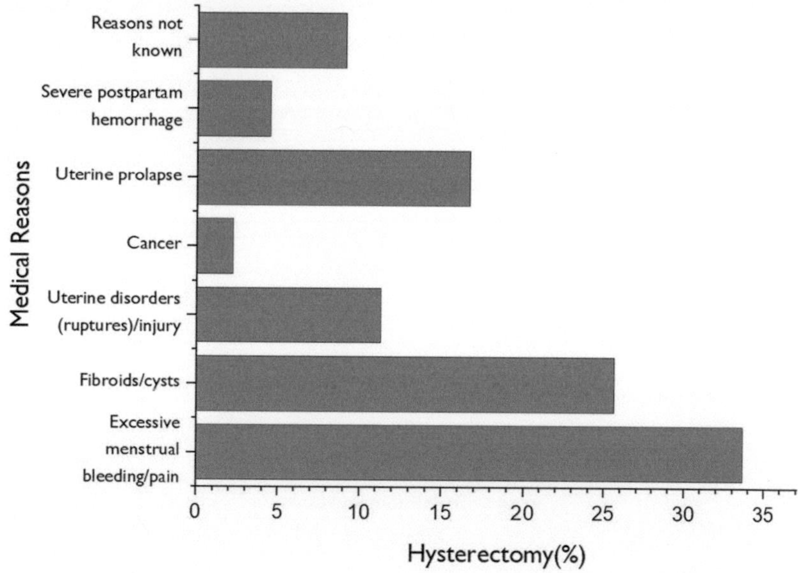

Fig. 9.3 Medical reasons for undergoing hysterectomy

9.4 Discussion

The study suggested that a significant percentage of women aged 40 and above have undergone a hysterectomy in India. However, even though the prevalence is comparatively low at the national level, Andhra Pradesh shows a higher prevalence than the national outcome.

In India, demographic factor age showed a peak in hysterectomy in the age group 40–50 years. Women residing in an urban area, with adequate levels of education, being married, working, and belonging to the affluent quintile, showed significant hysterectomy rates concerning their counterparts. The leading medical reason for undergoing hysterectomy was excessive bleeding constituting one-fourth of the hysterectomies. Keeping poor lifestyle behaviours and a high number of pregnancies or livebirths indicates a slight increase in the prevalence of hysterectomies in India. Additionally, the odds indicated the chance of hysterectomies is associated with wealth, proving a higher concentration in the wealthier quintile. The Rural–Urban differentials in undergoing are mainly contributed by pregnancy history and lifestyle changes between the two sectors.

Previous studies based on the National Family and Health Surveys have provided information on a hysterectomy in India for aged 15–49, claiming a low prevalence of hysterectomy in India till 2015–16. Our study primarily focused on the menopausal and post-menopausal women shows a prevalence that is quite significant. A similar trend was observed in rural areas of Northern India for a similar age group (Verma & Verma, 2021). Many studies have revealed that hysterectomy cases increase by age to a certain point and then decreases, that specific peak at the age group 40–50 years was also observed in our study (Desai et al., 2019; Prusty et al., 2018; Shekhar et al., 2019; Singh et al., 2020). This peak in the pre-menopausal stage of the menopausal stage can be due to the desire to complete the desired family size, children being old enough or the family commitments that might affect their routine life (Singh & Arora, 2008). Southern states like Andhra Pradesh reported high hysterectomy cases for the age group 40 and above, similarly, previous studies that only focused on under 49 years also reported a similar trend (Meher & Sahoo, 2020; Prusty et al., 2018; Singh & Govil, 2021). Socio-economic and demographic correlates like age, wealth, and education associated with hysterectomy were similar to the previous studies (Desai et al., 2019; Prusty et al., 2018; Shekhar et al., 2019; Singh et al., 2020). Meanwhile, association related to lifestyle behaviour and pregnancy history emerges as a new finding.

Table 9.1 Proportion of women undergone Hysterectomy (40 and above) by socio-economic and demographic characteristics, LASI Wave 1, 2017–18

Characteristics		Hysterectomy (%)	Goodman and Kruskal ɣ
Age	40–50	12.66	−0.078***
	50–60	12.51	
	60–70	11.94	
	70–80	7.78	
	80+	4.42	
Residence	Rural	9.76	0.099***
	Urban	14.78	
Living arrangements	Living alone	8.81	−0.123***
	Living with spouse and others	12.38	
	Living with spouse and children	12.24	
	Living with children and others	10.87	
	Living with others only	5.29	
MPCE quintile	Poorest	7.96	0.182***
	Poorer	8.78	
	Middle	10.61	
	Richer	13.72	
	Richest	16.99	
Education	Primary education or	12.57	−0.115***
	Middle school education	16.24	
	Secondary/higher seco	10.51	
	Graduate	12.42	
	Post graduate	10.05	
	Professional course	52.97	
	None	10.25	
Religion	No religion	3.98	−0.101***
	Hindu	11.7	
	Muslim	8.94	
	Christian	8.42	
	Others	15.61	
Caste	SC	10.21	0.081***
	ST	5.74	
	OBC	13.23	
	None	10.95	
Marital status	Currently married	12.24	−0.17***
	Widowed	9.95	
	Divorced/separated	10.91	
	Not married	4.64	
Currently working	No	11.06	−0.068***
	Yes	12.12	
Total frequency		**4479**	

*** Significant at 1% level ($p < 0.01$)

Table 9.2 Proportion of women undergone hysterectomy (40 and above) by health risk behaviour, LASI Wave 1, 2017–18

Characteristics		Hysterectomy (%)	Goodman and Kruskal γ
Currently smoke tobacco products	No	11.52	−0.345***
	Yes	6.6	
Currently consume smokeless tobacco	No	11.72	−0.209***
	Yes	9.44	
Ever smoked or consumed tobacco	No	11.9	−0.228***
	Yes	9.16	
Ever consumed any alcoholic beverage	No	11.45	−0.164***
	Yes	9.3	
Frequency of consumption of 5 or more drinks on one occasion	No	11.4	−0.242***
	Less than once a month	4.73	
	1–3 days per month	23.65	
	1–4 days per week	4.65	
	Almost daily	7.9	
Involvement in activities like yoga, asanas, meditation etc.	No/rarely	11.3	0.189***
	Yes	12.24	
Engage in vigorous physical activities	No/rarely	10.44	−0.002
	Yes	14.31	
Engage in moderate energetic physical activities	No/rarely	9	0.067***
	Yes	12.36	
Total frequency		**4479**	

*** Significant at 1% level ($p < 0.01$)

The primary reason for undergoing hysterectomy in the age group 40 and above was excessive menstrual bleeding, followed by fibroids/cysts, uterine prolapse, and uterine disorders. While previous studies conducted on age group of 15–49 years showed a similar pattern of reasons (Desai et al., 2019; Shekhar et al., 2019), whereas a study on women aged 35 and above stated the most common reason indicating hysterectomy were pelvic organ prolapse followed by fibroids, uterine bleeding (Verma & Verma, 2021).

Relatively inequality in hysterectomy cases was observed due to economic inequality. Hysterectomy is concentrated chiefly among the wealthier quantile of women showing a disadvantage among the poorer section of women. This inequality may be due to the unavailability or inaccessibility of healthcare facilities and the unaffordable burden of undergoing hysterectomy (Singh et al., 2020). Alternatively, higher rates of hysterectomy were found among women living in urban locations of India. Moreover, it may partly explain the urban slum population for some states but differs from previous studies of hysterectomies in India (Desai et al., 2011, 2019; Singh & Govil, 2021). Undergoing hysterectomy may be the not viable option for treating various gynaecological morbidities for rural women. Most of the women in rural areas lack adequate access to the treatment or can't afford to lose the number of days in the treatment for low-income working women (e.g. no hospitals nearby, no adequate resources, high expenditure on surgery) (Desai, 2016). Other explanations for the high rate of hysterectomy in urban locations could be hysterectomy, an easy solution for women for

Table 9.3 Proportion of women undergone hysterectomy (40 and above) by pregnancy history, LASI Wave 1, 2017–18

Characteristics		Hysterectomy (%)	Goodman and Kruskal γ
Number of pregnancies	0	7.22	−0.091***
	1–3	13.86	
	4–9	10.19	
	10 or more	5.07	
Number of medical termination of pregnancy (MTP)	0	11.41	0.0868
	1	13.3	
	2	6.67	
	3	14.18	
	4 or more	16.79	
Number of live births	0	9.65	−0.075***
	1	10.45	
	2	16.16	
	3	13.27	
	4 or more	9.21	
Number of stillbirths	0	11.31	0.123***
	1	12.76	
	2	12.03	
	3	8.53	
	4 or more	9.6	
Number of spontaneous abortions or miscarriages	0	10.74	0.071
	1	17.99	
	2	14.2	
	3	12.12	
	4 or more	26.26	
Total frequency		**4479**	

*** Significant at 1% level ($p < 0.01$)

all the menstrual and post-menstrual problems, or the commercial gain than a medical necessity by the healthcare institutions (Chaudhuri, 2013). Variation in hysterectomy rate by place of residence is not just an issue of access and available choice, the pregnancy history and various lifestyle factors could also be contributing to the differentials.

The study's main strength is the availability of data of women aged 40 and above, as previously national data was available on hysterectomy only for the 15–49 age group. Secondly, the data also provides reasons for which they have undergone hysterectomy, which is valuable for the study as it provides backup in medical terms. However, the study has limitation that the data does not provide information about the healthcare provider, the expenditure incurred and age in undergoing hysterectomy, as they could have given better insights to the health departments about an upcoming health problem, relationship with age and its effect on the poor population respectively. Secondly, all the data on medical reasons and other socio-demographic determinants were self-reported, indicating bias or recall error.

Table 9.4 Adjusted multivariate logit model for undergoing hysterectomy (40 and above) as the outcome, LASI Wave 1, 2017–18

Outcome variable: undergone hysterectomy		AOR (95% confidence interval)
Residence	Rural®	
	Urban	1.225*** (1.127, 1.333)
Living arrangements	Living alone®	
	Living with spouse	1.231 (0.836, 1.812)
	Living with spouse	1.219 (0.833, 1.784)
	Living with children	1.023 (0.837, 1.25)
	Living with others	0.684** (0.506, 0.925)
Wealth quintile	Poorest®	
	Poorer	1.225*** (1.07, 1.403)
	Middle	1.437*** (1.259, 1.64)
	Richer	1.753*** (1.54, 1.996)
	Richest	2.162*** (1.896, 2.465)
Age		0.996** (0.991, 1)
Education	Primary education or less®	
	Middle school education	0.73*** (0.625, 0.853)
	Secondary/higher secondary	0.73*** (0.635, 0.838)
	Graduate	0.503*** (0.382, 0.663)
	Post graduate	0.308*** (0.174, 0.544)
	Professional course	0.232*** (0.103, 0.527)
	None	0.944 (0.858, 1.038)
Religion	No religion®	
	Hindu	1.291 (0.466, 3.578)
	Muslim	0.843 (0.302, 2.354)
	Christian	1.347 (0.482, 3.768)
	Others	1.73 (0.618, 4.847)
Caste	SC	
	ST	0.47*** (0.397, 0.556)
	OBC	1.183*** (1.062, 1.317)
	None	0.969 (0.861, 1.09)
Marital status	Currently married®	
	Widowed	0.994 (0.704, 1.403)
	Divorced/separated	0.745 (0.461, 1.205)
Currently working	No®	
	Yes	0.957 (0.877, 1.045)
Currently smoke tobacco products	No®	
	Yes	0.737* (0.515, 1.055)
Currently consume smokeless tobacco	No®	
	Yes	0.924 (0.702, 1.216)
Ever smoked or consumed tobacco	No®	
	Yes	0.867 (0.669, 1.122)
Ever consumed any alcoholic beverage	No®	

(continued)

Table 9.4 (continued)

Outcome variable: undergone hysterectomy		AOR (95% confidence interval)
	Yes	1.264** (1.018, 1.571)
Involvement in activities like yoga, asanas, meditation etc.	No/rarely®	
	Yes	1.132** (1.012, 1.268)
Engage in moderate energetic physical activities	No/rarely®	
	Yes	1.03 (0.945, 1.123)
Number of pregnancies		0.96 (0.862, 1.068)
Number of medical termination of pregnancy (MTP)		0.932 (0.785, 1.106)
Number of live births		0.977 (0.878, 1.087)
Number of stillbirths		1.139** (1.017, 1.276)
Number of spontaneous abortions or miscarriages		1.113* (0.989, 1.252)
Constant		0.075*** (0.024, 0.23)

®: Reference category; *$p < 0.10$; **$p < 0.05$; ***$p < 0.01$

9.5 Conclusion

The study on hysterectomy points us to the future new-age reproductive health problem in the country. Presently India's public healthcare services like primary health centres, community health centres are more focused on pregnancy and maternal health-related care. Lack of appropriate gynaecological care in the rural area and public health enterprises calls for an intervention focusing on all services for women's health in the lifetime. Secondly an adequate knowledge provider should be made available to the women to provide gynaecological health education. The less educated or illiterate women with similar problems relating to hysterectomy might choose not to go for hysterectomy as they might be scared or ignorant without understanding the risk associated with it, which might have an impact on their future health. Similarly, women with less knowledge about the procedure or the alternative options available goes for surgery falling under the spells of private hospitals who works in money minded way.

Although national surveys like LASI and NFHS collect data on hysterectomy, giving us basic information, a thorough in-depth and medical study with proper medical information and any other long-term or short-term effect can bring light to the health planners. Women's health is among one of the factors in achieving Sustainable development Goals. Government-supported plans with low cost and primary care should be made available in the general hospitals, which can be helpful to the common women in rural and urban India.

Table 9.5 Concentration index depicting economic inequality with respect to undergoing hysterectomy, comparing between groups by demographic factors

Variables	Concentration index	Standard error
Place of residence		
Rural	0.198***	0.012
Urban	0.097***	0.014
Marital status		
Currently married	0.163***	0.011
Widowed	0.131***	0.018
Divorced/separated	0.325***	0.083
Not married	0.216**	0.102
Age		
40–50	0.129***	0.017
50–60	0.168***	0.016
60–70	0.171***	0.018
70–80	0.141***	0.031
80+	0.235***	0.061
Living arrangements		
Living alone	0.241***	0.046
Living with spouse	0.192***	0.023
Living with spouse	0.147***	0.012
Living with children	0.107***	0.019
Living with others	0.303***	0.055
Education		
Primary education or less	0.156***	0.019
Middle school education	0.046	0.031
Secondary/higher seco	0.1***	0.029
Graduate	0.128**	0.063
Post graduate	0.066	0.115
Professional course	0.571***	0.086
None	0.164***	0.012
Religion		
No religion	−0.507	0.358
Hindu	0.149***	0.011
Muslim	0.22***	0.031
Christian	0.144***	0.029
Others	0.159***	0.037
Caste		
SC	0.145***	0.023
ST	0.169***	0.029
OBC	0.165***	0.014
None	0.132***	0.017
Currently working		
No	0.156***	0.011
Yes	0.169***	0.016
Overall	**0.159*****	**0.01**

* $p < 0.10$; ** $p < 0.05$; *** $p < 0.01$

Table 9.6 Percentage contribution of selected characteristics towards rural–urban difference in proportion women (40 or above) undergone hysterectomy

Characteristics	Coefficient	Contribution (%)
Living arrangements	0.00022	−1.54
Wealth quintile	−0.00187***	12.86
Age	−0.00001	0.09
Education	0.00007	−0.48
Religion	0.00000	−0.01
Caste	−0.00144**	9.90
Marital status	0.00054***	−3.71
Currently working	−0.00068	4.67
Currently smoke tobacco products	−0.00018	1.23
Currently consume smokeless tobacco	−0.0001	0.69
Ever smoked or consumed tobacco	−0.00143**	9.82
Ever consumed any alcoholic beverage	0.00000	0.02
Involvement in activities like yoga, asanas, meditation etc.	−0.00091***	6.26
Engage in moderate energetic physical activities	−0.00002	0.13
Number of pregnancies	−0.00623***	42.85
Number of live births	0.00418**	−28.73
Number of stillbirths	0.00209***	−14.36
Total	**−0.00617*****	**42.42**

* $p < 0.10$; ** $p < 0.05$; *** $p < 0.01$

9.6 Availability of Data and Materials

The data used for the study i.e. LASI Wave-1 cannot be shared publicly as it is collected and stored by International Institute for Population Sciences, Mumbai, India. https://iipsindia.ac.in/lasi/. However, if researchers wish to access the data, they can fill-up the data request form (https://iipsindia.ac.in/lasi/) and send a request to the director of the institute at datacenter@iipsindia.ac.in.

Acknowledgements The authors cordially acknowledge International Institute for Population Sciences (IIPS) for providing us the LASI Wave 1 dataset for conducting the study.

References

Chaudhuri, M. (2013). Women's groups and fertility experts campaign to reduce prevalence of hysterectomy in India. *BMJ, 347*, Article f7551. https://doi.org/10.1136/bmj.f7551

Desai, S. (2016). Pragmatic prevention, permanent solution: Women's experiences with hysterectomy in rural India. *Social Science and Medicine, 151*, 11–18. https://doi.org/10.1016/j.socscimed.2015.12.046

Desai, S., Shukla, A., Nambiar, D., & Ved, R. (2019). Patterns of hysterectomy in India: A national and state-level analysis of the Fourth National Family Health Survey (2015–2016). *BJOG: an International Journal of Obstetrics and Gynaecology, 126*(Suppl 4), 72–80. https://doi.org/10.1111/1471-0528.15858

Desai, S., Sinha, T., & Mahal, A. (2011). Prevalence of hysterectomy among rural and urban women with and without health insurance in Gujarat, India. *Reproductive Health Matters, 19*(37), 42–51. https://doi.org/10.1016/S0968-8080(11)37553-2

Domingo, S., & Pellicer, A. (2009). Overview of current trends in hysterectomy. *Expert Review of Obstetrics and Gynecology, 4*(6), 673–685. https://doi.org/10.1586/eog.09.51

Fairlie, R. W. (2005). An extension of the Blinder–Oaxaca decomposition technique to logit and probit models. *Journal of Economic and Social Measurement, 30*(4), 305–316. https://doi.org/10.3233/JEM-2005-0259

International Institute for Population Sciences (IIPS) and ICF. (2017). *National family health survey (NFHS-4), 2015–16: India.* IIPS.

International Institute for Population Sciences (IIPS), National Programme for, Health Care of Elderly (NPHCE), MoHFW, & Public Health (HSPH) and the University of Southern California (USC). (2020). *Longitudinal Ageing Study in India (LASI) Wave 1, 2017–18, India Report*. International Institute for Population Sciences, Mumbai. https://www.iipsindia.ac.in/lasi/

Meher, T., & Sahoo, H. (2020). Changing trends in the preference of health care facility and reasons for hysterectomy in India. *Health Care for Women International, 41*(7), 802–816. https://doi.org/10.1080/07399332.2019.1683847

Murray, L., & Munz, P. (2015). *Binomial link functions*. 30.

Pokras, R., & Hufnagel, V. G. (1988). Hysterectomy in the United States, 1965–84. *American Journal of Public Health, 78*(7), 852–853. https://doi.org/10.2105/ajph.78.7.852

Prasetyo, R. B., Kuswanto, H., Iriawan, N., & Ulama, B. S. S. (2019). A comparison of some link functions for binomial regression models with application to school drop-out rates in East Java. *AIP Conference Proceedings, 2194*(1), Article 020083. https://doi.org/10.1063/1.5139815

Prusty, R. K., Choithani, C., & Gupta, S. D. (2018). Predictors of hysterectomy among married women 15–49 years in India. *Reproductive Health, 15*(1), 3. https://doi.org/10.1186/s12978-017-0445-8

Shekhar, C., Paswan, B., & Singh, A. (2019). Prevalence, sociodemographic determinants and self-reported reasons for hysterectomy in India. *Reproductive Health, 16*(1), 118. https://doi.org/10.1186/s12978-019-0780-z

Singh, A., & Arora, A. K. (2008). Why hysterectomy rate are lower in India. *Indian Journal of Community Medicine: Official Publication of Indian Association of Preventive and Social Medicine, 33*(3), 196–197. https://doi.org/10.4103/0970-0218.42065

Singh, A., & Govil, D. (2021). Hysterectomy in India: Spatial and multilevel analysis. *Women's Health, 17*, 17455065211017068. https://doi.org/10.1177/17455065211017068

Singh, S. K., Sharma, S. K., & Siddhanta, A. (2020). Major correlates and socioeconomic inequalities in hysterectomy among ever-married women in India. *Indian Journal of Community Medicine: Official Publication of Indian Association of Preventive and Social Medicine, 45*(1), 12–17. https://doi.org/10.4103/ijcm.IJCM_12_19

Verma, D., & Verma, M. L. (2021). Trends of hysterectomy in the rural tertiary level teaching hospitals in Northern India. *Indian Journal of Obstetrics and Gynecology Research, 3*(3), 212–215.

Vessey, M. P., Villard-Mackintosh, L., Mcpherson, K., Coulter, A., & Yeates, D. (1992). The epidemiology of hysterectomy: Findings in a large cohort study. *BJOG: an International Journal of Obstetrics and Gynaecology, 99*(5), 402–407. https://doi.org/10.1111/j.1471-0528.1992.tb13758.x

Wright, J. D., Herzog, T. J., Tsui, J., Ananth, C. V., Lewin, S. N., Lu, Y.-S., Neugut, A. I., & Hershman, D. L. (2013). Nationwide trends in the performance of inpatient hysterectomy in the United States. *Obstetrics and Gynecology, 122*(201), 233–241. https://doi.org/10.1097/AOG.0b013e318299a6cf

School Education, Health, and Sanitation 10

Shazia Farooq Fazli

Abstract

Health and Sanitation are interrelated with Education. School hygiene education aims to improve behaviour by teaching appropriate hygiene practices, and thus it is an urgent need. The government of India and UNICEF have identified school sanitation as a key area of collaboration. School Sanitation and Hygiene Education (SSHE) is globally recognized as a key intervention to promote children's right to health and a clean environment. A focus on school sanitation stems from the fact that children have a right to basic facilities such as school toilets, safe drinking water, clean surroundings, and information on hygiene. In the urban regions, there is a growing disparity between the number of students on campus and the corresponding sanitation on facilities available has raised health concerns. The National Education Policy (NEP, 2020), the government hopes to transform India into a "global knowledge superpower," but this can only be accomplished by improving the flexibility, holistic nature, and multidisciplinary nature of the education system for schools and colleges, which will highlight each student's talents. Preschool education, disabilities, access to a bathroom, and menstrual hygiene practices are some of the new topics covered in NFHS-5. Unfortunately, there is also a great deal of ambiguity on whose responsibility it is to ensure functional toilets with adequate water facilities in schools. At present, there is no provision in Sarva Shiksha Abhiyan (SSA) for the cleaning of toilets. In addition to adequate funding for cleaning, sanitation training, and toilet maintenance, the issue of accountability must be addressed. Otherwise, we will keep returning to the fundamental issues, reformulating strategies, and recommissioning funds. Moreover, the implementation of government programmes still has flaws.

10.1 Introduction

It is important to inculcate a sense of responsibility in young minds towards basic hygiene and cleanliness practices. Developing health literacy entails fostering the advantages of education and learning that contribute to overall personal growth. School life lays the groundwork for development; Whatever is learnt in school is unconsciously assimilated and becomes a habit or practice, contributing to the growth of a prosperous society and nation. As a result, schools play an essential role in a community's health. There are various ways in which children learn in and outside the classroom (UNICEF & IRC, 2002).

S. F. Fazli (✉)
Department of Sociology, Faculty of Social Sciences, Aligarh Muslim University, Aligarh, India
e-mail: shaziafarooqfazli@gmail.com

S. S. Acharya et al. (eds.), *Paradigm Shifts in Population and Health in India*, Sustainable Development Goals Series, https://doi.org/10.1007/978-981-95-1719-0_10

Education is just one of a variety of social practices that embraced the power of psychotherapeutic values and where a variety of health interventions were administered and politicized (Petrina, 2006). Hence, schools have a pivotal role to play in the overall health of a community. It is important to note that there is clear evidence that the level of an individual's education is related to health outcomes in adulthood and clear evidence that healthier children learn better and are more likely to be academically successful than those with health issues (Allensworth, 2015; Basch, 2011; Bradley & Greene, 2013; Freudenberg & Ruglis, 2007; Wallen, 2015; Woolf et al., 2007). Schools are the best place to educate children about the importance of basic hygiene practices, and effective hygiene education must be compulsorily imparted to all in primary schools. Attitudes and habits acquired during childhood can help to prevent a large proportion of the diseases which afflict so many people and cause death in developing countries (Karlin, 1988). We all want to improve health outcomes for individuals of all ages in all communities through health education and promotion (Birch, 2017). After evaluating several studies, we find a strong correlation between education and health. To order to better comprehend this, we have certain objectives to look into.

1. To understand the relationship between School health education vis a vis student's personal health and school attendance
2. To comprehend the features of quality health education and sanitation programmes
3. To review strategies designed for enacting school reforms as a public health strategy

10.2 Health and Hygiene

The World Health Organization (WHO) defines health as a state of complete physical, mental, and social well-being and not merely the absence of disease or infirmity (WHO, 1948). This is consistent with the biopsychosocial model of health, which considers the physiological, psychological, and social factors in health and illness, as well as their interactions. Contrary to the traditional medical model, which defines health as the absence of illness or disease and emphasises clinical diagnosis and intervention, this model defines health as the presence of wellness. The WHO definition explicitly links health with well-being and conceptualises health as a human right that requires physical and social resources to attain and maintain. The term "wellbeing" refers to a positive state as opposed to a neutral one, framing health as a positive goal. This definition was adopted by the Ottawa Charter of 1986, which defines health as "a resource for daily life, not the purpose of living." From this perspective, health is a means to a good life, highlighting the connection between health and social participation (Jakab, 2011).

Social structure and cultural practices have tangible effects on the lives of individuals. The sociological analysis emphasises that illness is not a random occurrence. Different types of societies produce their own health and disease patterns. The sociology of health examines such topics as how social and cultural factors affect health and people's perceptions of health and healing, as well as how healing is practised in various societies. The health and well-being of individuals and communities are influenced by multiple factors. Illness is a state of poor health resulting from a disease of the body or mind. The health status of individuals is determined by their circumstances and environment. Significant impacts on health and well-being are exerted by factors such as where we live, the environment we live in, genetics, diseases, employment and income, education, and relationships with friends and family, whereas access to and use of health care services often have less of an effect.

Individuals have a specific and distinct relationship with the society or structure in which they reside. Giddens provides a useful illustration of how structure (society) influences the actions and experiences of individuals. This concept refers to a collection of ideas about the capacity of individuals to determine their lives, alter their surroundings, and ultimately affect the larger structure. Therefore, the concept of agency enables us to comprehend how society shapes us and how we in turn shape society. If the subject matter of sociology is human society and behaviour is primarily explained in terms of "structure," then this logically denotes specific components of the discipline's explanatory framework. Sociological explanations of what determines our health will inevitably differ from biological explanations, for instance. Disease is a biological and physical entity that manifests itself through the body. Although the cause of the disease is biological, social and structural factors can also be considered. The immediate cause of a disease may be an infection, but there may be multiple contributing factors. We may refer to these as the social determinants of health. The social determinants of health are the circumstances under which individuals are born, raised, reside, and age. The distribution of money, power, and resources at the international, national, and local levels shapes these conditions. The social determinants of health are primarily responsible for health disparities—the unequal distribution of health (Giddens, 2006).

Hygiene is a series of practices and rituals used to keep one's health in check. It refers to behaviours that can lead to good health. It mainly includes proper cleanliness, waste and sewage disposal, and safe drinking water. The term "hygiene" comes from the Greek word "Hygeia," which means goddess of health, cleanliness, and sanitation (AI-Rifaai et al., 2018). Hygiene refers to practices associated with ensuring good health and cleanliness (Temitayo, 2016).

Many diseases and conditions can be prevented or controlled through appropriately and regularly washing parts of the body. Good hygiene is essential for preventing the spread of infectious illnesses and assisting children living healthy lives. Hygiene is a series of practices performed to preserve health. According to the World Health Organization (WHO), "Hygiene refers to conditions and practices that help to maintain health and prevent the spread of diseases." (WHO, 2020).

It also keeps students from missing school, which leads to better learning. Good hygiene means staying healthy and spending less on health care for families.

While hygiene is about personal cleanliness through individual actions and preventing the spread of illness, sanitation, on the other hand, is about creating an environment safe from pathogens. It is the process of keeping places free from dirt, infection, disease, etc., by removing waste, trash, garbage, sewage, etc. Sanitation is a prerequisite for hygiene.

As a result, school hygiene is one of the most important requirements of any educational facility. A successful school is always the one that offers its students a clean and safe environment. School hygiene is reflected in a variety of ways, including trash management, cleaning services, clean water and general student and staff health.

10.3 Education and Health Relationship

Is education often related to good health? There is a growing amount of research investigating the impact of education on health. Even in highly developed countries like the United States, it has been observed that adults with lower educational attainment suffer from poor health when compared to other populations (Zajacova & Lowrencw, 2018). A good quality education is the foundation of health and well-being. For people to lead healthy and productive lives, they need the knowledge to prevent sickness and disease. For children and adolescents to learn, they need to be well-nourished and healthy (UNESCO, 2023). Education is a catalyst for development and a health intervention in its own right. The Incheon Declaration confirms that education develops the skills, values and attitudes that enable citizens to lead healthy and fulfilled lives, make informed decisions, and respond to local and global challenges (Incheon Declaration, 2015). A focus on school sanitation stems from the fact that those children have a right to basic facilities such as school toilets, safe drinking water, clean surroundings and information on hygiene. The National Education Policy (NEP, 2020) has considered health an indispensable and integral element for educational attainment. It acknowledges the provision of functional toilets and clean drinking water (NEP, Chapter 5.9). Education and health are co-dependent. Dirty facilities can make children sick. Improved hygiene and sanitation at school are critical to the health of school children (Snel & Shordt, 2005). School hygiene education aims to improve behaviour by teaching appropriate hygiene practices, and thus it is an urgent need. The New Education Policy [NEP] envisages creating a conducive environment for preparing "good, successful, innovative, adaptable, productive human beings" (NEP 4.23, p. 15). If these conditions are met, students will attend class, enjoy it, learn more, and bring concepts and behaviours related to sanitation and hygiene home to their families, particularly their siblings. From the schools, hygiene education will automatically be extended to the children's families, and further, the whole community will benefit from proper hygiene practices. Hygiene habits and hand-washing practices among all children improve their overall health. (Snel & Shordt, 2005). Such conditions have an even greater positive outcome for girls who often stay away from or drop out of schools which do not have toilet facilities. Therefore, school hygiene education, especially at the primary level, can help prevent many diseases in developing countries. Lack of proper hygiene and sanitation facilities increases the burden of communicable diseases among developing countries. (Vivas et al., 2010). The hygiene habits developed in school days go a long way in the prevention of diseases that afflict people and even cause deaths as important for learning in schools. Gene Carter, former Executive Director and CEO of ASCD emphasized the importance of recognizing this relationship at the 2014 SOPHE Annual Meeting by stating, Health and education are related. They are interrelated. They are symbiotic. There is a connection between the two sectors. When one fails, so does the other. When one succeeds, that success feeds the other. We do not just have an isolated duty to want the child to be healthy and educated—we have a moral imperative (Birch, 2017). Schools provide an excellent opportunity to create lifelong changes in hygiene behaviour. In Africa and Southeast Asia, 62% and 31% of all deaths are caused by infectious diseases. (Curtis et al., 2009). Children who learn what personal hygiene is and how to follow adequate hygiene practices will usually sustain those habits into their adulthood too. Numerous studies have illuminated that effortless acts of hand-washing and basic hygiene behaviour could prevent diarrhoea, acute respiratory infection and skin infections (Luby et al., 2005; Shahid et al., 1996).

Diseases associated with an inadequate water supply and poor sanitation and hygiene are especially common within developing countries. Many schools in developing and developed countries lack adequate water and sanitation services, with associated potential detrimental effects on health and school attendance (Mathekgana et al., 2001; Haines et al., 2000). Most diarrheal diseases are caused by inadequate and unsafe water supply and poor sanitation and hygiene facilities. Schoolchildren in the Least Developed Countries (LDCs) and fragile contexts are the most affected, and emerging data shows that few schools have disability-accessible WASH services (UNICEF/WHO, 2022).

Children who have adequate water, sanitation and hygiene facilities at school are more able to integrate hygiene education into their daily lives and are effective behaviour-change communicators in their communities. According to the World Health Organization, 11% more girls attend school when sanitation is available (WHO, 2002). While communities whose school children have been exposed to disease risk due to inadequate supply of water, sanitation, and hygiene services are more at risk. Many children in both developing and developed nations spend time absent from school due to diseases contracted within the school environment (Koopman, 1978).

In the urban regions also, the growing disparity between the number of students on campus and the corresponding sanitation facilities available has raised health concerns among parents. It is estimated that 88% of diarrhoeal disease is caused by unsafe water supply and inadequate sanitation and hygiene (WHO, 2004). Health problems are prevalent among the students of such schools that lack sufficient water supply, sanitation and hygiene. If everyone in the world had access to a regulated piped water supply and sewage connection in their houses, 1863 million days of school attendance would be gained due to less diarrhoeal illness (WHO, 2004). Not just in government schools, but the condition of sanitation facilities in colleges and universities run by the government is deplorable. "Access to water, sanitation and hygiene is not only essential for effective infection prevention and control but also a prerequisite for children's health, development and well-being," said Dr Maria Neira, WHO Director, Department of Environment, Climate Change and Health (UNICEF/WHO, 2022).

The lack of clean and well-maintained toilets is a problem not only in government schools but also in most public/private schools, except for a few. "Far too many children go to schools without safe drinking water, clean toilets, and soap for handwashing—making learning difficult," said Kelly Ann Naylor, UNICEF Director of Water, Sanitation, Hygiene, and Climate, Environment, Energy, and Disaster Risk Reduction (UNICEF/WHO, 2022).

Students in Public schools come from sound economic and social backgrounds and are reluctant to use school washrooms. They refuse because of the stench and soiled toilets and washrooms. "Schools should be settings where children thrive and not be subjected to hardship or infections due to lack of, or poorly maintained, basic infrastructure" (UNICEF/WHO, 2022). The combination of adequate water and sanitation facilities, correct behavioural practices and education are critical for securing children's good health, learning, and overall development.

10.4 Girls-Specific School Sanitation and Hygiene

The education of girls is recognised as an investment with many valuable returns, including the health and economic prosperity of women, their families and their nations (Herz & Sperling, 2004).

Investing in girls' education is just work half done. Investing in sufficient sanitation for females at their educational institutions is also critical. By overlooking this essential component, developing-country governments are expanding the gender gap and depriving millions of girls of the fundamental right to education and valuable quality health care.

The lack of separate bathrooms for girls jeopardizes gender-sensitive distinctions. According to Red Cross research in Senegal, girls are encouraged not to use unclean school latrines. For obvious reasons, girls must "hang on" to pee during school hours and refrain from drinking. This forced habit impairs focus and causes a slew of health issues. According to UNICEF, more than 15% of females in 70 developing nations are routinely absent from school. Lack of sufficient sanitation is one of the fundamental reasons why so many schoolgirls are denied an education, good health, and a dignified existence.

Of the 113 million children not in school, 60% are girls. Water and sanitation are some of the key issues preventing girls from enrolling in schools. According to an Indian citizen-led survey published in January 2019, 11.5% of India's rural schools lack separate toilets for girls, and 11.7% of those that do have them are locked and inoperable. Schools with separate toilets for boys and girls are not enough, as they do not facilitate the girls in their periods. Even if toilets are separated for male and female students, sufficient hygiene conditions, running water and soap are absent. Toilets with proper locking doors for privacy, proper disposal facilities, and sanitary products are lacking. According to a Bank research, a survey of 62 primary schools in rural western Kenya discovered that while 84% of the schools had separate latrines for females, 77% did not have a lock and just 13% had water in or near the latrine. Furthermore, only 10% of schools reported always giving sanitary pads to female students. Most schools' sanitary pad disposal arrangements were inadequate.

Menstruation influences adolescent girls' school dropout, which is a big issue in most nations. Menstrual Hygiene Day (28 'May) was initiated by German-based NGO WASH in 2013, in collaboration with the World Bank and other partners to address and promote knowledge about menstrual hygiene management among teenage females in schools and beyond. Strong cultural taboos around menstruation, which are present in many societies, coupled with a lack of Menstrual Hygiene Management services in schools, results in girls staying away from school during menstruation (UNESCO, 2014).

In 2012, the WHO and UNICEF decided to "add MHM in schools and health facilities as a global advocacy issue in the lobbying effort for the post-2015 sustainability goals" (Sommer et al., 2015).

Plan International's Stefanie Conrad says that "Menstruating girls face extreme challenges without adequate sanitation facilities, and often just stay at home during their period." Many adolescent girls experience the humiliation of having to maintain their hygiene during menstruation without water and in dark areas, with the fear of being watched. Conrad adds, "Girls reported harassment through boys and teachers when having to use the open to relieve themselves."

Sanitary disposal facilities and single-sex toilets are important requirements-as Richard Jolly at the Institute of Development Studies says, "Unless there are separate facilities for girls many parents don't want their girls to be in school—especially when the girls are starting menstruation." Parents of adolescent girls are sometimes unwilling to expose their daughters to risk due to a shortage of toilets in schools. When menstruation begins, families take out their daughters from school because they have reached "reproductive age." Withdrawal from school may result in early marriage, teenage pregnancies, increased risk of sexually transmitted infections, and loss of opportunities (Baird et al., 2012; Jukes et al., 2008). The majority of females who dropped out of school owing to poor sanitation ended up in early marriages and pregnancies.

A recent WaterAid research in Nepal discovered that almost half of the girls polled had missed school due to menstruation, mostly owing to a lack of privacy for cleaning and washing. Another research by UNESCO found that one out of every ten females in Sub-Saharan Africa misses school when on their period. Girls are predicted to skip 4 days of school every month in Kenya, losing them 165 learning days during 4 years of high school and one in four girls does not complete primary school. According to studies, a quarter of all girls in India took time off when menstruation due to insufficient gender-specific school toilets and the unavailability of sanitary pads in schools. According to an Ethiopian survey, half of all girls miss 1–4 days of school each month due to menstruation. A Plan International study found that in an advanced country such as the United Kingdom, 64% of girls aged 14–21 missed part or all of their school day due to their period, and 13% of girls missed an entire day of school at least once a month. A survey in Indonesia reported 11% of adolescent girls missed school during their last period (Davis et al., 2018) in Niger, Burkina Faso, and Nigeria, 15%, 17%, and 23% of girls aged 15–24 years reported missing school in the past year due to menstruation (Tegegne & Sisay, 2014); In Ethiopia, 43–50.7% of students reported being absent from school due to menstrual-related problems (Tegegne & Sisay, 2014). Regular school absenteeism can affect school performance, self-esteem, and ability to pursue higher levels of education (Biddlecom, 2008).

The evidence through research supports the idea that a lack of water and sanitary facilities in schools to manage menstruation causes discomfort and avoidance of school during menstruation. Freeman et al., have shown a decrease in absenteeism among girls after water and hygiene interventions (Freeman, 2012). This is particularly significant in light of high drop-out rates among young women in many developing countries (Herz & Sperling, 2004). The relationship between education and women's health, economic success and educational status has been documented (Fahimi & Moghadam, 2003). Measures that encourage women and girls to stay in school are critical to reaching the Millennium Development Goals of universal education and fostering women's gender equality and empowerment. Data from over 10,000 schools in Zambia was analyzed in 2017 and confirmed that improved sanitation provision in schools was correlated with high female-to-male enrolment ratios, and reduced repetition and drop-out ratios, especially for girls (Agol et al., 2018). The study thus confirmed the linkages between adequate toilets in schools and the educational progression of girls (Agol et al., 2018).

The lack of restrooms in schools has a particularly negative impact on females when they enter puberty. They eventually drop out because they are unable to keep up with the classwork. Every year, around 23 million girls in India drop out of school owing to menstruation. Another research in India discovered that up to one in every five females drop out of school after getting their period. According to one study, females in the menarche group had a 12% drop in school enrolment.

Girls bear a disproportionate share of the burden of a lack of toilets. When a girl hits puberty, the lack of separate restrooms for her might be the determining factor in whether or not she continues her education, lowering her chances of a brighter future. Studies globally, have shown an extra year of secondary school can increase a girl's potential income by 15–25%, and a 1% increase in a girl's secondary school attendance can boost a country's GDP by 0.3% (Fiske, 2012). Better-educated women are more likely to be healthier and have better health status for their children than uneducated women, they also tend to have formal employment, earn higher wages, marry later, have fewer children, and prioritise their children's education.

10.5 Health Education and Sanitation Programmes

When every child is promised the right to quality education; moreover, it is also their right to safe water, sanitation and hygiene (WASH) facilities at school. Therefore, water, sanitation, and hygiene (WASH) in schools has received widespread recognition for its major contributions to the achievement of the ambitious Sustainable Development Goals (SDG), also known as the Global Goals. The United Nations established these goals in 2015 as a global call to action to eradicate poverty, safeguard the environment, and guarantee that by 2030, all people enjoy peace and prosperity. UNICEF works with over 100 countries to develop and rehabilitate WASH facilities in schools.

WASH is the acronym for Water, Sanitation and Hygiene and each is dependent on the presence of the other. For example, without clean water, basic sanitation and hygiene practices are not possible. (UNESCO, 2016) Access to water and sanitation is one of the major challenges for the twenty-first century. World Health Organization (WHO) estimates that still "2.5 billion people-more than one-third of the global population live without basic sanitation facilities" (WHO & UN, 2014).

As children spend a considerable amount of time on the school campus, WASH services have a significant impact on their learning and healthy growth. It further contributes immensely to school attendance and upholds the dignity, especially of female students. Lack of WASH facilities can prevent students from attending school, particularly female students (UNICEF, 2015).

WASH in schools promotes hygienic behaviours and good health by improving access to and management of clean, gender-friendly, and inclusive sanitation facilities. WASH in Schools thus improves the health and well-being of children, their families and the community.

More than half of all primary schools in the developing countries with available data do not have adequate water facilities and nearly two-thirds lack adequate sanitation (UNESCO, 2012). Even where facilities exist, they are often in poor condition. Children can more fully participate in school when there is improved access to water (World Bank, 2015: 24).

UNICEF, in collaboration with its partners, advises governments, NGOs (non-government organizations) and donors, on how to improve WASH services in schools while also facilitating knowledge sharing and learning.

10.6 Methods to Improve WASH in Schools

Methods to improve the situation of WASH infrastructure at schools include on a policy level: broadening the focus of the education sector, establishing a systematic quality assurance system, and distributing and using funds wisely. Other practical recommendations include: having a clear and systematic mobilization strategy, supporting the education sector to strengthen intersectoral partnerships, establishing a constant monitoring system which is located within the education sector, educating the educators and partnering with the school management (Dauenhauer, 2016).

10.7 The Role of NGOs in Hygiene and Sanitation

NGOs have a vital role in the field of sanitation and hygiene. Whereas the governments have to play a significant role, NGOs (non-governmental organisations) active involvement is necessary to deliver sanitation and hygiene programmes. They work as a link between the people and government planning.

The goal of NGO programme interventions is to educate school students, teachers and staff. They address infrastructural deficiencies in WASH and encourage inclusive designs and menstrual hygiene facilities. The NGOs give technical support and help the local administration and schools to integrate the operation and maintenance of water, sanitation, and hygiene systems.

NGOs continue to play an important role in achieving results for children, both via cooperative programmes and campaigning. UNICEF has created several coordination structures to aid in the development of partnerships with NGOs, both international (INGOs) and national/local, as well as other civil society players. However, there is always room for development and more participation to increase the effectiveness of these relationships.

The Office of Emergency Programmes (EMOPS) recognises that deeper partnerships with NGOs play a crucial role in the delivery and enhancement of UNICEF interventions in the context of UNICEF's Strategic Plan 2018–2021 and increasing efforts to provide humanitarian results for children. UNICEF and the International Council of Voluntary Agencies (ICVA) have decided to work together to reach out to the NGO sector in the hope to receive feedback and perceptions of the current partnership with UNICEF in this manner and to explore ways to improve the partnership, including the establishment of a formal mechanism for regular consultations. The initiative's overarching goal is to provide a dedicated safe place for debate and exchange to strengthen collaboration between UNICEF and NGOs to progress results for children in humanitarian contexts.

With a tradition of local-level community engagement, non-government organizations (NGOs) have a comparative advantage in addressing some of these critical components of successful sanitation initiatives. NGOs play a variety of roles in the sanitation sector and have been credited with developing, trailing and promoting many innovative and locally-appropriate approaches. They are known for being advocates of equitable, sustainable and cost-effective development and for playing a critical role as intermediaries, for example between communities and utilities or other service providers. Building on the foundations of successful approaches, there is potential for the range of actors in the sanitation sector to engage more closely with NGOs drawing on their strengths and collaborating to achieve more successful and sustainable sanitation outcomes.

The International Water Centre and the Institute for Sustainable Futures at the University of Technology, Sydney, conducted a study and found that the majority of NGOs have significant strengths and play an important and diversified role in the sanitation industry. NGOs have aided in improving poor people's access to sanitation services, and they generally provide on-the-ground influence in boosting access to services in relatively short timeframes through established community ties.

NGOs are versatile and can be seen playing multiple functions in response to local community and policy conditions. Simultaneously, NGOs may rely on worldwide expertise through their practitioner networks, promoting the interchange of fresh ideas from one region to the next. NGOs in the sanitation sector build partnerships and promote networking between different sector actors including representing community views to governments and service providers and translating and communicating national policies and regulations at the local level. They also participate in policy discussion, which includes supporting tried-and-true ideas and technology, articulating lessons learned, communicating community needs, pushing for gender parity, and assessing the success of programmes and government efforts.

10.8 Conclusion

The chapter sheds light on the crucial aspects of health and hygiene at the school level. One of the key areas discussed in the chapter is the provision of WASH facilities in schools. Adequate access to clean water, sanitation, and hygiene facilities is essential for maintaining a healthy and safe learning environment. The study emphasizes the importance of well-maintained school toilets and proper sanitation practices to prevent the spread of diseases and to promote overall hygiene among students. Moreover, the study highlights the alarming issue of girls' dropout rates due to insufficient toilet facilities and the challenges faced by them while managing their menstrual hygiene at school.

It also delves into the efforts of international organizations such as the World Health Organization (WHO) and the United Nations Children's Fund (UNICEF). Their initiatives focus on capacity building, policy development, and advocacy to raise awareness and encourage the implementation of best practices in school health and hygiene.

Further, the chapter discusses various government programs to improve WASH facilities and implement hygiene education campaigns. These initiatives reflect the recognition of the government's responsibility in ensuring the well-being of students and fostering a conducive learning environment.

In addition, the instrumental role played by non-governmental organizations (NGOs) in addressing health and hygiene challenges in schools is discussed. Their involvement complements the efforts of governments and international organizations, bridging gaps and ensuring the effective delivery of health and hygiene education programs.

In conclusion, the chapter on "School Health and Hygiene Education" emphasizes the critical importance of addressing and promoting hygiene education, for fostering the healthy growth and development of future generations.

References

Agol, D., Harvey, P., & Maíllo, J. (2018). Sanitation and water supply in schools and girls' educational progression in Zambia". *Journal of Water Sanitation and Hygiene for Development., 8*(1), 53–61.

Al-Rifaai, J. M., Al Haddad, A. M., & Qasem, J. A. (2018). Personal hygiene among college students in Kuwait: A Health promotion perspective. *Journal of Education and Health Promotion, 7*, 92.

Alam, M. U., Luby, S. P., Halder, A. K., Islam, K., Opel, A., Shoab, A. K., Ghosh, P. K., Rahman, M., Mahon, T., & Unicomb, L. (2017). Menstrual hygiene management among Bangladeshi adolescent schoolgirls and risk factors affecting school absence: Results from a cross-sectional survey. *British Medical Journal Open, 7*(7), 1.

Allensworth, D. D. (2015). Historical overview of coordinated school health. In D. A. Birch & D. M. Videto (Eds.), *Promoting health and academic success* (pp. 13–25). Human Kinetics.

Basch, C. E. (2011). Healthier students are better learners: High-quality, strategically planned, and effectively coordinated school health programs must be a fundamental mission of schools to help close the achievement gap. *Journal of School Health, 81*, 650–662.

Bradley, B. J., & Greene, A. C. (2013). Do health and education agencies in the United States share responsibility for academic achievement and health? A review of 25 years of evidence about the relationship of adolescents' academic achievement and health behaviours. *Journal of Adolescent Health, 52*, 523–532.

Baird, S. J., Garfein, R. S., McIntosh, C. T., & Ozler, B. (2012). Effect of a cash transfer programme for schooling on prevalence of HIV and herpes simplex type 2 in Malawi: A cluster randomised trial. *Lancet (London, England), 379*(9823), 1320–1329.

Biddlecom, A., Gregory, R., Lloyd, C. B., & Mensch, B. S. (2008). Associations between premarital sex and leaving school in four sub-Saharan African countries. *Studies in Family Planning, 39*(4), 337–350.

Birch, D. A. (2017). Improving schools, improving school health education, improving public health: The role of SOPHE members. *Health Education and Behavior, 44*(6), 839–844.

Curtis, V. A., Danquah, L. O., & Aunger, R. V. (2009). Planned, motivated and habitual hygiene behaviour: An eleven country review. *Health Education Research, 24*(4), 655–673.

Davis, J., Macintyre, A., Odagiri, M., Suriastini, W., Cordova, A., Huggett, C., Agius, P. A., Faiqoh, Budiyani, A. E., Quillet, C., Cronin, A. A., Diah, N. M., Triwahyunto, A., Luchters, S., & Kennedy, E. (2018). Menstrual hygiene management and school absenteeism among adolescent students in Indonesia: Evidence from a cross-sectional school-based survey. *Tropical Medicine and International Health: TM and IH, 23*(12), 1350–1363.

Dauenhauer, K., Schlenk, J., & Langkau, T. (2016). *Managing WASH in schools: Is the education sector ready? A thematic discussion series hosted by GIZ and SuSanA*. Sustainable Sanitation Alliance.

Fahimi, R. F., & Moghadam, V. M. (2003). Empowering women, developing society*: Female Education in the Middle East and North Africa*; Population Reference Bureau: Washington, DC, USA, 1–7.

Field Guide: Hardware for Group Handwashing in Schools. Deutsche Gesellschaft für *Internationale Zusammenarbeit (GIZ), Philippines. ISBN 978-3-95645-057-0*

Fiske, E. B. (2012). *WORLD of gender equality in education of gender equality in education* (p. 8).

Freeman, M. C., Greene, L. E., Dreibelbis, R., Saboori, S., Muga, R., Brumback, B., & Rheingans, R. (2012). Assessing the impact of a school-based water treatment, hygiene and sanitation programme on pupil absence in Nyanza Province, Kenya: A cluster-randomized trial. *Tropical Medicine and International Health, 17*(3), 380–391.

Freudenberg, N., & Ruglis, J. (2007). Reframing school dropout as a public health issue. *Preventing Chronic Disease, 4*(4), 1.

Giddens, A. (2006). *Sociology* (5th ed.). Polity Press.

Haines, L., & Rogers, J. (2000). A study of drinking facilities in schools. *Nursing times, 96*(40), 2.

Hargreaves, J. R., Morison, L. A., Kim, J. C., Bonell, C. P., Porter, J. D., Watts, C., Busza, J., Phetla, G., & Pronyk, P. M. (2008). The association between school attendance, HIV infection and sexual behaviour among young people in rural South Africa. *Journal of Epidemiology and Community Health, 62*(2), 113–119.

Hennegan, J., OlaOlorun, F. M., Oumarou, S., Alzouma, S., Guiella, G., Omoluabi, E., & Schwab, K. J. (2021). School and work absenteeism due to menstruation in three West African countries: Findings from PMA2020 surveys. *Sexual and Reproductive Health Matters, 29*(1), 1915940.

Herz, B., & Sperling, G. (2004). What works in girls' education: Evidence and policies from the developing world: A report by barbara herz and gene sperling.

"Hygiene: Overview". World Health Organization (WHO). 2020

Jakab, Z. (2011). *Public health: Investing in a healthier future*. World Health Organisation, Regional Office for Europe.

Jukes, M., Simmons, S., & Bundy, D. (2008). Education and vulnerability: The role of schools in protecting young women and girls from HIV in southern Africa. *AIDS (London, England), 22*(Suppl 4), S41–S56.

Karlin, B. (1988). Hygiene education in primary Schools. *International Journal of Water Sanitation and Waste, 6*(3), 1.

Koolwal, G., & Van de Walle, D. (2010). *Access to water, women's work and child outcomes*. The World Bank.

Koolwal, G., & van de Walle, D. (2013). Access to water, women's work, and child outcomes. *Economic Development and Cultural Change, 61*(2), 369–405.

Koopman, J. S. (1978). Diarrhoea and school toilet hygiene in Cali, Colombia. *American Journal of Epidemiology, 107*(5), 412–420.

Luby, S. P., Agboatwalla, M., Feikin, D. R., Painter, J., Billhimer, W., Altaf, A., & Hoekstra, R. M. (2005). Effect of handwashing on child health: A randomised controlled trial. *Lancet (London, England), 366*(9481), 225–233.

Mathekgana, M. A., Chauke, L. K., & Otieno, F. A. (2001). Improvement of environmental health and hygiene practices–a case study in the Northern Province. *Water Science and Technology: A Journal of the International Association on Water Pollution Research, 44*(6), 109–117.

National Education Policy (NEP). (2020). *National education policy 2020*. Ministry of Education, Government of India.

Petrina, S. (2006). The Medicalization of Education: A Historiographic Synthesis. *History of Education Quarterly, 46*(4), 503–531.

"Puberty Education and Menstrual Hygiene Management". *UNESCO. 2014.*

Raising Even More Clean Hands: Advancing Learning, Health and Participation through WASH in Schools. (2010). New York: UNICEF, United Nations C*hildren's Fund.*

Raising Even More Clean Hands: Advancing Health, Learning and Equity through WASH in Schools, Joint Call to Action. (2012) UNICEF.

Rodríguez Martín, J. A., del Holgado Molina, M. M., & Salinas Fernández, J. A. (2015). An index for quantifying female education and child health in emerging economies. *Archives of Disease in Childhood, 100*(Suppl 1), S10–S12.

Scaling Up Group Handwashing in Schools—Compendium of Group Washing Facilities Across the Globe (2016). New York, USA; Eschborn, Germany: UNICEF, GIZ.

School Community Manual—Indonesia (Formerly Manual for Teachers), Fit for School. (2014). GIZ Fit for School, Philippines. ISBN 978-3-95645-250-5.

School Sanitation and Hygiene Education—India, UNICEF and IRC International Water and Sanitation Centre, The Netherlands, 2002.

Shahid, N. S., Greenough, W. B., 3rd., Samadi, A. R., Huq, M. I., & Rahman, N. (1996). Hand washing with soap reduces diarrhoea and spread of bacterial pathogens in a Bangladesh village. *Journal of Diarrhoeal Diseases Research, 14*(2), 85–89.

Snel, M., & Short, K. (2005). The evidence to support hygiene, sanitation and water in schools. *School Sanitation and Hygiene Education, 23*(3), 1.

Sommer, M., Caruso, B. A., Sahin, M., Calderon, T., Cavill, S., Mahon, T., & Phillips-Howard, P. A. (2015). Managing menstruation in the workplace and educational settings: A global review. *Waterlines, 34*(2), 137–154.

Tegegne, T. K., & Sisay, M. M. (2014). Menstrual hygiene management and school absenteeism among female adolescent students in Northeast Ethiopia. *BMC Public Health, 14*, 1118.

Temitayo, I. O. (2016). Knowledge and Practices of Personal Hygiene among Senior Secondary School Students of Ambassadors College, Ile-Ife, Nigeria. *Texila International Journal of Public Health, 4*(4), 648–660.

The Importance of Water and Sanitation. (2015). UNICEF.

Tiberghien, J. E. (2016). *School WASH research: India country report*. WaterAid.

Tiberghien, JE (2016). *School WASH research: Pakistan country report*. WaterAid.

Tiberghien, J. E. (2016c). *School WASH research: Nepal country report*. WaterAid.

Tiberghien, J. E. (2016d). *School WASH research: Bangladesh country report*. WaterAid.

UNESCO. (2012). *Education for sustainable development sourcebook*. United Nations Educational, Scientific and Cultural Organisation.

UNESCO. (2014). *Teaching and learning: Achieving quality for all (Education for all global monitoring report 2013/4)*. United Nations Educational, Scientific and Cultural Organisation.

UNESCO. (2016). *Education 2030: Incheon declaration and framework for action towards inclusive and equitable quality education and lifelong learning for all*. United Nations Educational, Scientific and Cultural Organisation.

UNESCO. (2023). *Reimagining our futures together: A new social contract for education*. United Nations Educational, Scientific and Cultural Organisation.

Vivas, A. P., Gelaye, B., Aboset, N., Kumie, A., Berhane, Y., & Williams, M. A. (2010). Knowledge, attitudes and practices (KAP) of hygiene among school children in Angolela, Ethiopia. *Journal of Preventive Medicine and Hygiene, 51*(2), 73–79.

Wallen, M. (2015). Linking health and academic success. In D. A. Birch & D. M. Videto (Eds.), *Promoting health and academic success* (pp. 65–74). Human Kinetics.

Woolf, S. H., Johnson, R. E., Phillips, R. L., Jr., & Phillipsen, M. (2007). Giving everyone the health of the educated: An examination of whether social change would save more lives than medical advances. *American Journal of Public Health, 97*, 679–693.

World Bank. (2015). *World development report 2015: Mind, society, and behaviour*. World Bank Group.

World Health Organisation (WHO). (2004). *Promoting mental health: Concepts, emerging evidence, practice (Summary Report)*. World Health Organisation.

Water, Sanitation and Hygiene. (2016). UNICEF.

Water, Sanitation and Hygiene for Populations at Risk. (2005).

Water, Sanitation, and Hygiene: Introduction, UNICEF. 2015.

World Health Organization. Better Health for Poor Children. (2009).

World Health Organization (WHO). The World Health Report. (2002). *Reducing risks, promoting healthy life*.

World Bank Group. Education Global Practice: Smarter Education Systems for Brighter Futures. (2022).

World Health Organization & UN-Water. (2014). *UN-water global analysis and assessment of sanitation and drinking water (GLAAS) 2014 report: Investing in water and sanitation: increasing access, reducing inequalities*. World Health Organization.

Zajacova, A., & Lawrence, E. M. (2018). The relationship between education and health: Reducing disparities through a contextual approach. *Annual Review of Public Health, 39*, 273–289.

Water, Sanitation, and Hygiene Practices Among Slums Population in Bhubaneswar City, Odisha

11

Ajit Kumar Lenka and Rajshree Chanchal

Abstract

Water sanitation and hygiene plays very crucial role in public health. Without proper water supply, sanitation, and inadequate hygiene practice leads to infectious diseases. Every year, around 37.7 million people in India get waterborne infections. In 2015, diarrhea killed over 117,000 children under the age of five, accounting for 13% of all under-five mortality in the country and 22% of the global total. Water-related diseases also cause the loss of almost 73 million workdays each year, resulting in an estimated economic loss of approximately $600 million (United Nation in Health, Water and Sanitation | United Nations in India, 2022). The Swachh Bharat Mission and all sanitation-related metrics from NFHS 5 show that sanitation coverage has increased in the county. Uttar Pradesh, Bihar, Madhya Pradesh, Odisha, and Jharkhand are the states with the worst performance, according to the Swachh Bharat Mission. These states alone account for 37% of the Indian population, or 448 million people (NFHS, 5). Diarrhea is India's third biggest cause of death. Odisha will meet the MDG target within the next century. Madhya Pradesh planned to fulfil the goal in 2105, but Odisha did so in 2116 (Bhagat in Rural and urban sanitation in India, 2014. https://www.researchgate.net/publication/269702342_Rural_and_Urban_Sanitation_in_India). The current paper discusses the condition of water supply and sanitation facilities and the hygienic practices among slums population in Bhubaneswar city. Mixed method approach has been used to understand the issues of access to sanitation and hygiene practices in two slums of Bhubaneswar city. The findings suggest that limited duration of piped water supply forces slum dwellers to fetch water from the public hand pump. The handpump water quality is poor due to contamination which makes it unfit for drinking. Respondents said that many times they have to carry drinking water from far off places. Majority of the household don't have toilet facilities and they practiced open defecation. Those HHs have toilet facility they did not have the running water connectivity in the toilets. They small dimension of the toilets makes it difficult for regular use. Both slum areas do not have drainage facility hence majority of households are forced to drain the waste water on the streets which leads to breeding of mosquito and contamination of water and generate foul smell. People

A. K. Lenka (✉)
Department of Public Health, Noida International University, Delhi, India
e-mail: ajitlenka.lenka@gmail.com

R. Chanchal
School of Education Studies, Dr. B. R. Ambedkar University Delhi, Delhi, India
e-mail: rajshree07raj@gmail.com

S. S. Acharya et al. (eds.), *Paradigm Shifts in Population and Health in India*, Sustainable Development Goals Series, https://doi.org/10.1007/978-981-95-1719-0_11

are experiencing various issues due to poor drainage facility. Most of the HHs were not using garbage bin and they throw HHs garbage in open space. Some of the places the garbage bin is damaged. Majority of the people are not using any type soap for handwashing and less awareness about benefits of handwashing practice in preventing certain diseases. Another reason for not washing hands is lack of access to sufficient water for household use. Thus, there is need to provide basic safe drinking and sanitation facilities to all slum dwellers. Spread awareness about benefits of hygienic practices and garbage management at community level.

11.1 Introduction

Adequate water supply and sanitation are essential to ensure human health (Eid, 2015). Globally, 844 million of people are living without access to safe water supply. More than two billion of people are accessing drinking water from contaminate sources. Poor water supply and lack of sanitation facilities is the main reason for spread of diarrhoea, malaria, fluorosis, guinea worm diseases, trachoma, typhoid (Acharya, 2015; Buttenheim, 2008; Bhunia, 2009). Every year 502,000 deaths happen due to contaminated water (WHO, 2018). Improved water supply and sanitation facilities are critical to economic growth and health in developing countries. Over 10% of diseases at global level occur because of inadequate water supply and poor sanitation (Min & Hung, 2011). In a study Tiwari and Nayak (2015) found that, households who do not get sufficient public taps or hand pumps water as a result of suffering from waterborne diseases.

Inadequate access to safe drinking water and poor sanitation can result in malnutrition, waterborne illnesses, gastroenteritis, diarrhoea, and dysentery (Kuberan et al., 2015). According to WHO estimates, insufficient drinking water and sanitation were responsible for 58% of diarrhoea deaths in 2012, totalling 840,000 deaths in low and middle-income countries. Safe, appropriate water supply and sanitation minimize infections, promote health, and lower family expenditures (Karan & Harada, 2002; Howard & Bartram, 2003; Government of India, 2012).

Evans (2007) in his study shows that millions of urban dwellers are excluded for getting water supply and sanitation service delivery by formal system. Galiani et al. (2005) study reflected that the improper water supply and poor sanitation cause of communicable diseases in overcrowded slums.

11.2 Urban Water Policy in Odisha

In 2013, Odisha introduced its first urban water supply policy. The policy's primary goal is to handle the complex, technical, institutional, social, and environmental difficulties that urban water supply agencies face, as well as to ensure universal access to drinkable water for all individuals living in urban areas at an affordable price. The policy emphasized the improvement of infrastructure, institutions, monitoring mechanisms, and regulatory frameworks for providing water services at all levels. Individual performance recognition was proposed as a way to ensure greater service provision incentives, such as development funding. It is also recommended that suitable training and skill development programs be organized for individuals participating in water provision services on a regular basis (H & UDO, 2013).

11.3 Urban Sanitation Policy in Odisha

According to the government of India, "sanitation is a state subject ground on implementation and sustenance of public health and environmental outcomes require strong city level institutions and stakeholders" (GoO, 2016). To improve sanitation conditions in Odisha, the first Urban Sanitation Strategy (USS) was launched in 2011, with the goal of making Odisha's cities and towns completely sanitized, safe, healthy, and liveable. The Housing and Urban Department of the Government of Odisha launched the National Urban Sanitation Policy (NSUP) in 2008.

Water supply and sanitation in urban Odisha are in poor condition, and access to safe drinking water is a big issue. Almost half of the households did not have access to safe drinking water, and just 42% had access to treated drinking water, with fewer than 57% having sources on their premises. According to sanitation data, more over 35% of urban households did not have access to any form of toilet facility. According to the 2011 census, urban Odisha has the second highest rate of open defecation in India. Odisha ranks second among the five most critical states (Chhattisgarh, Odisha, Jharkhand, Bihar, and Madhya Pradesh) with the highest urban open defecation (RGI, 2011). The first graph depicts the district-by-district average urban population, Open Defecation (OD) percentage of the district urban population, and the proportion of district urban population to total urban population in Odisha. In Khordha district, roughly 48% of the population resides in cities. The findings also suggest that more than half of the urban population (53%) engages in OD. Odisha's capital city, Bhubaneswar, is located in the Khordha district. Despite the fact that the majority of government and non-government financing is being earmarked for infrastructure development, more than half of the population is opting for OD Which has had a negative impact on the capital's development and progress (Graph 11.1).

11.4 Condition of Water Supply and Sanitation in Bhubaneswar City

The population of Bhubaneswar is rapidly rising. According to the 2011 census, the population density in Bhubaneswar city is 6533 people per square kilometre, which is greater than the state's average population growth. Figure 11.1 illustrates that Bhubaneswar's population increased 50 times between 1951 and 2011. The city's geographical area has also expanded throughout the same period (Office of the Registrar General & Census Commissioner, 2011).

11.5 Urban Slums

In slums, people live in compact area in temporary built settlement in the cities. Slums are characterized by inadequate housing, overcrowding, and deplorable living conditions. NSSO (2001) defines slum as a "*compact settlement with a collection of poorly built tenements, mostly of temporary nature, crowded together usually with inadequate sanitation and drinking water facilities in unhygienic conditions*". As per the 2011 census, slums are mainly three types such as: Notified, recognised and identified. In case of Bhubaneswar, as per the special state government act slum are categorised on the basis of land rights such as authorised[1] and unauthorised.[2] Authorised slums are approved by the BMC, existing within BMC boundaries and dwellers retain their land rights. Unauthorised Slums are illegal settlements, on the government land and BMC do not approve of these and the dwellers do not have any land right (BMC, Officials).

Slums have expanded in the city as a result of urbanization, and 30% of the population now lives in them (Praharaj, 2021). The data also said that there are 436 slums in the city, with just 116 slums authorized by the state government and being under the jurisdiction of the Bhubaneswar Municipal Corporation. Slum neighborhoods continue to have poor water and sanitation amenities. More than 80% of the population practices open defecation for a variety of reasons, including poor economic conditions and a lack of space to build a

[1] The present study uses the define the Odisha property right to slum dwellers and prevention of new slum Bill, 2012 to defines authorised as "Competent Authority means the Authority empowered under the Odisha Public Premises Act, 1972 and the Odisha Prevention of Land Encroachment".

[2] The present study uses the define the Odisha property right to slum dwellers and prevention of new slum bill, 2012 to defines unauthorised as "Act, 1972 to exercise power of eviction and demolition over the land on which such encroachment or construction of illegal structure or building has been reported".

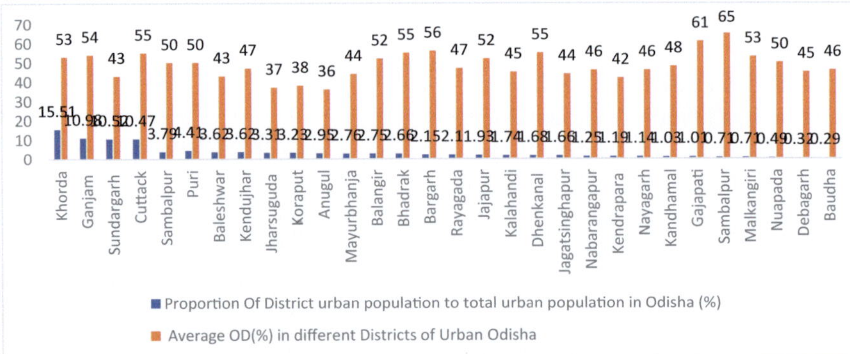

Graph 11.1 Urban population and the prevalence of open defecation in the districts of Odisha. *Source* Office of the Registrar General & Census Commissioner, India 2011, https://urban.odisha.gov.in/sites/default/files/2021-05/Policy_Manual_Guidelines_OUSP%20Policy%202017%20%281%29.pdf

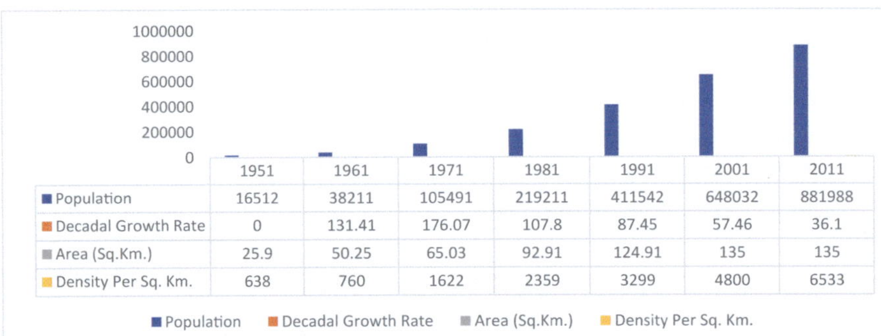

	1951	1961	1971	1981	1991	2001	2011
Population	16512	38211	105491	219211	411542	648032	881988
Decadal Growth Rate	0	131.41	176.07	107.8	87.45	57.46	36.1
Area (Sq.Km.)	25.9	50.25	65.03	92.91	124.91	135	135
Density Per Sq. Km.	638	760	1622	2359	3299	4800	6533

Fig. 11.1 Decadal population growth patterns in Bhubaneswar City. *Source* Census report 2011, CDP, Bhubaneswar (2006)

toilet within the home. In slum regions, just 18% of the population utilizes in-house toilets, whereas 2% use community toilets (USAID, 2012).

In Bhubaneswar, the PHEO and BMC have taken the effort to provide water supply facilities. The primary sources of drinking water in the city are surface and ground water. Data shows that 75% of daily requirement of potable water are from "*Manhanadi*" and "*Daya*" rivers and rest of the water requirement is fulfilled by open wells and tube wells. In the city presently water supply is 275 lpcd. Data shows that everyday 206 Million Litres Daily (MLD) (surface: 166 MLD + groundwater 40 MLD) water supply for nearly 7.50 lakhs population in 2005. Currently, water supply per capita is 181 lpcd but demand is 242 lpcd per capita. The pipe water supply covers 911 km and it covers about 55% of the total road length of 1600 km by PHED in other words Only 17 wards are fully covered by piped water supply and 26 wards out of 46 wards are partially covered while rest of wards do not have water supply facilities. Other wards are mainly covered by Tube wells and wells for fulfilling their everyday water needs. The coverage of water supply does not fully cover the majority of the population. Especially in urban poor (slum) areas, water coverage of local point distribution of network, public stand post tube wells details are not available. Even in peripheral areas, water supply information in terms of distribution where the water supply is weak, where is water distribution inequitable, where is water supply services connection is illegal/uncountable is not available. In these areas there is a need for equitable system of water supply facilities and cost also needs to be recovered (USAID, 2012).

Figure 11.2 shows that the current water supply is insufficient to meet the people's demand for maintaining their day-to-day life activities. Every year population grows rapidly in the city and the demand for water supply is increases. Data also highlights that two third of slum areas do not have access to safe drinking water facilities (BMC, n.d.; USAID, 2012). Only 17% of the slum areas have access to pipe water supply facilities through public stand posts in their locality and one fourth of slums depend upon both public stand post and hand pump/tube wells across the city. The duration of water supply is a major problem for accessing water facilities, data reported that water accessed only two hours a day in 69 slums while 17 slums reported that they accessed water an hour a day and some of the slums accessed for less than that. Data also mentioned that 10% of the sources are from open wells and ponds. Eight per cent of slums did not have access drinking water facilities (Satpathy, 2011).

11.6 Sanitation Facilities in Bhubaneswar City

In Bhubaneswar City, BMC is taking most challenging role to provide city dwellers a healthy life and clean city. Availing central assistance under the Central Pollution Control Board, BMC prepared a Detailed Project Report (DPR) for management of solid waste in corporation area with a total project cost of Rs. 23.68 crores. Sanitation workers have been engaged in cleaning work to provide healthy life and clean city. Sanitation worker is mainly engaged to provide sanitation services such as segregation of waste at the source of generation, house-to-house collection of wastes, cleaning of roads, night cleaning on busy and important roads, market areas and transportation of waste from different areas up to the selected disposal site, collection of wastes from a particular area/lane in a fixed time by using wheel barrows/pedal bicycles etc. For providing better sanitation services to citizens, BMC has privatized sanitation/cleaning services in respective 57 wards out of 67 wards and rest of 10 wards are under the BMC supervision for sanitation/cleaning work. Number of wards taken by three private agencies such as Jagruti, PMR and Ramky are 28, 14, and 15 to start initiatives for providing sanitation service facilities in city under the supervision BMC (BMC, n.d.; USAID, 2012). From Table 11.4 we can see that there are Sulabha Sauchalya (11), Public Toilet (6) and Public Urinal (9) in the city. The condition of public toilets is very poor and majority of population do not use public toilets due to lack of water supply and cleanliness, most of the people do not use as there are high chances of infection (BMC, n.d.).

In Bhubaneswar city, BMC is mainly taking responsibility of solid waste collection, transportation and disposal within the city municipal limits which is mainly handled by the municipal organization body. Every day, the city generates roughly 300 MT of municipal solid waste (biodegradable and non-biodegradable). Every day, 400 g of garbage are generated per person, which exceeds the normative threshold of 250 g per capita. Domestic chores, fruit and vegetable markets, hotels and restaurants, fish/meat shops, markets, street sweeping, hospitals, offices, and institutions all contribute to the city's solid waste generation. The report stated that a scientific and well-developed procedure of source segregation and waste storage at sources was frequently absent, resulting in a haphazard and ad hoc primary collection. The report also noted the possibility of initially implementing source segregation in a few places, particularly in the city's commercial and high-class well-developed residential neighbourhoods. Otherwise, most areas did not have bin storage for domestic, commerce, or institutional garbage, and relatively few households used buckets, plastic bins, or plastic bags to keep their waste. Most residential areas toss rubbish on streets, sewers, or public and private open spaces, which degrades the overall quality of the environment (USAID, 2012).

Many private organisations have also taken part in solid waste management, which is promoted by ULB. In the city, the BMC is implementing steps to collect rubbish from houses and establishments that store waste so that it does not end up on the street or in other open areas, and put it in the community storage bin. Another major issue that must be addressed is the necessity for

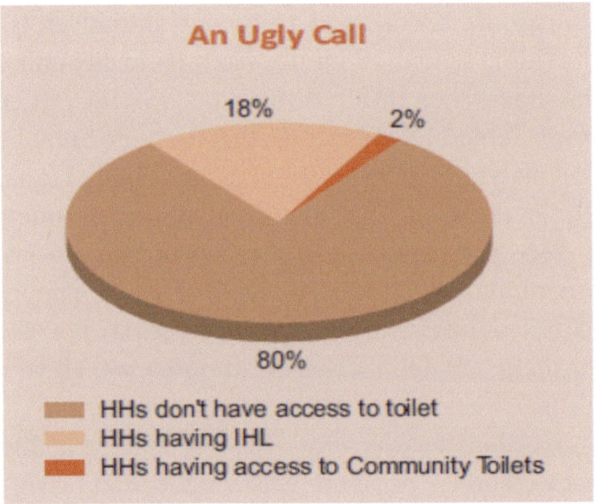

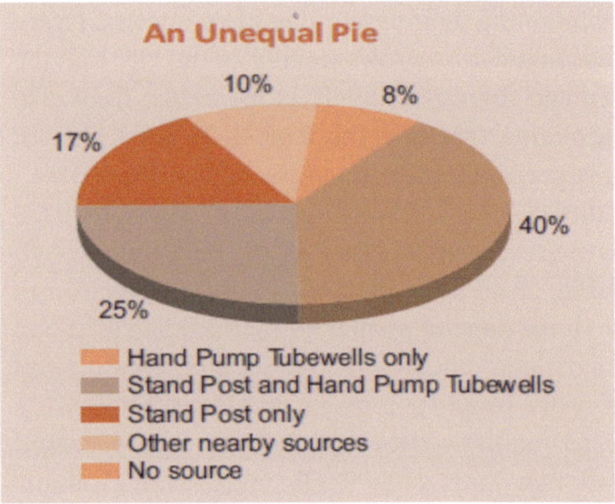

Fig. 11.2 Slums' access to water supply and sanitation facilities in Bhubaneswar City. *Source* USAID 2012, http://populationfoundation.in/wp-content/uploads/2015/09/WASH-Fact-n-Factors-Bhubaneswar.pdf Accessed 13/05/2017

guidelines for the type of storage, receptacles, and waste segregation so that people involved in this activity can do their jobs easily. Sanitation personnel gather debris from streets and other sources, but non-biodegradable waste is not separated, compromising uniformity with biodegradable waste (USAID, 2012).

Bhubaneswar is the fastest growing city in Odisha and due to city growth; rural areas are being incorporated under the urban areas. In these "new" areas, coming under the urban areas, the situation of water supply and sanitation is not abysmal. In urban Odisha, average piped water supply is 127 L per capita per day (lpcd) from Public Health Engineering Organization (PHEO)[3] and pipe which varies from town to town. In Bhubaneswar, 265 lpcd from PHEO but after that majority of the population is still not getting the adequate with amount of water supply. The majority of households have poor water supply and sanitation compared to the city's central neighbourhoods. The government has introduced various schemes and policies of water supply and sanitation but still the water supply and sanitation facilities remain poor (USAID, 2012). Due to poor water supply and sanitation facilities number of disease occurred among people. Nearly half of the population have no latrine facilities and the condition of water supply is very poor (USAID, 2012). Thus, the current study aims to investigate the state of water supply and sanitation, as well as hygiene practices among Bhubaneswar's slum population.

11.7 Methodology

It is a cross-sectional research. The study collected both qualitative and quantitative data. Interviews, observations, and questionnaires were utilized to obtain qualitative and quantitative information from research participants. The data was collected using purposive sampling. Qualitative data was acquired through a semi-structured interview schedule, case studies, and Focus Group Discussions (FGD). Quantitative data was acquired using a standardized interview schedule. A total of 290 houses were chosen by easy sampling.

11.8 Results

Table one data shows that in both study areas a total 290 of households. Male responses were higher than female responses. Both study locations had a higher percentage of Hindu households. In terms of educational achievement, approximately one-third (29.7%) of respondents

[3] The main aim and objective of the organisation, Public Health Engineer Organisation (PHEO), is the inspection and Monitoring of Water Supply and Sewerage System of all Urban Local Bodies and Census towns of Odisha.

were illiterate. Thirty percent of the respondents had finished primary education, followed by middle school (19.7%) and matriculation or higher (18.6%).

According to the data, SC had the highest percentage of households (39.7%), followed by OBC (35.9%), Others (23.1%), and ST (1.4%). Data also shows that in the Bhimpur area, nearly half of the homes belonged to the SC community, compared to the Naharkanta area (32.9%). Similarly, in Nahrkanta, a bigger number of respondents (45.3%) belonged to the OBC community than in Bhimpur (22.5%). Regarding the marital status of the survey population. The findings suggest that a higher percentage of the study group was married (88.3%). While 4.5% of survey respondents were divorced, 3.8% were unmarried, and 2.8% lived apart from their families (Table 11.1).

Table 11.2 contains information about household characteristics. According to data, the majority of households (77.6%) belonged to nuclear families, while just 22.4% belonged to joint families. In terms of home ownership, data show that a higher percentage of households reported not having any house records with them. While 32.8% of households carried their home documents with them. According to data, Nahrakanta had a greater percentage of households having household records (47.6%) than the Bhimpur area (11.7%).

In terms of dwelling types available to the surveyed population, more than half (51.7%) lived in semi pucca houses, followed by pucca houses (31%), and 17.2% lived in kutcha houses. According to data, Nahrakanta has a higher number of people living in pucca houses (42.4%) than the Bhimpur area (15%). Similarly, in Bhimpur, a higher proportion of respondents lived in semi-pucca dwellings than in Naharkanta (37.6%). When it comes to the types of ventilation facilities accessible in the study population's homes, data show that more than one-third of the families did not have any. While 57.6% of households had window facilities, only 12.1% of households had skylights (Table 11.2).

About the availability of a separate space for cooking, data show that 66.2% of households have one, while 33.8% do not. In Bhimpur, a higher proportion of homes (66.7%) lacked a separate cooking area than in Naharkanta. In terms of power availability, records show that the majority of households (97.6%) have it in their homes.

Table 11.3 shows information about water supply facilities in individual homes. According to data, around 35.2% of homes had access to tap residence water, followed by public tap stand posts (29.7%) and public handpumps (24.8%). While 6.9% of households received water from unprotected wells, 2.1% used tube wells, and 1.4% used municipal tanks. In Bhimpur, the highest percentage of houses (30.8%) obtained water from public tap standposts, followed by tap dwelling

Table 11.1 Socio-demographic profile of the study population

Respondents	Bhimpur *N* (%)	Naharkanta *N* (%)	Total *N* (%)
Male	96 (80)	137 (80.6)	233 (80.3)
Female	24 (20)	33 (19.4)	57 (19.7)
Religion			
Hindu	119 (99.2)	170 (100)	289 (99.7)
Muslim	1 (0.8)	0 (0)	1 (0.3)
Education attained			
Illiterate	35 (29.2)	51 (30)	86 (29.7)
Primary school complete	48 (40)	45 (26.5)	93 (32.1)
Middle school	22 (18.3)	35 (20.6)	57 (19.7)
Matriculation above	15 (12.5)	39 (22.9)	54 (18.6)
Social identity			
SC	59 (49.2)	56 (32.9)	115 (39.7)
ST	4 (3.3)	0 (0)	4 (1.4)
OBC	27 (22.5)	77 (45.3)	104 (35.9)
Non-SC, ST, and OBC	30 (25)	37 (21.8)	67 (23.1)
Marital status			
Married	108 (90)	148 (87.1)	256 (88.3)
Unmarried	2 (1.7)	9 (5.3)	11 (3.8)
Divorce	0 (0)	2 (1.2)	2 (0.7)
Separated	3 (2.5)	5 (2.9)	8 (2.8)
Widowed	7 (5.8)	6 (3.5)	13 (4.5)

Source Fieldwork

Table 11.2 Household characteristics

Household types	Bhimpur *N* (%)	Naharkanta *N* (%)	Total *N* (%)
Nuclear family	106 (88.3)	119 (70)	225 (77.6)
Joint family	14 (11.7)	51 (30)	65 (22.4)
Record of the house			
Yes	14 (11.7)	81 (47.6)	95 (32.8)
No	106 (88.3)	89 (52.4)	195 (67.2)
Type of the house			
Pucca	18 (15)	72 (42.4)	90 (31)
Semi-Pucca	86 (71.7)	64 (37.6)	150 (51.7)
Kuccha	16 (13.3)	34 (20)	50 (17.2)
Type of ventilation facilities			
Window	44 (36.7)	123 (72.4)	167 (57.6)
Skylight	13 (10.8)	22 (12.9)	35 (12.1)
No ventilation	63 (52.5)	25 (14.7)	88 (30.3)
Separate space for cooking			
Yes	40 (33.3)	152 (89.4)	192 (66.2)
No	80 (66.7)	18 (10.6)	98 (33.8)
Electricity facilities			
Yes	117 (97.5)	166 (97.6)	283 (97.6)
No	3 (2.5)	4 (2.4)	7 (2.4)

Source Fieldwork

(28.3%), public hand pump (22.5%), and public unprotected well (16.7%). While in Naharkanta, the majority of houses (40%) received water from their own taps, followed by public tap stand-posts (28.8%), public handpumps (26.5%), and 2.4% from tube wells and municipality tanks (Table 11.3). Some of the main informants, community leaders, and respondents from both research areas had the following views:

The Key Informants (KI6) Bhimpur area mentioned that-

> The population of Bhubaneswar depends on Daya river water for fulfilling their day to day needs. In the community people are depending on pipe supply water, public hand pump, and municipality water tank. In the area people are mostly used hand pump pipe water. Most of the households in the area did not take pipe water supply and they mainly take water from public stand post and public hand pump. A year ago the local government pressured water consumers and now they need to register, according to the local government rules. Some of the households also registered in the area. The public stand posts were removed by the PHDE officials. The pipe water supply is working properly and people face various problem for getting water (KI6, Bhimpur Area)

Table 11.3 Water supply facilities

Source of water supply	Bhimpur *N* (%)	Naharkanta *N* (%)	Total *N* (%)
Tube well	2 (1.7)	4 (2.4)	6 (2.1)
Public hand pump	27 (22.5)	45 (26.5)	72 (24.8)
Tap dwelling	34 (28.3)	68 (40)	102 (35.2)
Public tap standpost	37 (30.8)	49 (28.8)	86 (29.7)
Public unprotected well	20 (16.7)	0 (0)	20 (6.9)
Municipality tank	0 (0)	4 (2.4)	4 (1.4)
Treatment of drinking water			
Electric purifier	2 (1.7)	5 (2.9)	7 (2.4)
Filter	0 (0)	20 (11.8)	20 (6.9)
Bleach	1 (0.8)	0 (0)	1 (0.3)
Without treatment	117 (97.5)	145 (85.3)	262 (90.3)
Duration of water supply in the morning time			
Don't come	46 (38.3)	22 (12.9)	68 (23.4)
Half an hour	74 (61.7)	148 (87.1)	222 (76.6)
Duration of water supply in the evening			
Don't come	98 (81.7)	3 (1.8)	101 (34.8)
Half an hour	22 (18.3)	91 (53.5)	113 (39)
One hour	0 (0)	76 (44.7)	76 (26.2)
Perception of drinking water supply			
Clean	99 (82.5)	91 (53.5)	190 (65.5)
Dirty	9 (7.5)	79 (46.5)	88 (30.3)
Satisfied	12 (10)	0 (0)	12 (4.1)

Source Fieldwork

This was also evident form the group discussions:

> In the area pipe water supply is irregular, people face problems in getting water. Only three public hand pumps are operational; one is not used due to poor quality of water. In absence of pipe water supply, most households depend on public hand pump. There are many conflicts over water supply.

> Many cases were registered at police station (FGD1, Bhimpur area)

In Naharakanta the FGD2 also reflected similar issues:

> for water, people mainly depend on supply water, public hand pump and well water. Pipe water covers more than fifty-five percent of the area and rest of the area need to work. Supply water generally comes in the mornings and evenings. When there is a lack of it, people mainly use public hand pump for drinking purpose. Some households have their own water bowring in the area (FGD2, Naharakanta Area).

The KI4 also corroborated:

> The main problem in the area is lack of water. Without water people face many problems, especially children, women and the elders. Women take the responsibility of collecting water, while men generally work outside. The pipe water never reaches households due to the poor pressure. People collect drinking water from outside of their colony. The situation is very difficult, especially in the summers (KI4, Bhimpur Area).

Another KI4 from Naharakanta said:

> The community mainly depends on well water. Most of the households in our community do not have access to pipe water supply or public hand pump. We demanded access to proper water facility many times, but the local councillors never paid any heed to our requests. People use well water, while the other community uses supply and public hand pump water (KI4, Naharakanta area).

Sankar, a 39-year-old also expressed similar ideas:

> ...people are now being more politicised on basics facilities provided by the government, including water supply. Nowadays, particularly lower caste people are targeted and disbarred from using basic facilities provided by the government. In the community, majority of the household's dependent on well water for drinking, while others use canal water (Naharakanta Area).

According to study, the majority of households drank untreated water. Only 6.9% of households used filters, while 2.4% used electric purifiers to treat drinking water. According to data, Bhimpur has a larger percentage of families consuming untreated water than Naharkanta (Table 11.3). It was discovered that water was treated in a variety of ways before ingestion. Those who cannot afford to buy packaged drinking water are compelled to consume unsafe water. Some of the responders stated their views as follows:

Sasmita a 35-year-old woman stated:

> The supply water quality not good, as more amount of bleaching powder is used. It is not drinkable. My family use hand pump water for drinking purposes. During winter seasons we did boil water for drinking purposes (Bhimpur Area).

The discussions in the FGD 1 supported the issues and is evident as follows:

> In the area, majority population are dependent on public hand pump. Only three hand pump are workable and rest of hand pump unworkable. The quality of water in the area not good. in the area one of the hand pump water undrinkable due to iron contain more. So majority of the population are dependent on two hand pump in the area. Most of time crowdedness happened to get water. Sometime water coming very slow and more than half an hour take to get full bucket of water (FGD 1, Bhimpur area).

Regarding the duration of water delivery in the morning, around 76.6% of homes said that it was for half an hour. While 23.4% of families reported not receiving any water delivery in the morning. In Bhimpur, a higher percentage of families (38.3%) reported no water supply at all compared to Nharkanta. Similarly, during the evening, more than one-third of the houses reported no water supply. Furthermore, 39% of households stated that they only had access to water for 30 min. While 26.2% of responders received water for only one hour (Table 11.3). Some of the responders stated their views as follows:

The KI6 leader said:

> When both the amount and duration of water reception are severely limited, people are not able to collect water from public stand posts. Sometimes there are conflicts over these issues" (KI6, Bhimpur area). Sasmita, a 39-year-old, reported: "Pipe water comes with very low pressure and for a limited time, which causes difficulties in water collection. The crowd around the stand posts does not make it easier (Bhimpur Area, Site 2).

Another respondent stated:

> The duration of water supply is a major problem in the case of pipe water. Every day they are conflicts over water, people use slang language during water collection. The main reason is short time of water reception. There are more conflicts among women during the time of water collection. Many case have registered in police station. In the area women are running all the direction to fetch water for drinking

purposes (Monalisha 37-year-old, Bhimpur Area, Site 2).

Data was collected on people's perceptions of water supply quality. According to data, 65% of respondents believed that water was clean. In both research locations, 30% of households reported having bad drinking water. Only 4% rated the water quality as satisfactory. More people of Bhimpur (82%), than Naharakanta, thought drinking water was clean. More respondents in Naharakanta (46% vs. 7% in Bhimpur) considered drinking water unsafe. A higher percentage of families (10%) in Bhimpur felt that drinking water was satisfactory (Table 11.3). Some responders expressed their views:

One of the respondents reported:

> The quality of water so poor in the area. We have no better option and belonged from poor socio-economic background we need to be struggling every day for accessing basic facilities. The struggle will never end it will continue. Because the situation remains same and the problems happen in the area increase day by day (Bhimpur Area, Bidulata, 42 year old, Site 1).

Bibek 37-year-old supported as follows:

> The quality of water very poor in the area. To get water we are facing more struggle then who will care about the quality of water. Either the water good or bad quality. We just use the water to fulfil our need (Bhimpur Area, Site 2).

Table 11.4 emphasizes the availability of toilet facilities in both study locations. According to the survey, 62.8% of households did not have a latrine. Only 37.2% of households had a toilet. It was also discovered that the Naharakanta area has a larger percentage of households (38.8%), while the Bhimpur area has the lowest percentage of households (35%), indicating that they have a toilet facility in their home.

Table 11.4 Toilet facility

Toilet of facilities	Bhimpur *N* (%)	Naharkanta *N* (%)	Total *N* (%)
Yes	42 (35)	66 (38.8)	108 (37.2)
No	78 (65)	104 (61.2)	182 (62.8)
Toilet of location			
Inside house	1 (2.4)	15 (22.7)	16 (14.8)
Outside for one HHs	34 (81)	51 (77.3)	85 (78.7)
Outside sharing HHs	7 (16.7)	0 (0)	7 (6.5)
Specification toilet			
Fully concrete structure	2 (4.8)	60 (90.9)	62 (57.4)
Only base is concrete	37 (88.1)	6 (9.1)	43 (39.8)
Septic tank	3 (7.1)	0 (0)	3 (2.8)
Water supply toilet			
Tap water with flush	1 (2.4)	62 (93.9)	63 (58.3)
No water supply	41 (97.6)	4 (6.1)	45 (41.7)
Don't water supply			
Bucket water	41 (97.6)	4 (6.1)	45 (41.7)
Pipe water	1 (2.4)	62 (93.9)	63 (58.3)
Aware about the government schemes			
Yes	6 (5)	18 (10.6)	24 (8.3)
No	114 (95)	152 (89.4)	266 (91.7)

Source Fieldwork

Table 11.4 summarizes the availability of toilet facilities in both study locations. According to the survey, 62.8% of households did not have a latrine. Only 37.2% of households had a toilet. It was also discovered that the Naharakanta area has a larger percentage of households (38.8%), while the Bhimpur area has the lowest percentage of households (35%), indicating that they have a toilet facility in their home. Data show that the majority of homes (78.7%) had a toilet outside their home. While 14.8% of homes had a toilet inside the house, 6.5% had one outside the house for sharing. According to the data, 88.3% of houses in the Bhimpur region had a toilet, while 77% of households in the Nahrkanta area had one outside their home. In the Bhimpur area, 16% of households shared toilet facilities located outside the house.

In terms of toilet facility specifications, data show that 57.4% of homes had a fully constructed toilet, 39.8% had a concrete base, and 2.8% had septic tank toilets. In Naharkanta, the majority of houses had entirely concrete toilet facilities, whereas in Bhimpur, 88.1% of families had only base-level concrete facilities (Table 11.4). Regarding the availability of water supply facilities in toilets, data show that in Bhimpur, the majority of households used bucket water, whereas in Naharkanta. It was discovered that in both research regions, female members had more problems than male members. Females are more vulnerable than male members. Some of the respondents' views are listed below.

Another respondent reported:

> We moved to this place eight year back. When we moved here, at that time my whole family went outside for open defecation. In urban area, it is very difficult to defecate open. Especially for women it very huge task. Having the toilet is very comfortable and you can go at any time when you want. Otherwise it is very difficult. In night time you always feel fear, many times snakes beaten when you go for open defecation. In the area, two to three incidents already happened. I also suffered from snake bite once. Since then I am scared to go for open defecation (Sandhyarani 39-year-old, Bhimpur area, Site 1).

Rasmita 46-year-old also supported this as follows:

> In the area, majority of the population are going for defecate in open area. In my childhood I seen people are going at river site and defecate open and wash their hand with sand. Still majority of the male members are going open defecation then the female member. Female members in the area are facing more problem than male members in the area. The government should constructed toilet facility (Naharakanta Area, Site-2).

Sarita 31-year-old respondents reported:

> I am staying in a rent house. More than three to four families are using one latrine. I do not like to share latrine and defecate open. Every day early morning me and my friend go together near at filed so that we have time to talk and get some fresh air. Now it is habituated for me and I can't feel comfortable when I used toilet. So I feel comfortable and get relax to defecate open (Naharakanta Area. Site-1).

11.9 Drainage and Garbage Bin Facilities

Table 11.5 shows that 55 percent of households had the draining facilities. While 45% of households did not have any drainage facility in front of their house. In Bhimpur area, there were no closed drainage in front of the house while in Naharakanta area 20% households replied that they had closed drainage outside the house. In Bhimpur a higher percentage of households 53% and Naharakanta the least percentage of households 40% reported that they had no drainage facilities outside their households. It was also observed that in Bhimpur a higher percentage of households 47% and Naharakanta the least percentage of households 44% reported they had open drainage facilities outside the house.

About dispose household waste, data shows 83% of households were reported they disposed households waste at open space outside their house. While 14% of households were reported they used garbage bin and 3% households were reported they had thrown garbage open space away form their house. About the often garbage collection by municipality workers (Table 11.5).

In Bhimpur the data shows that a higher percentage 58% of households reported that the sanitation workers never came to their localities for garbage collection. Only 30% of households reported that sanitation workers were coming twice a week for garbage collection. The data shows that only 8% of the households reported that sanitation workers came once a month for garbage collection. In Naharakanta the data shows that 74% of the households reported that sanitation workers never entered their localities for garbage collection. A total of 20% of households reported that twice a week and 4% of households reported that more than once a month sanitation workers came to their locality for garbage collection. It can be observed that one per cent of households reported that the BMC workers collected garbage regularly in their locality. The

Table 11.5 Having drainage and garbage bin facilities

Having drainage facility	Bhimpur *N* (%)	Naharkanta *N* (%)	Total *N* (%)
Yes	56 (46.7)	102 (60)	158 (54.5)
No	64 (53.3)	68 (40)	132 (45.5)
Types of drainage facility			
Closed	0 (0)	31 (30.3)	31 (19.6)
Open drainage	56 (100)	71 (69.7)	127 (80.4)
Dispose HHs waste			
Open space outside HHs	102 (85)	140 (82.4)	242 (83.4)
Open space away from HHs	8 (6.7)	0 (0)	8 (2.8)
Garbage bin	10 (8.3)	30 (17.6)	40 (13.8)
Often collection HHs garbage by municipality			
Not coming	61 (50.8)	126 (74.1)	187 (64.5)
Daily	14 (11.7)	0 (0)	14 (4.8)
More than twice a week	0 (0)	3 (1.8)	3 (1)
Twice a week	36 (30)	34 (20)	70 (24.1)
Once a week	0 (0)	1 (0.6)	1 (0.3)
Once a month	9 (7.5)	6 (3.5)	15 (5.2)

Source Fieldwork

data also shows that (12%) of households reported that twice week sanitation workers were coming to the locality for garbage collection. In both study areas the data shows that a higher percentage of households (65%) reported that sanitation workers never came to their localities for garbage collection when BMC had introduced schemes for door-to-door garbage collection. Only (24%) of households reported twice a week and (5%) of households reported more than once a month for garbage collection by the BMC workers.

It observed in both study areas the garbage collection was not happened properly. Some of the respondents are mentioned expressed their views as mentioned below:

One of the Key respondents reported:

> The sanitation workers are not coming to the area for garbage collection. They are complaining sanitation inspector but the nature of sanitation workers is not changing (KI7, Bhimpur Area).

Another Key Informant state:

> Most of time conflicts occur between sanitation workers and local people for garbage collection, road cleaning and drainage cleaning. Sometime councillor also intervene in to the matter and solve the problem but after one week or two weeks the saturation same again (KI9, Naharakanta Area).

Hand cleanliness is considered one of the most efficient ways to prevent the spread of infectious diseases. Every year, 1.8 million children under the age of five die as a result of diarrheal infections. Diarrhoeal illness is projected to cause 72.8 million disability adjusted life years (DALYs) lost each year owing to incapacity and premature death, with the majority of cases occurring in low and middle-income nations. The cause of diarrhoea is transmitted from person to person by contaminated food and water. According to some research, contaminated food and water account for more than 75% of all diarrhea cases. Hand washing after defecation or cleaning, as well as before preparing and eating food, can lower the incidence of diarrhoea (Ejemot et al., 2021).

Table 11.6 provides information about types of substances use for handwashing. Data shows higher percentage households reported that they were not using any substance for hand washing. While 47% households reported they are using substances such as soap, liquid and detergent powder for handwashing. Data further shows that those were using substance among them 54% households are used soap for handwashing as followed by liquid (27%) and detergent powder

Table 11.6 Handwashing behaviour and types of substances use for handwashing

Handwashing	Bhimpur *N* (%)	Naharkanta *N* (%)	Total *N* (%)
Yes	39 (32.5)	97 (57.0)	136 (46.9)
No	81 (67.5)	73 (43.0)	154 (53.1)
Types			
Soap	23 (59.0)	49 (50.5)	72 (54.4)
Liquid	5 (12.8)	32 (33.0)	37 (27.2)
Detergent powder	5.5 (14.1)	8 (8.2)	13.5 (9.9)
Both soap/liquid and detergent powder	5.5 (14.1)	8 (8.3)	13.5 (9.9)

Source Fieldwork

(10%). While 10% households were using both soap/liquid and detergent for handwashing.

11.10 Discussion and Conclusion

In both the study areas water supply and sanitation problem exists different levels. The accessibility and availability of water supply and sanitation also exists at different levels. In both areas due to various issues such as economic, political, socio-cultural, educational, administrative, structural, technology, lack of awareness and environmental factors are create barriers to access water supply and sanitation. The duration of water supply very less and majority household's dependent on hand pump water. When there is no water supply, most of the households travel long distance to collect water. Sometimes they would collect water from nearby colonies, temple and government official's premises. The quality of drinking water supply in the area was not good and majority of the people take water directly without any purifying treatment. The drinking water was highly contaminated of bleaching powder so most of the time the water could not be used for drinking purposes. Without water supply the higher percentage of households faced problems such as: drinking, cooking and bathing etc.

Regarding toilet facilities, in both study areas a higher percentage of households did not have toilet facilities and most of the households went outside for open defecation. Those who have toilets did not have water supply connectivity in the toilet. Most of the households use water buckets. Majority of households throw garbage in open space outside the house. The higher percentage households did not have drainage in front of their houses. The sanitation workers are not regular in terms of garbage collection, road and drainage cleaning in the study area. In the area people are face sanitation problem and for that they gave complaints to different levels like: registration of complain at community level, local level, and municipality. The distance to the complaint office was far from the study area which restricted people from registering complains. In the study area people faced registration problem like: no time, more distance, less education, lack of awareness and did not receive helpline number. A majority of the households were not aware about the government schemes on sanitation. Lack of awareness and less education are the main reasons people are unaware of the government schemes.

References

Acharya, S. S. (2015). Access to water and sanitation facilities-missing linkages with the providers and manifestations on health'. In S. B. Nimse & M. K. Agarwal (Eds.), *Public health and development in India* (pp. 26–45). London: New Delhi Northern Book Centre.

Bhagat, R. B. (2014). Rural and urban sanitation in India. *Kurukhetra*, 11–14. Retrieved from https://www.researchgate.net/publication/269702342_Rural_and_Urban_Sanitation_in_India

Bhunia, R., Ramakrishnan, R., Hutin, Y., & Gupte, M. D. (2009). Cholera outbreak secondary to contaminated pipe water in an urban area, West Bengal, India, 2006. *Indian Journal of Gastroenterology, 28*(2), 62–64. https://doi.org/10.1007/s12664-009-0020-5

Buttenheim, A. M. (2008). The sanitation environment in urban slums: Implications for child health. *Population and Environment, 30*(1–2), 26–47. https://doi.org/10.1007/s11111-008-0074-9

Eid, U. (2015). *The importance of water, sanitation, and hygiene as keys to national development* (pp. 1–5). Retrieved from https://www.issuelab.org/resource/importance-of-water-sanitation-and-hygiene-as-keys-to-national-development.html

Ejemot-Nwadiaro, R. I., Ehiri, J. E., Arikpo, D., Meremikwu, M. M., & Critchley, J. A. (2021). Hand-washing promotion for preventing diarrhoea. *Cochrane Database of Systematic Reviews, 1*, 1.

Evans, B. (2007). *Understanding the urban poor's vulnerabilities in water supply and sanitation.* Retrieved from http://eprints.whiterose.ac.uk/42852/

Galiani, S., Gertler, P., & Schargrodsky, E. (2005). Water for life: The impact of the privatization of water services on child mortality. *Journal of Political Economy, 113*(1), 83–120.

Government of Odisha, Housing & Urban Development Department. (2016). *Odisha urban sanitation strategy 2017*. State Secretariat Annex-B, Bhubaneswar, Odisha. https://urban.odisha.gov.in/sites/default/files/2023-09/Constitution%20of%20City%20Sanitation%20Task%20Force%20under%20OUSS%202017%20%288%29-pages-2.pdf

Housing & Urban Development Department, Government of Odish. Activity Report 2012–2013. Housing & Urban Development Department, Government of Odisha. http://www.urbanodisha.gov.in/(S(mmsysc45j1g52d55er0ffn45))/pdf/annual_activity_report/Annual_Activities_Report_2012-13.pdf. Accessed on 20/5/2025.

Howard, G., Bartram, J., & World Health Organization. Water, Sanitation and Health Team. (2003). *Domestic water quantity, service level and health/Guy Howard and Jamie Bartram.* World Health Organization. https://apps.who.int/iris/handle/10665/67884

Karan, S. K., & Harada, H. (2002). Field survey on water supply, sanitation and associated health impacts in urban poor communities.pdf. *Water Science and Technology, 46*(12), 279–275.

Kuberan, A., Singh, A. K., Kasav, J. B., Prasad, S., Surapaneni, K. M., Upadhyay, V., & Joshi, A. (2015). Water and sanitation hygiene knowledge, attitude, and practices among household members living in rural setting of India. *Journal of Natural Science, Biology, and Medicine, 6*(Suppl 1), S69–S74. https://doi.org/10.4103/0976-9668.166090

Minh, M., & Hung, N. V. (2011). Economic aspects of sanitation in developing countries. *Environmental Health Insights.* https://doi.org/10.4137/EHI.S8199

NSSO. (2001). *Concept and definiation used in national sample survey organization ministry of statistics and programme implimentation govt of India.* NSS. Golden Jublee Publication https://mohfw.nic.in/WriteReadData/l892s/6960144509Annual%20Report%20to%20the%20People%20on%20Health.pdf. Accessed on 19/5/2016

Office of the Registrar General & Census Commissioner, India. (2011). *House listing and housing census data, census of India 2011.* Ministry of Home Affairs, Government of India. https://censusindia.gov.in

Praharaj, S. (2021). Area-based urban renewal approach for smart cities development in India: Challenges of inclusion and sustainability. *Urban Planning, 6*(4), 202–215.

Tiwari, R., & Nayak, S. (2015). Drinking water, sanitation and waterborne diseases. *Economic and Political Weekly, 52*(23), 7–8.

United Nation, I. (2022). *Health, water and sanitation | United Nations in India.* Health, Water and Sanitation. https://india.un.org/en/171844-health-water-and-sanitation. https://india.un.org/en/171844-health-water-and-sanitation

USAID. (2012). *Water and sanitation state serise 2012 Odisha: After baby steps, run.* Health of the urban poor programe population foundation of India. https://www.academia.edu/12765890/Water_and_Sanitation_STATE_SERIES_2012_ODISHA_AFTER_BABY_STEPS_RUN_

World Health Organization. (Eds.). (2018). Water. https://www.afro.who.int/health-topics/water#:~:text=Globally%2C%20at%20least%201.8%20billion,000%20diarrhoeal%20deaths%20each%20year

Part IV
Towards Well-Being

12 Discourse on Climate Change and Well-Being: Examining Through the Lens of Political Ecology

Debayanti Bhowmick

Abstract

Political ecology is a theoretical approach in the discipline of geography which tries to look at the structural factors and units of an ecological phenomenon. It takes an interdisciplinary outlook on a given subject matter and tries to unravel the overlapping greys. This study is an attempt to review the climate change phenomenon through the theoretical lens of 'Political Ecology of Health', aiming to identify the strategic implications of climate change mitigation policies on health and well-being. In doing so, the paper also ponders upon the various discourses on climate change and well-being as observed across different global spaces and populations. The author uses a narrative review approach to examine a list of 285 articles. Out of these, 40 articles were shortlisted for the purpose of review. The articles were then thematically arranged and analysed.

12.1 Background

It was as early as 1935 that editor Frank Thone used the term "political ecology" in his article published in Science Service. Its usage became rampant post-1970s when the recurrence of this term was observed in the works of Eric Wolf (1972), Bryant and Bailey (1997) and many more. The discourse was based on the conditional relationship between culture and the political economy of the State. Hence, political ecology helps us see one's way of life through the lens of the unequal distribution of wealth and power in society. The theoretical concept of political ecology questions the role that power dynamics, one's social positioning and wealth play in impacting the health status of an individual. Lastly, political ecology presents us with the interlinkages between politics, economic reasonings and the existing environmental resources. These interlinkages remain very much ingrained and open in the questions and methods adopted in health geography.

In a similar context, the rising concerns about climate change and its impacts are not a one-dimensional issue. Climate change-induced health vulnerabilities are a serious cause of concern which links itself to multiple socioeconomic and political factors, taking place around us (Warner et al., 2010). The distribution and severity of these impacts seem to

The paper is based on the author's MPhil dissertation submitted to Jawaharlal Nehru University, New Delhi, under the supervision of Dr. Sanghamitra Acharya.

D. Bhowmick (✉)
University of New South Wales, Sydney, Australia
e-mail: d.bhowmick@unsw.edu.au

S. S. Acharya et al. (eds.), *Paradigm Shifts in Population and Health in India*, Sustainable Development Goals Series, https://doi.org/10.1007/978-981-95-1719-0_12

be region-specific, population-specific and situation/cultural-specific. Exposure of the geographic space to climate-induced health impacts is also dependent on the region-specific healthcare system, the governance and its resilient capacity (Roy et al., 2016). Hence political ecology approach could be an insightful method to dig into the various structural understanding behind climate-induced health vulnerabilities and vis a vis the well-being of the population.

12.2 What is Political Ecology?

Political ecology is an interdisciplinary approach, drawing its principle from the discipline of human geography. Human geography further overlaps with anthropology, sociology, economics, environmental studies and political science. Political ecology emphasizes the human factor of the larger socio-political/physical environment and fathoms the under-rooted causes of the existing social fabric (Watts, 2017). Human societies are complex, hence conceptualizing their behaviour takes one back to their cultural and social histories. Anthropological findings may help trace the pathway to their present condition. Thus, political ecology aims at looking into the current lifestyle, cultural relations, social positioning and organization of a specific population group belonging to a specific space, by reflecting on the emerging traditions over time and their simultaneous interaction with their immediate spaces in action (Jackson & Neely, 2015).

Coming to the association of ecology with health, it was May (1959) who initially articulated the idea of disease ecology, binding the understanding of disease and pathology with geography. Disease ecology evolved as a sub-head under medical geography, later known as health geography (Jackson & Neely, 2015), which includes an explanation of disease causation in the cultural, political, social and physical context. It is important to mention that context in the case of public health is extremely important in identifying the systemic gaps in well-being (Mayer, 1996). Health geography when disintegrates to coalesce with questions of political interest, and methodology triangulating "medical anthropology, history of science and science and technology studies", the outline for "political ecology" emerges (Jackson & Neely, 2015). Contextual analysis via political ecology throws light on multiple factors which tend to impact population health as well as the effectiveness of a health policy. Basing arguments solely on biological factors in the past has often missed out on critical dimensions like climate, economy, politics, society etc. Missing out on these multifaceted contexts leaves us with unproductive health system outcomes. Political ecology of health got prominence with the gradual consideration of preventive medicine over curative since the early seventeenth century. Public health understanding of illness superseded medical sciences based on the arguments of "economic rationality of health" and instrumentality of health" put forth by the Government of every State. The life of the "labour force" was prioritized by the Government to stabilize the existing economic losses. Preventive measures in health advocated "economic justification of good health" (Choudhary, 2014) through investments in living conditions, hospitals, and associated public health efforts, including all socio-economic aspects directly or indirectly affecting individual well-being. Understanding disease, illness and public health needed study of the social fabric, distribution of health-related knowledge and observing the accessibility of different population groups. Distribution pattern of knowledge, health care services and resources have been produced by speckled rationality and uneven social factors which needs in-depth analysis. Political ecology of health centres on ecology and delves within the outcomes of human activity on the environment and vice versa in context of the existing type of administration, economy and polity. It is to be noted that politics in particular and ecology are intertwined at varied levels of operation. The structure of the Government, the policies it announces and the administrative calls are single headedly impacting the concerned environment. With the inception of the neoliberal era, State-led Government are rapidly privatizing the economy including health systems. Regulations and objectives thus proposed under this private–public partnership, often sabotages the ecology for profit-oriented benefits (mostly overlooking welfare). The way people perceive Sate or the State perceives people are different, based on one's social identity. In this context, political ecology vehemently questions the persistent gender gap in the daily social functioning. It shares its scope with the feminist theories of social understanding questioning the power relations which shape woman's eco-political agency (Resurrección, 2017). The politics around environment and society tends to answer this unevenness of "production and reproduction of healthy and unhealthy people", and which group is persistently put under what condition and why. This unevenness, discrimination and inequality seeks attention towards articulation of ecology-specific health practices, awareness and policies. The U.S. Centres for Disease Control and Prevention (CDC)'s Climate-Ready States and Cities Initiative (CRSCI) are few of the important bodies who have started using pollical ecology as a solution to the administrative gaps in climate-change risk management. Both the bodies prioritize local government as an active agent in handling the public health crisis as imposed due to climate change. The bodies work with the idea that with the health agencies being under-prepared and poorly associated to climate change assessment plans, their addressal to the adverse health impacts on population health has been inadequate. Identifying vulnerable population, the possible risk zones and health consequences are a part of the political ecology of the area and the CRCSI have approached it along similar lines. Partnership with relevant programmes, cross-disciplinary tactics, networked partnership between health and climate and recognition of qualitative methods to demarcate vulnerable demography are few of the steps proposed and executed by the bodies to prepare climate-ready states and cities (Sheehan et al., 2017).

12.3 Feminist Political Ecology

With the surging rise of debates around environmental issues since 1970s, scholars also started questioning the gender roles within these discourses. In the post-colonial era, the world witnessed the rise of ecofeminists and environmental feminists marking the third wave of feminism. The theories of feminist political ecology made a place in academia in the 1990s, critiquing the sustainable development goals and associated literature which did not include the gender standpoints within their scopes (Petchesky, 2014). The early works of Vandana Shiva marked the conceptualization of Women, Environment and Development (WED) and Women in Development (WID) infusing, the gender dimension to the developmental plannings functioning and decision-making. However, feminist political ecology rose to prominence as a critique to this. While the former recognizes women as a mere homogenous group in need and situated at a subordinate end in all the police reforms, the latter conceptualizes the gendered relationship from the perspective of culture and society as well. Examples could be drawn from the heavily critiqued paternalistic climate regulations imposed in Nicaragua, where though gender is considered while policy formulation, the reproduction of their subordinate roles in daily lives continue to render the outcomes ineffective (Gonda, 2019) Feminist political ecology holds the potential to "re-politicize" the techno-centric interventions which has very less translational impacts in the daily positioning of women's roles.

The study by Ylipää (2018) on climate change adaptation in Thai Binh also take a closer look at the gendered perspectives within the political ecology standpoint. The paper reveals that with rights and responsibilities selectively favouring the mobility and opportunities only among male farmers, the aforesaid Province is facing a strike outflow of young and male farmers, leaving the agrarian responsibility of the province mostly in the hands of elderly female farmers. It was only through the approach of feminist political ecology that the light was thrown on the unchecked ageing and feminisation of farming, pushing the population group to the probable risks of climate change adaptation, environmental vulnerabilities, wraths of poor profit inflow, constant devaluation of their knowledge and the avid fear of an unsustainable farming culture in the near future. The migratory impact on livelihood is thus directly and indirectly associated to the type of individual livelihoods, well-being and probable risks of climate change on the exposed population. It is unfortunate that these underlying issues has yet not been integrated within the Vietnamese strategies of policy analysis and continues to add to an incomplete climate change adaptation strategy.

Similarly, geographic insights from a study based in South Asia (Sultana, 2014) talks how the changing water dynamics in a region impacts the locals both in terms of physical vulnerabilities as well as by inducing psychosocial concerns. Findings suggest that women in the households tend to bear the larger brunt of the household vulnerabilities. They are responsible in the procurement of safe drinking water amidst the dearth, suffer poor reproductive health care needs and are also subjected to domestic violence owing to the wrath of adverse psychosocial condition within the family. Women also tend to reap lesser benefits out of a project owing to their lower positioning in the status quo (Nyantakyi-Frimpong, 2019) which are largely influenced by their marital status, ownership rights, decision-making power (Elmhirst et al., 2017) and knowledge reservoir. In the process their participation within beneficiary cooperatives is also hindered owing to the low proportion of representation in the decision-making markets or lack of knowledge regarding the formal business undertakings. Mainly because of their pre-assigned gender roles, restricting them to tasks primarily within the boundaries of a household.

Hence, it can be stated that, analysis of the climate crisis through a gendered lens can bring out the policy gaps, causes behind programme failures and the differences of climate induced impacts among genders.

12.4 What is Politics of Well-Being?

The concept of "Well-being" underwent multiple modifications in the past decade owing to governmental interests. Well-being was often explained as leading a "good life" which would to some extent benefit the economy by being able to extract the optimum human potential. The idea was thus for a long time centred around the GDP indicator of a society until Simon Kuznet stated that "The welfare of a nation can scarcely be inferred from a measurement of national income". It was then during the 1970s that social indicators were introduced in developmental politics, challenging the one-dimensional orthodox economic approach (Bache & Scott, 2018).

Perceptions of well-being are extensively found in the writing of Engels (1990), who was one of the few early pioneers of looking at public health through the societal lens of well-being. He wrote about the political sway which was in favour of the Bourgeois, and how every other individual was stripped down to a wage labourer or a commodity. The labour was sold to the leaders with a price tag round the collars. The price determined individual cost of production inclusive of the minimal means of subsistence which pushes the labourer to work. Hence the market which was being built under such a circumstance ensured the minimal requirement for the maintenance of life and labour. Social science's role is to identify these imbalances of everyday life and their interacting processes between the various levels of society which ultimately shapes the health and well-being situation of individuals. The contemporary world has its own modern problems of daily dealings. Though the idea of well-being has gone through intense modification of understanding, the process to attain the same has added complicated layers of obstacles. The methodology thus involves deeper knowledge and structural questions to thoroughly place the issues at an organizational level (Nyman & Nilsén, 2016).

Health equality and health well-being are the optimum situation of life. However, coming in way are the varied demographic attributes, culturally unique and differently abled population groups, unequal income levels and individual placings in the society which determines their level of exposure to risks and vulnerability. These differences call for priority specific interventions and policy targets. Health disparities among the marginalized sections, needs "coping and pedagogy of tolerance as an educational approach for mitigating stigmatization as well as the blame and guilt for health deviant minorities within the field of health disparities" (Karlsson et al., 2018).

Well-being when placed within the context of environmental issues, climate risks are most dreadful among the marginalized sections enjoying the least agency. Their livelihoods and living surroundings are positioned in the most vulnerable fronts which are too fragile to face the hazardous outcomes of climate change. Climate change risks massively attack the economic side of the population well-being. Hence, climate change adaptation calls for policy supporting solutions to ensure development and public welfare. Under the new paradigm as explained by Krishnaprabu (2020), "adaptation is fostered by a process of sustainable development and vulnerability reduction, rather than explicit adaptation policies. Though this approach of vulnerability reduction seems to be an efficient framework, the pathway to achieve it requires proper understanding of region-specific political ecology". Poor lifestyle adds on to their existing illnesses, impairments and any other recurring diseases. Attaining well-being for them are related to their access to healthcare which lacks even the minimum coverage. Addressing to these vulnerable communities need qualitative methodologies with interdisciplinary approach. Identifying the vulnerable zones is one of the ways forward to identify the structural entry points of possible threats. This may help address the gaps at their very roots. Well-being can only be achieved through effective support and care giving policies through appropriate identification of the causalities (Jormfeldt, 2016).

It thus can be said that, well-being should be approached through multiple perspectives. The methodology to do so is the adoption of an appropriate tool to fathom the structural causalities of well-being. However, in WHO's "Health 2020" framework the concerns of well-being are very much objectively determined (estimating GINI, availability of social support, unemployment rates, proportion of children not enrolled in school and population percentage with improved sanitation facilities) except individual take on 'satisfaction'. The concern here lies the lack of subjective concerns which are unique individual experiences within the health care system. Hagtvedt Vik and Carlquist (2018) extensively points out the extreme necessity of a subjective take on well-being and augments his argument with relevant sources. He refers to Campbell and Converse and says "Ultimately, the quality of life must be in the eye of the beholder".

Subjective interpretations of well-being can only be drawn through real-life consequences, self-perceived emotions and critical evaluation. Personal take on the idea of well-being will help form a more integrated policy framework where the invisible \drivers of well-being can also be addressed. The current health care system of the country have started to prioritize well-being post the year 1990. Introduction of the well-being therapy to increase the level of mental health recovery is an important part of ensuring effective health care (Fava, 2016). Thus, associating well-being to the subjective nature of individual health state.

12.5 The Intersectional Impact of Political Ecology, Well-Being and Climate Change/Environmental Issues

Post the 1960's wave of environmentalism, climate change discourses have positioned itself in an area of interdisciplinarity, claiming the process to be intricately linked to political, social and cultural realms. An interdisciplinary approach has made it possible to study the subject matter through the lens of social sciences including public health. The approach of interdisciplinarity has been triggered from the idea that addressing a problem might need suggestions from relevant knowledge disciplinaries beyond the parent subject matter. In case of the climate change, the field of relevance expanded to politics and the wide arena of social sciences. By the year of 1990, climate change had totally placed itself within the ambit of wider politics of geography, natural sciences and society. Integrated disciplines invited funds from every aspect to address the wider agenda of global environment change. The whole intention of this gradual progress in the discipline is to build a progressive theoretical approach towards dealing the issue. In the process, the researches successfully exposed important socio-ecological concepts and debates around climate change through objective questioning about the "processes and effects" (Bulkeley, 2019).

The works of Ylipaa et al. (2019) has been fundamental in questioning few essential loops regarding the local, priority-specific adaptation needs, identifying the gendered nature of rights and responsibilities triggering the behavioural change in a specific area and of course understanding the different ways in which climate change is being perceived among the different genders. The politics of ecology and well-being significantly aim to re-strategize the plans of environmental adaptation and in the process identifies the gendered responsibilities and power relations framing the household realities and community behaviour. Choudhary et al. (2019) has Intricately studied the cities in poor countries. The findings of their study could be extrapolated to the overall vulnerable conditions which the cities and urban spaces around the world are facing. With the growing vulnerabilities, inhabitable spaces have been inviting increasing number of climatic risks which seems too difficult to adapt. Though multilevel interventions are an immediate need, there lies regional disparities which separate the needs of different communities as per their social positioning. As a result, location specific vulnerabilities have been an important field of concern especially among the poorer section. These vulnerabilities could be seen through both "biophysical" and "social" lenses. With the inpouring adversities of climate change, urban cities in particular are being transformed into urban heat islands. The unchecked rise in photochemical smog poses as a great threat to the population health especially among the elders and the poor. Habitable spaces generate a huge proportion of waste as a result of increased consumption, unchecked urbanization, pollutive emissions and the constant alteration of land cover. These uncontrolled changes have been very impactful when it comes to human health, their livelihoods and their immediate living environment. The theoretical concept of political ecology comes to play when we look to find a solution for the crisis. The institutional scenario of each country is responsible in painting personalised pictures of consequences. Whereby, the maximum challenges are imposed upon the countries and population facing the blunts of economic marginalization. Governance looking into climate change adaptation must also look into the underlying region-specific vulnerabilities which forms potential hurdles towards mitigation. In this context, Vietnam's lengthy water management history can be cited as a strong political ecology scenario where the country's governance system was closely observed and interpreted. The authorities of Vietnam for long, have been responsible to problematize the issues pertaining to health, poverty and sexuality in the country. These authoritative controls and political manipulation have starkly framed the rationalities behind every climate change adaptation technique, and other governance policies. In case of Vietnam's water management policies, political ecology played a huge role in establishing the management system in each era. The system witnessed striking shifts from early periods of programmes addressing food security and well-being, to the gradual change into prioritizing domestic control of security and territory expansion. Finally, it was during their colonial period that programme priority shifted its focus to exploitative profit-making intentions; *"The canals enabled both exploitation and purported development by providing transport and drastically expanding access to land which could be used for agriculture"*. (Lindegaard, 2020). Soon after this high modernist approach, the management system was again reinstated for agriculture recovery under the communist regime of the newly formed Democratic Republic of Vietnam (1945). In this period the programmes were focused around social stability, food security and economic government.

In 2013–14, IPCC had been vividly transparent in mentioning the Anthropocene nature of the environmental process; "—any change in climate over time, whether due to natural variability or as a result of human activity". Human dimensions of climate change are a major factor why the concept of political ecology and politics of well-being comes to play in understanding the multi-causal drives of climate-change crisis. Multitude studies have been performed to establish the relation between political ecology, well-being and health. The studies have been a gateway towards understanding the multiple socio-economic causations associated to health situations of population groups. Researches far and wide have proved modernization and governance to be the frontline actors impacting and modifying the health consequences of climate change. Empirical evidences show rising dominance of technocentric advancements on ecological dynamics. These changes have mostly focussed on the macro-level economic developments which are in stark conflict with environmental exploitation (Adua & York, 2015).

In another instance it was observed that with the increase use of pesticide, Zimbabwe's small holding cotton farmers were exposed to the public health hazards of chemical pollution (Zinyemba et al., 2018). Increased pest-control not only impacted on the climate variability, but also to the wraths of economic fluctuations as perceived by the government and private actors. Political ecology plays a massive role here to determines the behaviour and perception of the farmers using pesticide. The decision-making surrounding it, strongly relies upon its past of government monopoly over the cotton production and manufacturing. As a result, the governing bodies had massive influence on the farmers regarding pesticide use, popularised by the integrated pest management approach. Hence, even post liberalization the cotton companies have failed to break free from the traditional culture of excessive pesticide use; "Despite liberalization, the government of Zimbabwe remains responsible for key research and regulatory issues which impact on the usage through the Ministry of Agriculture's Cotton Research Institute (CRI)". Secondly, with the private contractors coming into play, farmers are left with very minimum agency when the private units fail to supply the pesticide timely, as per the contract. This have led to lengthy waiting periods or "resistance due to lengthy exposure to increasing amounts of the same pesticide". Lastly, with all these systematic gaps, the changing climate increases the risk of pesticide induced adversities. Unfortunately to combat, farmers resorts to more pesticides for maximum yield from a degraded quality of land; "the pesticides which we receive from the companies will be sufficient, but if the season is bad, we are obliged to purchase more pesticides".

Chandra et al. (2017) in his work had taken up the political ecology perspective to introduce the concept of "climate-smart agriculture". He reviews the troubles of climate risk as perceived by the smallholder farmers owing to multiple socio-political processes of inequal power relations and social injustice. His work comments on the global and local level institutions and actors directly influencing the property rights, knowledge and security of smallholder farmers, the gendered dynamics of climate vulnerability as well as the challenges to mitigation and adaptation of climate induced risks. The paper documents that the regional unevenness of risks is mostly in line with food insecurity, rural livelihood in accordance to demographic attributes, daily coping with climatic and non-climatic shocks, power play of the authorities imposing on marginalised and disadvantaged groups and the structural determination of adaptation capabilities.

Ajibade et al.'s (2019) paper looks into the political economy and political ecology perspective of Nigeria and Qatar in their dealings with the Millennial Development Goals. These insights are necessary to identify the gaps of policy formation and implementation, so that the similar consequences are not felt upon the upcoming and ongoing SDGs. Sustainability is an important concept in both the ideas of development and environment (Choudhary, 2016). The multi-faceted issues which come in the way of policy implementation and sustainability includes the changing ownership of agricultural seeds, trade conflicts, border politics, fluctuating commodity market prices, food wastage related to varying taste preferences, land rights reformation across states, technological innovations and weak geopolitical coherence. Though Qatar and Nigeria share the same responsibilities of the policies, their areas of improvement vary as per their specific geopolitical location and relationship with neighbouring countries. On one hand, Qatar had much amendments to make along the lines of technological improvements, reduction of unchecked food wastage and conflict arising in trade, agricultural and regional investments. While, Nigeria needed to address the issues of exploitation among smallholder farmers, food security, technological upgradation, domestic conflicts and institution cooperation on agro-based problems. Political ecology comes into play when the effectiveness of SDGs is identified as crucial determinant of political and legal frameworks of operation, government's method of financing, private sector involvement, agricultural programmes and several other large-scale investments.

Mbereko et al. (2018) had also conducted a case study in Gwanda district to understand the climate change adaptation of the locals through the lens of political ecology and tried interpreting the well-being status there. His study hypothesis was based on the IPCC report claiming "climate change will benefit some regions and disadvantage others". The coping strategies in Gwanda mostly varied owing to the differences in wealth situation and adaptive capacity. Thus, material well-being was a prominent factor of determination to understand vulnerability at the face of climate catastrophes. Wealthier population groups were found to be better equipped with alternative livelihoods and coping mechanisms in times of extreme losses. The locals of Gwanda had also based their adaptation behaviour as per the regulations of risk management promoters. Since NGOs were more effectively responsive than Government bodies, people were more reliant on their social capital and NGO doners.

In the works of Brisbois et al. (2018), it is mentioned that "political ecological approaches, typically situate present-day environmental conditions in historical context, and especially seek to understand how particular places and populations are affected by forces operating at multiple scales". Hence, political ecology is perceived as an ongoing practice rather than just a methodological approach. The practice involves borrowing multi-layered contexts from perspectives of gender, historical past and narratives, political governance and the associated health situation and of course the human–environment relationship. At the end of the practice is the ultimate objective of "long-term well-being and individual agency". The paper cites example from the lived experiences of the communities working in the banana industry of Southwestern Ecuador. The extensive exposure of the banana farmers in this region have left them with extensive respiratory and skin related health complications, whose exposure were again very gendered and socially determined. However, as the historical discourse unfolds, the issues of the competing North America, past authoritative clashes within the production companies, hurricane attacks in Central America, government's involvement of aerial fumigation for developing multi-scaler relationships, unevenness of resources among the rich and poor farming class and many other politically infused triggers came to light.

Martin et al. (2019) throws light on the ways political ecology operates in Western America. The geopolitics of energy, soaring prices and technocentric advancement has been the forces behind extraction of non-renewable energies. These climate exploiting activities call for urgent legislative actions. However, it is rightly concluded by the author that "efforts to govern contentious extractive activities through simple spatial strategies, leave unresolved deeper conflicts over power, jurisdiction, and procedural fairness". Additionally, the participatory governance for decision making and resource management are aimed for positive social and environmental outcomes. However, the tension between community participation and management are greatly influenced by the regional power dynamics, leaving the communities in conflict with each other along the lines of knowledge production, perceived differences and exclusionary practices; "Tensions between these expert and local knowledges and the stymying of stakeholder engagement (also) comes to a critical political ecology perspective".

In similar context, Hoffmann (2018) studies Egypt's exploitation of the cold war geopolitical rifts to achieve its hydro-civilisational mission of the Nile. Egypt's "hydro-hegemony" caused adequate damage on the ecology as well as displaced the Native Nubian tribes to continue to compete over the waters of Nile. These imperial pasts have left deep impression on the postcolonial states which are still overcoming the postcolonial legacy of interrupted social development. This scenario, though holds as a prime example from the Middle East, is common in rest of the world too. Strong association of regional geopolitics to the ecological well-being as well as to the developmental visions has always been a historical reality.

Political ecology and well-being politics also tries to explain the morphology of human settlement and their impacts on the immediate environment. Rahman et al. (2019) explains in his paper the concept of urban ecology, which is the theory of political ecology placed within an urban context. He cites a very ordinary example of a conflict between the privileged community flooding the lower areas inhabited by the poorer community in Bandar Lampung city. The jammed-up drains in the poorer community are owing to their marginalized situation in terms of wealth ownership, access to health and education and low-income levels. Hence people with lesser resources are more exposed to the hazards of environmental issues like abrupt sea-level intrusion, flooding or shrinking drainage. These are the usual results of land reclamation leading to disrupted tidal patterns and the narrowing down of the estuaries. He termed vulnerability to be "a sectional issue" which is time and again being addressed via structural unearthing of socio-political set-ups. Chitewere et al. (2017) on the other hand identified "agency", "social construct" and structural operations involved in the formation of a neighbourhood. He established strong association between these causal forces with the health impacts as faced by the communities residing in it. The research well documents the differences as perceived by different communities dwelling in common or separate neighbourhoods and the way they are separated along the lines of culture, personal agency, housing provisions, social location, and other factors. Bulkeley et al. (2014) uses the same framework to question the changing housing patterns in response to the changing climate in Philadelphia. His paper questions the housing authority, the process of this change, and lastly the consequences of the change as perceived in the community. He takes up Philadelphia's "The Coolest Block Contest", which is an urban housing governance public–private partnership, as a case study to bring out the association of housing with climate change. In the process he identifies a variety of actors who are influencing the housing patterns in the area. The paper notes that in the entire governance, community participation happens to be an important mobilizer to build the individualized responsibilities of dealing with climate change, without which the entire programme holds absurd.

Most of the discourses dealing with health ecologies points at the poor health of the marginalised, underprivileged communities associated to the different politico-socially triggered causalities. Though many infections are emerging over the time, the process to tackle them have also traversed a long journey. However, as Farmer (2000) points out, the solutions to these emerging diseases often doesn't "involve the consideration of poverty". The community at risk are exposed to the stings of victim-blaming, subjugated expression and restricted representation. It is important to mention that ensuring individual well-being revolves around the concept of "*Homo capax*". *Homo capax* as the name suggests talks about the capability which an individual owns in the society with respect to their power position, resource possession and capacity. *Homo capax* is also dependent on one's socio-cultural and economical capital which promotes individual agency, accessibility and validation. It is evident that all humans are not privileged enough to attain the top most power positions, but are definitely influenced by the ones who are in control of the system and relations. Power dominance of one sect on the other compromises on the health needs of the underprivileged as well as hinders individual agency of personal knowledge, experiences and strengths.

Well-being thus depends on how judiciously the power relations are in play (Larsson & Jormfeldt, 2017) and the extent to which voices are covered to extend care, support, security and benefits.

The study on HEAP (Household Economy and Poverty trajectory) model in Bangladesh was an exemplary work by Adams et al. (2007) to present us with the economic inequalities as identified through political ecology approach. He gave insights on the association of household well-being with the dynamics of poverty and poor adaptation agency. His paper revolves around the argumentative clash between poverty reduction targets of the SDGs, and the current natural resource management around the globe. It is to be noted, that treatment of natural resources only as income sources has not been an effective sustainable approach to deal with poverty. This gap has been addressed by presenting the effects of ecosystem services on economic change and also representing the natural resources as a safety net for the proper health of population groups. The paper uses the political ecology paradigm to build a relevant model showing the long-term poverty trajectories of different livelihoods. The livelihoods in this case are exposed to the adversities of climate change. As Lazar et al. (2020) puts it; "*influenced by processes at the regional and national scales that directly affect hazards, environmental quality and the economy for households themselves*".

Instances of power inequality could be cited from the work of Bodomo (2020) in which he studied the perspective of well-being among Africans living in China. The unequal treatment of the Africans living in China along the lines of health accessibility and quality of life in general is researched through a political ecology approach, where historical and contemporary perspectives are drawn to address the situation. The history of the Tang Dynasty had degraded the African identity to that of slaves, marginalizing them from every aspect of quality living. Their well-being still, is compromised due to the instilled narrative of non-inclusive treatment and unfair dominance. Discrimination at times of pandemic or during usual health care utilization reflects the racially profiled nature of the country's understanding, which is nothing but driven due to the past narratives. However, the contemporary picture has shown improved agency and resilience in the attainment of well-being among African locals owing to updated policy frameworks against the relational "asymmetries" of health governance.

"*Homo capax*" also determines the way a public health crisis is reported. The reporting of crises is also associated to the political ecology of the situation and the population being addressed. Communication often involves multiple socio-political driven factors working in favour of a broader authority-oriented purpose. Belfer et al. (2017), in their paper writes how representation of indigenous people in context of climate change crisis can be manipulated, misinterpreted and wrongly represented. His study reviews newspaper articles published in the countries of Canada, USA, Australia and New Zealand shows how the impact narratives of climate change on indigenous communities lacks discussion relating to their subjugated past of colonial marginalization, whose repercussions are still strongly felt on their social positioning, knowledge system and adaption practices. Media reports often fails to highlight the underlying politics of an existing crisis to cover up the structural roots of vulnerability. Disparity in coverage among communities, denial of the long-term colonial impact legacies, biased tone of coverage is the culmination of a corrupt politicised regime. Biased representation of vulnerable voices is the gateway towards environmental injustice. Communities whose voices have been conspicuously subdued tend to face the maximum repercussions of the climate crisis with very minimal resources to fall back upon.

London (2016) in his paper "Environmental justice and regional political ecology converge in the other California" questions the role political ecology plays in regional planning and environmental justice. His study was based in the San Joaquin Valley of California, where he found that multiple forms of conflict may arise while delivering environmental justice and regional planning. The study area had suffered several issues in executing planning strategies owing to the largely fragmented planning areas which contributes in impeding coordinated action of addressal. San

Joaquin Valley had identified regionalisation as an important framework for climate change mitigation. But the approach to regionalization in the area is different among the local government and the disadvantaged community seeking for environmental justice. Political ecology has played an important role here to identify the interactions between the social movements and the government responses. A conflicting nature of the regional planning has triggered the emergence of social and environmental inequality among the inhabitants. Hence in spite of meaningful investments pertaining to income, public participation and community knowledge being under process, the extent of evenness in delivering environmental justice is still under scrutiny by the public agencies.

12.6 Conclusion

Conservation of the habitat has reached the epitome of utmost priority. Hence the discourses surrounding it must also emerge and shift to appropriately address the concern at its very root. The viewpoints critiquing neo-liberal policies, affirmation of political ecology theory, well-being perspectives and ecofeminism are few of the emerging concepts which hold strong arguments to frame a more inclusive agenda of action.

It is through these concepts that we have started questioning the economically driven "Development paradigm" and the simultaneous cost which is being paid via environmental mishaps, poverty and social corrosion. The piling GNP are is in constant conflict with the impoverished ecosystem, over-exploitation, competitive market and the ever-polluting waterbodies and biological realm.

Political ecology also recognizes the climate crisis through a gendered lens. Unfortunately, women are still considered to be "marginal to food system" pushing them to the blunt of faulty pregnancies, undernourishment and higher percentage of deaths. As a result, children born are also undernourished, poorly fed and devoid of proper neo-natal care. Women's pre-assigned gender roles and poor representation in the decision-making processes have further restricted their agency and made them more vulnerable to the ongoing climatic shocks. The wide range of health indicators have revealed higher cases of morbidity, mortality, low hospital enrolment numbers among women especially among the marginalized communities.

Climate change and its associated risks on health is a serious public health issue, demanding immediate resolution. Collective responses to this cause would dig out the vulnerabilities of the crises. Political ecology is one such theoretical approach which leads to collective understanding, control and management.

References

Adams, W. M., & Hutton, J. (2007). People, parks and poverty: Political ecology and biodiversity conservation. *Conservation and Society, 5*(2), 147–183.

Adua, L., & York, R. (2015). *The human dimensions of climate change.* http://www.elsevier.com/open-access/userlicense/1.0/1

Ajibade, I., Egge, M., Pallathadka, A., & Babalola, A. (2019). Climate change and the sustainable development goal on food security: Barriers and opportunities for progressive realization in qatar and Nigeria Idowu. *Journal of Sustainable Development Law and Policy, 133*(11), 158–183. https://doi.org/10.4314/jsdlp.v10i2.2

Bache, I., & Scott, K. (2018). Wellbeing in politics and policy. *The Politics of Wellbeing.* https://doi.org/10.1007/978-3-319-58394-5_1

Belfer, E., Ford, J. D., & Maillet, M. (2017). Representation of Indigenous peoples in climate change reporting. *Climate Change, 145*, 57–70. https://doi.org/10.1007/s10584-017-2076-z

Bodomo, A. (2020). Historical and contemporary perspectives on inequalities and well-being of Africans in China. *Asian Ethnicity, 21*(4), 526–541. https://doi.org/10.1080/14631369.2020.1761246

Brisbois, B. W., Harris, L., & Spiegel, J. M. (2018). Political ecologies of global health: Pesticide exposure in southwestern ecuador's Banana industry. *Antipode, 50*(1), 61–81. https://doi.org/10.1111/anti.12340

Bulkeley, H. (2019). Navigating climate's human geographies: Exploring the whereabouts of climate politics. *Dialogues in Human Geography, 9*(1), 3–17. https://doi.org/10.1177/2043820619829920

Bulkeley, H., Edwards, G. A., & Fuller, S. (2014). Contesting climate justice in the city: Examining politics and practice in urban climate change experiments. *Global Environmental Change, 25*, 31–40.

Chandra, A., McNamara Paul Dargusch, K. E., Lecturer Karen McNamara, S. E., & Professor Paul Dargusch, A. (2017). The relevance of political ecology perspectives for smallholder climate-smart agriculture: A review. *Review: Political Ecology Perspectives on CSA Journal of Political Ecology* (Vol. 24). http://www.climatesmart agconcerns.info

Chitewere, T., Shim, J. K., Barker, J. C., & Yen, I. H. (2017). How neighborhoods influence health: Lessons to be learned from the application of political ecology. *Health and Place, 45*, 117–123. https://doi.org/10.1016/j.healthplace.2017.03.009

Choudhary. (2016). Sustainable urbanization: A conceptual discourse. *Espacialidades. Revista De Temas Contemporáneos Sobre Lugares, Política y Cultura, 6*(1), 6–36.

Choudhary, B. (2014). Health, illness and disease the enjoyment of the highest attainable standard of. *Economic and Political Weekly, 49*(45), 60–68.

Choudhary, B. K., Tripathi, A. K., & Rai, J. (2019). Can 'poor' cities breathe: Responses to climate change in low-income countries. *Urban Climate, 27*(January), 403–411. https://doi.org/10.1016/j.uclim.2019.01.001

Elmhirst, R., Siscawati, M., Sijapati Basnett, B., & Ekowati, D. (2017). Gender and generation in engagements with oil palm in East Kalimantan, Indonesia: Insights from feminist political ecology. *The Journal of Peasant Studies, 44*(6), 1135–1157. https://doi.org/10.1080/03066150.2017.1337002

Engels, F. (1990). Capital: Manifesto of the communist party. In *Encyclopedia Britannica.*

Farmer, P. (2000). Infections and inequalities: The modern plagues. *Medical Anthropology Quaterly, 14*(3), 448–451.

Fava, G. A. (2016). Well-being therapy: Current indications and emerging perspectives. *Psychotherapy and Psychosomatics, 85*, 136–145. https://doi.org/10.1159/000444114

Gonda, N. (2019). Re-politicizing the gender and climate change debate: The potential of feminist political ecology to engage with power in action in adaptation policies and projects in Nicaragua. *Geoforum, 1067*, 87–96. https://doi.org/10.1016/j.geoforum.2019.07.020

Hagtvedt Vik, M., & Carlquist, E. (2018). *Measuring subjective well-being for policy purposes: The example of well-being indicators in the WHO "Health 2020" framework*. Scandinavian Public Health.

Hoffmann, C. (2018). Environmental determinism as orientalism: The geo-political ecology of crisis in the middle east. *Journal of Historical Sociology, 31*, 94–104. https://doi.org/10.1111/johs.12194

Jackson, P., & Neely, A. H. (2015). Triangulating health: Toward a practice of a political ecology of health. *Progress in Human Geography, 39*(1), 47–64. https://doi.org/10.1177/0309132513518832

Jormfeldt, H. (2016). Perspectives on health and well-being in human vulnerability. *International Journal of Qualitative Studies on Health and Well-Being, 11*(1), 31477. https://doi.org/10.3402/qhw.v11.31477

Karlsson, S., Ziegert, K., & Kristén, L. (2018). Perspectives on equal health and well-being. *International Journal of Qualitative Studies on Health and Well-Being, 13*(1), 1679589. https://doi.org/10.1080/17482631.2019.1679589

Krishnaprabu, S. (2020). Climate change adaptation and development exploring the linkages. *Indian Journal of Pure and Applied Biosciences, 8*(2), 282–288. https://doi.org/10.18782/2582-2845.8038

Larsson, I., & Jormfeldt, H. (2017). Perspectives on power relations in human health and well-being. *International Journal of Qualitative Studies on Health and Well-Being, 12*, 2. https://doi.org/10.1080/17482631.2017.1358581

Lazar, A. N., Adams, H., Adger, W. N., & Nicholls, R. J. (2020). Modelling household well-being and poverty trajectories: An application to coastal Bangladesh. *PLoS ONE, 15*(9), 3–23. https://doi.org/10.1371/journal.pone.0238621

Lindegaard, L. (2020). A historical, scaled approach to climate change adaptation: The case of Vietnam. *Journal of Political Ecology, 27*, 105–124.

London, J. K. (2016). Environmental justice and regional political ecology converge in the other California Jonathan. *Journal of Political Ecology, 23*, 1.

Martin, J. V., Epstein, K., & Bergmann, N. (2019). Revisiting and revitalizing political ecology in the American West. *Geoforum, 107*, 227–230. https://doi.org/10.1016/j.geoforum.2019.05.006

May, J. M. (1959). The ecology of human disease. *The Ecology of Human Disease, 1959*, 1.

Mayer, J. (1996). The political ecology of disease as one new focus for medical geography. *Progress in Human Geography, 20*(4), 441–456.

Mbereko, A., Chimbari, M. J., & Mukaratirwa, S. (2018). The political ecology of stakeholder-driven climate change adaptation: Case study from Ntalale ward, Gwanda District, Zimbabwe. *Journal of Disaster Risk Studies, 10*(1), 1–10. https://doi.org/10.4102/jamba.v10i1.419

Nyantakyi-Frimpong, H. (2019). Visualizing politics: A feminist political ecology and participatory gis approach to understanding smallholder farming, climate change vulnerability, and seed bank failures in Northern Ghana. *Geoforum, 105*, 109–121. https://doi.org/10.1016/j.geoforum.2019.05.014

Nyman, C., & Nilsén, Å. (2016). Perspectives on health and well-being in social sciences. *International Journal of Qualitative Studies on Health and Well-Being, 11*(1), 31468. https://doi.org/10.3402/qhw.v11.31468

Petchesky, R. (2014). Feminist political ecology. In *The Oxford handbook of transnational feminist movements* (pp. 791–837).

Rahman, M. B., Nurhasanah, I. S., Nugraha, E., & Harahap, T. (2019). Applying the urban political ecology (UPE) framework to re-visit disaster and climate change vulnerability-risk assessments. *Journal of Regional and City Planning, 30*(3), 224–240. https://doi.org/10.5614/jpwk.2019.30.3.4

Resurrección, B. P. (2017). Gender and environment from "women, environment and development" to feminist political ecology. In *Routledge handbook of gender and environment* (pp. 71–85). https://www.routledge.com/Routledge-Handbook-of-Gender-and-

Roy, J., Ghosh, D., Mukhopadhyay, K., & Ghosh, A. (2016). Exacerbating health risks in india due to climate change: Rethinking approach to health service provision commercializing a scalable low cost arsenic remediation technology for societal impact view project vulnerability assessment of home-garden eco-syste. *Handbook of Research on Climate Chnage Impact on Helath and Environmental Sustainability*. https://doi.org/10.4018/978-1-5225-1674-3.ch051

Sheehan, M. C., Fox, M. A., Kaye, C., & Resnick, B. (2017). Integrating health into local climate response: Lessons from the US CDC climate-ready states and cities initiative. *Environmental Health Perspectives, 125*(9), 1–6. https://doi.org/10.1289/EHP1838

Sultana, F. (2014). Gendering climate change: Geographical insights. *The Professional Geographer, 66*(3), 372–381. https://doi.org/10.1080/00330124.2013.821730

Warner, K., Hamza, M., Oliver-Smith, A., Renaud, F., & Julca, A. (2010). Climate change, environmental degradation and migration. *Natural Hazards, 55*(3), 689–715. https://doi.org/10.1007/S11069-009-9419-7/FIGURES/4

Watts, M. (2017). Political ecology. *A Companion to Economic Geography, 2017*, 257–274.

Ylipää, J. (2018). *In the eye of the storm A gendered study on climate change adaptation in small-scale farming in Thái Bình, Vietnam.*

Ylipaa, J., Gabrielsson, S., & Jerneck, A. (2019). Climate change adaptation and gender inequality: Insights from rural Vietnam. *Sustainability (Switzerland), 11*(10), 1–16. https://doi.org/10.3390/su11102805

Zinyemba, C., Archer, E., & Rother, H.-A. (2018). Climate variability, perceptions and political ecology: Factors influencing changes in pesticide use over 30 years by Zimbabwean smallholder cotton producers. *PLoS ONE, 13*(5), 1–19. https://doi.org/10.1371/journal.pone.0196901

13 Well-Being of the Elderly Population in India

Trisha Mukhopadhyay and Sumanta Roy

Abstract

Ageing is a normal biological process that is a part of the life process. The way one defines aging differs depending on the various social constructions and varies according to culture. Usually, the age of retirement i.e., 60 or 65 years is considered as the starting of old age and on the basis of changing social roles and capabilities. The data points out that the elderly population is increasing globally. According to the India Ageing Report of 2017, the global old age population stood at 11.5% of the total population of 7 billion and it is projected to increase to 19% by the year 2050. Thus, most countries of the world are going through the demographic transition phase where there is continuous increase of elderly population which is the result of decrease in birth rate as well as death rate and increase in life expectancy. The changing family norms and the elderly family who are living alone are more vulnerable. The COVID-19 pandemic has aggravated the challenges being faced by the elderly. With the increase in age the elderly population has to face challenges in terms of physiology, mentally, economically, socially and emotionally. For a healthy ageing the well-being of the elderly population also has to be looked into. Well-being adds to the component of increasing longevity. Well-being is associated with reduction in monetary burden and rise in economic contribution. The paper focuses on analyzing LASI data to understand the ageing and well-being of the elderly population on the basis of various socio-economic indicators.

13.1 Introduction

Ageing is a part of the life phase which everyone has to go through. It is a part of the change in the life course. The World Health Organization states that the process of ageing a biological reality which begins with concepts and the terminating point of this process is death. Though this process is beyond the control of human but the conceptualization and defining of ageing differs with the various social construction. The percentage of elderly population to the total population globally is about 11.5% of the seven billion total population. The percentage of elderly population is expected to rise to 19% by the year 2050. According to the 2011 Census of India the percentage of elderly population in the country was 8.3% of the total population. The percentage

T. Mukhopadhyay (✉) · S. Roy
Doctoral Fellow, Centre of Social Medicine and Community Health, Jawaharlal Nehru University, New Delhi, India
e-mail: 28thtrisha@gmail.com

S. Roy
Doctoral Fellow, Department of Anthropology, Washington State University, Pullman, Washington, USA

S. S. Acharya et al. (eds.), *Paradigm Shifts in Population and Health in India*, Sustainable Development Goals Series, https://doi.org/10.1007/978-981-95-1719-0_13

of the elderly population may represent a small one but the absolute numbers are quite high. Most of the elderly population globally are from the less developed regions of the world. The World Population Prospects state that there is a rapid increase in the proportion of elderly population in the developing countries as compared to the developed countries of the world. The decline in fertility and mortality are the main reason for the increase in the elderly population. Increase in life expectancy has been leading to the continuous increase of the elderly population. The pattern of age in the decline of mortality favours the youth more than the elderly and the decline in the fertility leads to a faster change in the age distribution. The life expectancy of women is more than the male hence leading more number of female elderly population. The process of ageing is associated with physiological changes, neurological disorders, psychological changes, economic changes, social role changes. As the elderly population rises there is also rise in the old age dependency and more care giving. The changing demography of the country calls for changes in policy to keep up with the demographic transition. To understand the issues faced by the elderly population there is a need to understand their needs in terms of demography and economy.

13.2 Aging Concept

The old age population mainly comprises those in the age group of 60 and above. It is important to understand the concept of ageing due to the increasing elderly population. Though there is no specific definition to define old age, it is the age of retirement from the service in the organized sector which is usually taken as the initiation of old age. It is during which the Government of the country begins to provide social assistance in the form of pension to the people at old age. The usual age of retirement in most of the countries is 60 or 65. The understanding of old age is not only dependent on the economic terms but also the socio-cultural perceptions as well. It is also important to understand the concept of old age in the informal work setting. The decline in active social participation is a social construct as a benchmark for old age. Old age can be defined in terms of chronology i.e., the increasing age; social role changes and the reducing capabilities. One of the components of old age is the reduced capabilities, hence an increasing socio-economic dependence, as well dependence on others for completing daily activities. The well-being of the elderly population is affected by the surroundings in which they are living.

13.3 Well-Being Concept

World Health Organization defines well-being as, "Well-being is a positive state experienced by individuals and society. Similar to health, it is a resource for daily life and is determined by social, economic and environmental conditions. Well-being encompasses quality of life and the ability of people and societies to contribute to the world with a sense of meaning and purpose." The WHO definition of health also has one component of social well-being. Well-being can be applied at the individual level as well as the societal level. At the individual the two philosophical views are hedonic and eudemonic view. The Hedonic view explains the subjective aspect of well-being which is of feeling good; whereas the eudemonic view explains the meaning and purpose of life. There are factors like the daily life events which affect the individual often referred to as the subjective well-being. On the other hand, societal well-being is the population level well-being and is holistic in nature by taking into consideration the surrounding in which people live, physical, social, and economic aspects. Well-being is also contextual and may differ from individual to individual.

Ottawa Charter for Health Promotion has further dwelled on the concept of health and well-being by considering it as everyday resource. Eventually the Report of the Commission on Social Determinants of Health pointed the structural factors, intermediary factors which lead to differences in equitable differences in health and well-being. In 2011 the World Conference on Social Determinants of Health was held which promoted well-being concept. Well-being is determined by the individual quest, inter personal connections, pleasure, income, health and activities which are like breaks in the daily life (Drene, 2017). Recently the COVID-19 pandemic has demonstrated the relation of economic, social, physical, mental impacts with health, and well-being of the society as well as the individual level. Well-being does not comprise only of the mind but also the situations which are external in nature (Drene, 2017). Thus, we cannot separate health and well-being and in the process of ageing.

13.4 Aging and Well-Being

Ageing and health are two complex dynamics (Thiyagarajan et al., 2022). World report on Aging and Health was published by WHO in the year 2015 for taking up action on aging in a framework of public health and also gave the concept of 'Healthy Aging'. Healthy aging is defined as the 'process of developing and maintaining the functional ability that enables well-being in older age' (WHO, 2015). The elderly people are important human resource of the society who have experience of life, are holders of values and knowledge bundle of the traditions. The change in the family structure increases the neglect and loneliness in the elderly population. With ageing the social participation and social support becomes an important linkage and the decline in the social relationships affects the psychological and physical well-being of the older person (Clifton, 2009). Well-being of the elderly including subjective, psychological well-being and a positive attitude towards life will help in a better quality of life. The life expectancy has been increasing hence leading to a rise in the elderly population. Though the life expectancy has been increasing but the gain in life years has not been equally healthy (World Health Organization, 2020a, 2020b, 2021). The improvement in the life span of the elderly population is hindered by the chronic diseases associated with the ageing process, still the relation of age and health are affected by various other determinants (Scott et al., 2021; Beard et al., 2019). An action plan at the global level was declared by the WHO and United Nations i.e., The UN Decade of Healthy Ageing from 2021 to 2030. The plan aimed to provide for a healthy and greater longevity for not only the older people but also the family members, the communities and place of residence (United Nations, 2020; World Health Organization, 2020a, 2020b). In India various programmes and schemes have been launched which affect the health and well-being of the elderly population directly and indirectly. Some of the programmes to be mentioned are National Policy for Older Persons (1999); Maintenance and Welfare of Parents and Senior Citizens Act, 2007; National Social Assistance Programme, Integrated Programme for Senior Citizens, National Action Plan for Senior Citizens, National Initiative on Care for the Elderly (2004) and National Programme for the Healthcare of the Elderly (2011).

The objective of the current study is to understand the ageing and well-being of the elderly population in India by analyzing the socio-economic indicators from the LASI, Wave 1 data.

13.5 Methodology

The study is mainly based on secondary data analysis. Data has been taken from the Longitudinal Ageing Survey in India (LASI), WAVE-1 India Report 2020 (Longitudinal Ageing Study in India (LASI), 2020). As mentioned, well-being is a subjective concept and it is not only about the mind but the external factors as well which affect the well-being of the person. LASI WAVE-1 Report provides the health, economic and social well-being data of the elderly population in India. In the study we have taken certain proxy indicators to understand the well-being of the elderly population in India.

LASI has a huge variety of indicators of which the variables taken are-current living arrangement, major probable depression based on CIDI-SF (Composite International Diagnostic Interview-Short Form) Scale, Activities of Daily Life (ADL) limitation, Discrimination and Perceived satisfaction of life. Among the variables we have tried to look into the various background characteristics for a better understanding and comparison across groups. The background characteristics are-residence, sex, living arrangement, marital status, caste, work status, and MPCE (Monthly Per Capita Expenditure) quintile. Percentage of the elderly for the variables as given in the LASI data has been used for the analysis and graphical representation. The analysis of the data has been done variable wise with literature to support the findings.

13.6 Results

According to Census of India 2011 the percentage of the elderly population to the total population was 8.6% which has been an increase from the year 1961 when the percentage of elderly population stood at 5.6%. The difference between the percentage of rural elderly population and urban population has been always existing but a change in the trend can be seen with a reducing gap between the percentage of the elderly population in rural and urban area. Census of India 2011 records that the percentage of elderly population residing in rural area is 8.8% and in urban area it is 8.1% whereas in the year 1961 the percentage for elderly population in rural area was 5.8% and in urban area it was 4.7%. The youth used to migrate to the urban area for better opportunities and return to their native place after retirement from service but now the elderly prefer staying back in the urban area for the presence of better facilities. The percentage of female elderly population is more as compared to the male elderly population thus making the female elderly especially those living alone a vulnerable group.

13.7 Living Arrangement of the Elderly

Residence is one of the factors which affects the well-being of the elderly. Not only the place of residence but the environment and family structure play an important role in the well-being of the elderly. With the increase in age the elderly population are often isolated which affects their mental well-being. The family structure in India is going through changes where there is more nuclearization of family. As members of the household are into services the elderly person is often left alone at home. Those living with spouse have each other for support but the widowed and those living alone face the increased feeling of isolation and often leading them towards depression.

From the Fig. 13.1, it can be observed that the 6.3% of the elderly population in the rural area are living alone and in urban area the percentage is 4.1%. In the rural area the percentage of elderly population living with spouse is higher in rural areas as compared to the urban areas i.e. 21.5% and 17.5% respectively. The percentage of elderly population living with children and spouse is approximately same in both the rural and urban area. In urban the percentage of the elderly population living with children but without spouse in 32.6% and in rural area is 25.6%. The percentage of female elderly population living alone is higher as compared to the male elderly population and similarly the percentage of the female elderly living with children without spouse is higher (40.7%). For the male elderly population living with spouse (26%) and living with spouse and children (54.4%) is higher. It is the higher life expectancy of women and widowhood which leads to the elderly women living alone and living with children without spouse. Widowed living alone is 14.3% and living with children without spouse is 73.5%. On the basis of caste other backward class has the highest percentage of the elderly living alone (6.3%); 22.1% of the elderly population in scheduled tribe live with their spouse; highest percentage of the elderly live with spouse and children and the 28.7% of the elderly live with children without spouse. According the work status background 49.5% of the elderly population currently working are living with children and spouse has the highest percentage share. The richest category of the MPCE quintile has the highest elderly population living alone of 7.5%, similarly in the category of living with spouse the percentage by the richest quintile is 32.4% whereas in the category of living

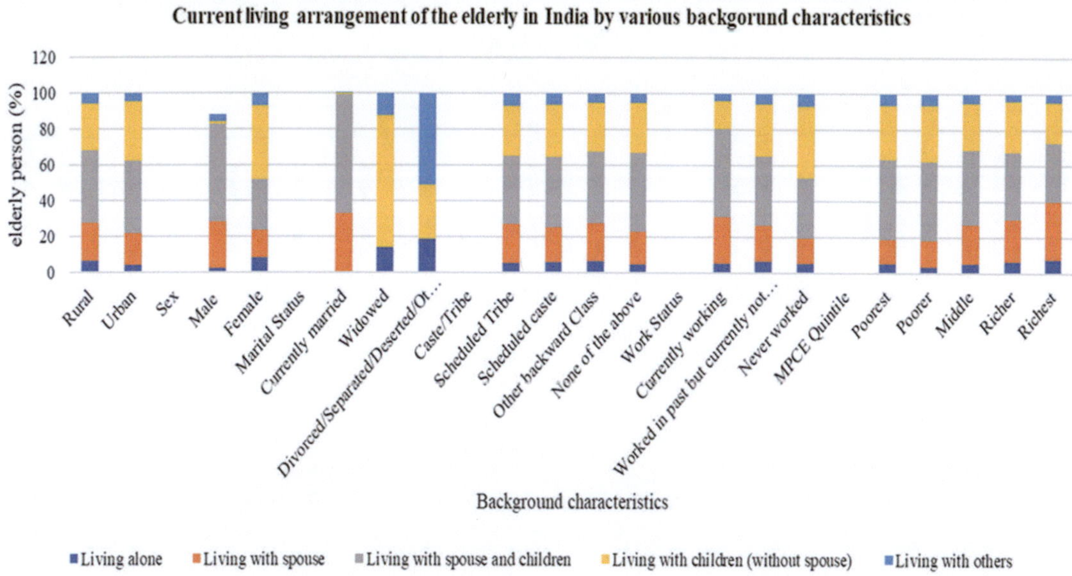

Fig. 13.1 Current living arrangement of the elderly in India by various background characteristics. *Source* LASI, WAVE 1–2020

with spouse and children the poorest MPCE quintile has a percentage share of 44.4% and the poorer MPCE quintile with 30.8% of the elderly population is for the elderly living with children without spouse. 51.4% of the elderly population who have either been divorced or separated or deserted have been living with others. Across the different background characteristics, it is extensively visible that the highest percentage of the elderly have been living with spouse and children followed by the category of living with children (without spouse) among which the widowed elderly has the greater proportion.

13.8 Elderly with Depression

With the increase in age there is weakening of the physiology, functional abilities as well the mental health of the elderly population. Well-being of the elderly is affected not only by the physical health but also the mental health thus making it an important determinant in the study of the well-being of the elderly. Decision making, decline in working ability, social interactions are impacted by the decreased cognitive functioning. With the increase in age there is increased isolation, lesser social interactions which leads to depression among the elderly population (Ofstedal et al., 2005; WHO, 2013).

Depression can have an impact on the daily activities of a person when there is loss of interest in the activities which were once enjoyed by the person. For the current study data by LASI validated Composite International Diagnostic Interview-Short Form (CIDI-SF) scale has been used to understand the major depression in the elderly population of India.

From the Fig. 13.2, given, it can be observed that the elderly persons living alone are the highest with probable major depression with 12.8% followed by the elderly persons who are living with others i.e., 11.1%. Elderly residing in rural areas are more prone to depression as compared to the urban area and female elderly are more depressed than the male elderly population. On the basis of marital status, the widowed have higher percentage of depression i.e., 9.7%. The elderly persons who had worked in the past but are currently not working have a higher chance to be depressed as after retirement they have to spend most of the time at home with reduced social interaction and other engagements. The richest MPCE quintile have the highest

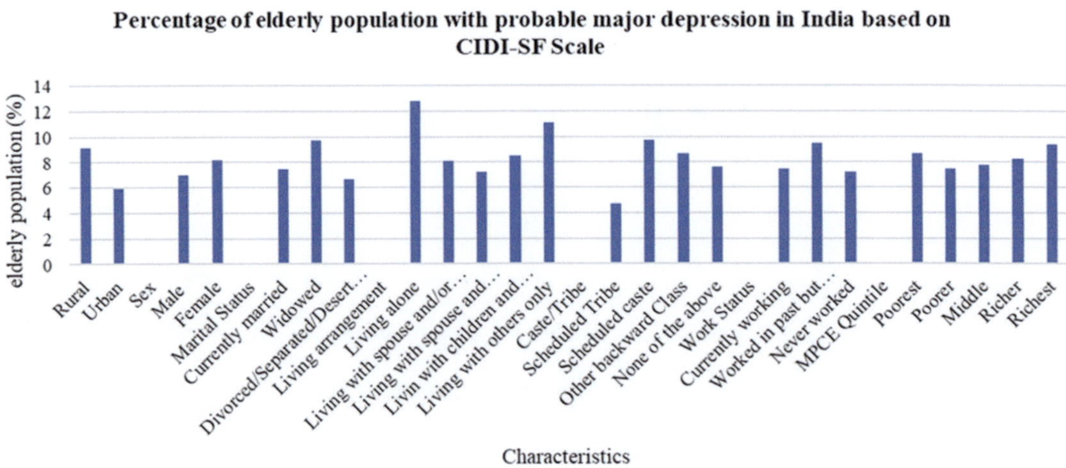

Fig. 13.2 Percentage of elderly with probable major depression in India based on CIDI-SF scale. *Source* LASI, WAVE 1–2020

percentage of elderly persons with depression of 9.4% persons.

13.9 Activities of Daily Life

The ageing process is associated with decline in the physical ability, increased chronic diseases which in turn increases the dependence on others requiring long term care and more medical expenditure. The graph explains the limitations in activities of daily life with either one limitation or more than two limitations. The elderly population living in the rural areas have more than one limitation (24.4%) as well as more than two limitation (14.7%) (Fig. 13.3) when compared to the urban areas having lower limitation. The female elderly population have more limitations thus making them more dependent on others for their daily activities with 26.4% female elderly having more than one limitation in the daily activities and 16.4% female elderly having more than two ADL. The widowed elderly persons have more limitation in both the categories. The elderly population having more than 2 ADL live with children and others requiring more care and dependency. The elderly population living alone have more than one ADL but lower 2 + ADL. The elderly population living alone have to be dependent on themselves for the daily activities. Elderly population belonging to the scheduled caste have more than one ADL. Those elderly persons who have worked in the past but is currently not working have more limitation in activities of daily life i.e., 29.9% with 1 + ADL and 18.8% with 2 + ADL. When they were a part of the labour market the dependency on others were less but with ageing the reduced physical activities somewhat makes them dependent on others. The poorest MPCE quintile have the highest number of elderly population with limitation in their daily life activities (25.6% with 1 + ADL; 15.5% with 2 + ADL). The higher life expectancy of the women enables them to live longer leading to greater period of limitation and more dependency.

13.10 Discrimination Against the Elderly Population

Elderly population have been facing discrimination and neglect which affects their well-being. Though 90% of the elderly face no discrimination, still the rest few face one kind or more than two kind of discrimination. Widowed elderly population with one kind of discrimination is 5.5% and 3.4% with two or more discrimination (Fig. 13.4). Elderly population living alone have been facing two or more kind of discrimination of 5.7% and those elderly population living with children but without spouse 5.8%. The other backward class and scheduled tribe have been facing

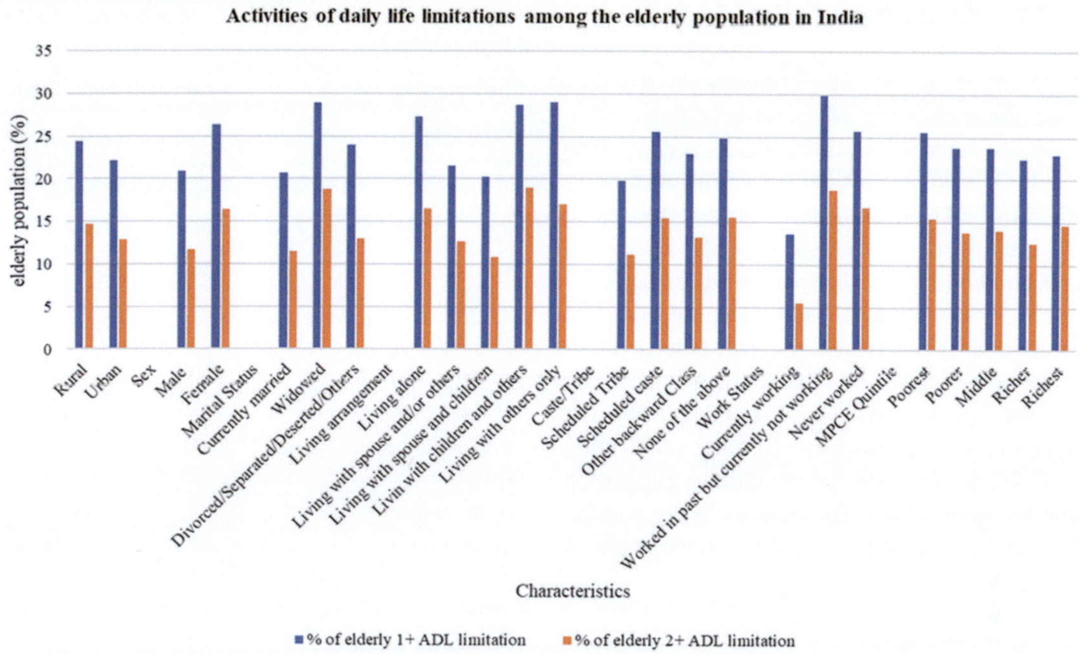

Fig. 13.3 Activities of daily life limitations among the elderly population in India. *Source* LASI, WAVE 1–2020

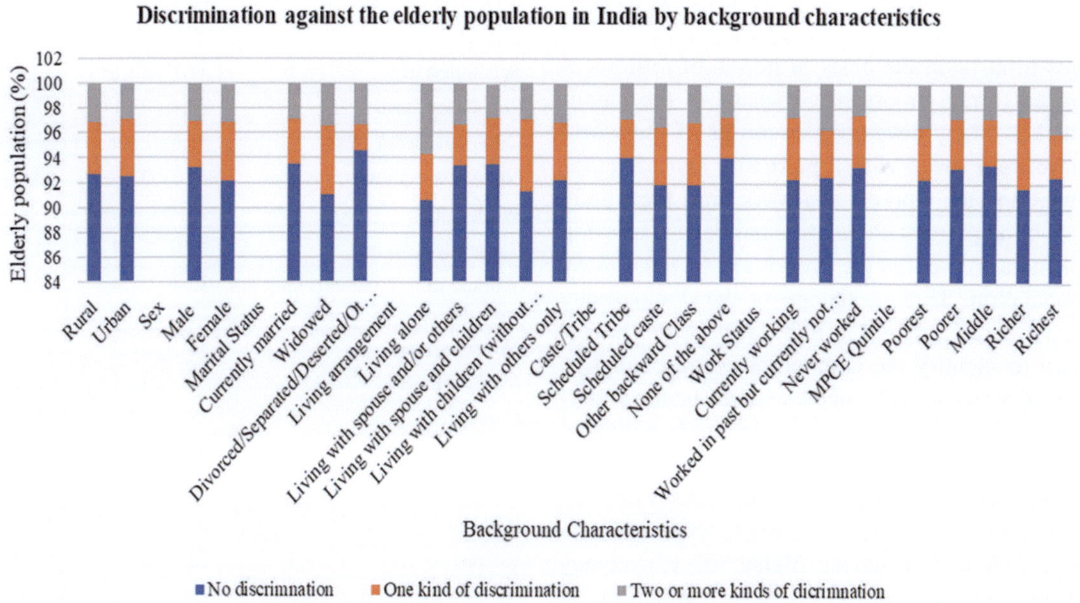

Fig. 13.4 Discrimination against the elderly population in India by background characteristics. *Source* LASI, WAVE 1–2020

one kind of discrimination i.e. 4.9% and 4.6% respectively. The richer elderly population does face one kind of discrimination (5.8%) and the richest elderly population in the MPCE quintile background have two and more discrimination (4%).

13.11 Perceived Life Satisfaction

Perceived life is one of the components to understand the well-being of the elderly population. Perceived satisfaction of life differs according to people depending on their experiences of daily life, surroundings, family structure and the way of life. Elderly population residing in the urban area have claimed for a higher perceived life satisfaction of 53.7% (Table 13.1). Among the male and female elderly population, the male elderly population have a higher life satisfaction of 47.2% and also the female elderly have a higher life satisfaction of 44%. Lower perceived life satisfaction of 47.7% is observed for the elderly population who are living alone. The richest elderly population have a highest perceived life satisfaction of 52.3%.

Table 13.1 Perceived level of life satisfaction among the elderly in India

Characteristics	Low	Medium	High
Residence			
Rural	34.4	23.5	42.2
Urban	26.7	19.6	53.7
Sex			
Male	30.4	22.5	47.2
Female	33.8	22.3	44
Marital status			
Currently married	29.7	22.9	47.4
Widowed	35.6	21.4	43
Divorced/separated/deserted/others	44.1	23.2	32.7
Living arrangement			
Living alone	47.7	19.3	32.9
Living with spouse and/or others	31.6	23.1	45.3
Living with spouse and children	28.6	22.8	48.5
Living with children (without spouse)	32.6	22	45.4
Living with others only	42.1	21.2	36.7
Caste/tribe			
Scheduled tribe	37.1	23.1	39.8
Scheduled caste	39.4	23.1	37.5
Other backward class	31.6	21.9	46.6
None of the above	26.7	22.5	50.9
Work status			
Currently working	31.9	23.7	44.4
Worked in past but currently not working	32.4	21.3	46.2
Never worked	32	22.4	45.7
MPCE quintile			
Poorest	38.4	24	37.6
Poorer	34.1	22.9	43
Middle	30.2	22.9	46.9
Richer	28.4	21.9	49.7
Richest	28.2	19.3	52.3

Source LASI, WAVE 1–2020

13.12 Discussion

In India the persons who have attained the age of 60 and above are considered as elderly and this limit is on the basis of norms of retirement in the formal or organized sector of the labour market. Many developed countries of the world have done away with a particular age of retirement and the workers can work until their body and mind permits. Population has been increasing in India as well as the proportion of the elderly population. Thus, a change in the demography and age sex pyramid in India. It becomes necessary to identify the demographic and economic characteristics of the aged so as to better understand the issues of ageing in India (Visaria, 2001).

The rise in the proportion of the elderly population is due to the increase in life expectancy at birth and with women having higher life expectancy there is feminization of the elderly population. As the Census of India 2011 notes the increase in the percentage of the elderly population from the year 1961 (5.6%) to 2011 (8.6%) and a reducing gap of the elderly population residing in rural area (8.8%) or urban area (8.1%). The reducing gap is mainly due to the preference of staying back in the urban areas with better facilities. The percentage of female elderly population is higher as compared to the male elderly population thus making them a more vulnerable group.

Well-being of the elderly is impacted by the place of residence, arrangement of family, the acceptance of the elderly in society, the mental health condition, limitation in the activities of daily life, discrimination faced by the elderly and the perceived life satisfaction. Family and the different relationships in family are relevant for the health and well-being of the elderly (Tesch-Romer et al., 2002). The family structure is changing in India with nuclearization of family. Family members are an important caregiver for the elderly persons (Liebar et al., 2020). With the changing family structure the elderly are often neglected and feel isolated, lack of assistance which in turn leads to poor outcomes in health (Hass, 2017; He, 2015). The percentage of the elderly population living alone or the elderly living with spouse is high in the rural areas as the children move out for job, education opportunities leaving behind the aged. Even while living with children the elderly can feel neglected if they have nobody to talk to and all these can lead them towards depression.

Elderly population living alone have the highest percentage share with probable depression (12.8%). Elderly residing in the rural areas, the widowed and the female elderly population are more depressed. With the increase in the elderly population in India the prevalence of non-communicable diseases is also likely to increase and hence the magnitude of depression (Kritiotis, 2007) (World Health Organization, 2012a, 2012b, 2012c). The change in the family structure with the children migrating and settling in the urban areas leaving the parents alone. The elderly have issues in adjusting to a new environment when they move out with their children which affects their psychological well-being. The elderly with age lose their significance at home and the feelings of neglect, loneliness leads them towards depression. A social divide is created when the society considers the elderly as valueless, with low energy, thus, decreasing their participation in various spheres of life (World Health Organization, 2012a, 2012b, 2012c). The presence of depression among the elderly is often not diagnosed properly, low treatment and is associated as part of the ageing process (Moussavi et al., 2007).

Depression impacts the day to day activities of the individual and hence an increase of dependency on others. The elderly living in the rural areas have one as well as more than two ADL. The female elderly population have more limitations thus making them more dependent on others for their daily activities with 26.4% female elderly having more than one limitation in the daily activities and 16.4% female elderly having more than two ADL. The widowed elderly persons have more limitation in both the categories. The elderly population having more than 2 ADL live with children and others requiring more care and dependency. Life satisfaction of the elderly becomes less with the presence of various problems and kind of social life (World Health Organization, 2012a, 2012b, 2012c) (World Health Organization, 2012a, 2012b, 2012c) (National Academy on an Aging Society, 2000). Coronary heart disease, hypertension, cancer, diabetes mellitus are at a higher risk among the elderly population with depression (World Health Organization, 2012a, 2012b, 2012c).

Widowed elderly population with one kind of discrimination is 5.5% and 3.4% with two or more discrimination. Elderly population living alone have been facing two or more kind of discrimination of 5.7% and those elderly population living with children but without spouse 5.8%. The decreased mobility with ageing process requires for long term care and greater dependency. The risk and vulnerability of the elderly towards discrimination, less care, lack of dignity and increased maltreatment towards the elderly increases due to their dependency on others (Pilania et al., 2013). Perceived life is one of the components to understand the well-being of the elderly population. Perceived satisfaction of life differs according to people depending on their experiences of daily life, surroundings, family structure and the way of life. The perceived life satisfaction is higher for the elderly population residing in the urban area and a lower life satisfaction among those elderly population living alone.

Thus, an interconnectedness is visible in between the variables selected for the present study. The well-being of the elderly is not just affected by the physical health but also the mental well-being is an important component. As the World Health Organization states that the well-being is determined by the social, economic and environmental conditions. The Ottawa Charter also focused on the well-being and considered as part of everyday resource. Sustainable development goal with Goal three talks about the health and well-being. Thus, be it young or elderly well-being is important and cannot be neglected.

13.13 Conclusion

Along with the basic health services there is requirement of mental health services for the elderly population. In India various programmes and schemes have been launched which affect the health and well-being of the elderly population directly and indirectly. Some of the programmes to be mentioned are National Policy for Older Persons (1999); Maintenance and Welfare of Parents and Senior Citizens Act, 2007; National Social Assistance Programme, Integrated Programme for Senior Citizens, National Action Plan for Senior Citizens, National Initiative on Care for the Elderly (2004) and National Programme for the Healthcare of the Elderly (2011). There has to be awareness of the needs, the physical dependency, social dependency of the elderly population on their family and others have to be taken into account while planning for the policies, welfare schemes and programmes for the elderly population in the country. With the demographic transition and the country moving towards a higher elderly population has to adjust to the changes for creating a healthy ageing environment.

References

Beard, J. R., Jotheeswaran, A. T., Cesari, M., & De Carvalho, I. A. (2019). The structure and predictive value of intrinsic capacity in a longitudinal study of ageing. BMJ open, *9*(11), e026119.

Clifton, J. (2009). *Ageing and well-being in an international context* (p. 1–36). Institute for public policy research.

Daatland, S. (2005). Quality of life and ageing. In V. Bengtson, P. Coleman, T. Kirkwood & M. Johnson (Eds.), *The Cambridge handbook of age and ageing: Cambridge handbooks in psychology* (pp. 371–377). Cambridge University Press. https://doi.org/10.1017/CBO9780511610714.038

Drene, S. (2017). What have we learned about well-being? In D. Steve (Ed.), *Sociology of well-being: Lessons from India* (pp. 217–248). SAGE Publications.

Hass, Z. (2017). Unmet need for help with activities of daily living disabilities and emergency department admissions among older medicare recipients. *The Gerontologist, 57*(2), 206–210.

He, S. (2015). Unmet need for ADL assistance is associated with mortlity among older adults with mild disability. *The Journals of Gerontology Series a: Biological Sciences and Medical Sciences, 70*(9), 1128–1132.

Kritiotis, L. (2007). *Depressive disorders and chronic comorbid diseaase states: A Pharmaco-epidemiological Evaluation.* Nelson Mandela University.

Liebar, J., Clarke, L., Timaeus, I. M., Mallinson, P. A., & Kinra, S. (2020). Changing family structures and self-related health of India's older population (1995–96 to 2014). *SSM-Population Health, 11*, Article 100572.

Longitudinal Ageing Study in India (LASI). (2020). Wave 1, 2017–18, India Report. *International Institute for Population Sciences (IIPS)*, Pdf. LASI 2017–18. https://www.iipsindia.ac.in/lasi

Moussavi, S., Chatterji, S., Verdes, E., Tandon, A., Patel, V., & Ustun, B. (2007). Depression, chronic diseases, and decrements in health: Results from the World health Surveys. *Lancet, 370*, 851–858.

National Academy on an Aging Society. (2000). *Depression: A treatable disease.* National Academy on an Aging Society.

Pilania, M., Bairwa, M., Kumar, N., Khanna, P., & Kurana, H. (2013). Elderly depression in India: An emerging public health challenge. *The Australian Medical Journal, 6*(3), 107–111.

Scott, A. J., Ellison, M., & Sinclair, D. A. (2021). The economic value of targeting aging. *Nat Aging, 1*, 616–623.

Tesch-Romer, C., Motel-Klingebiel, A., & Kondratowitz, H. J. (2002). Importance of family for quality of life of the elderly in a social and cultural comparison. *Zeitschrift fur Gerontologie und Geriatrie, 35*(4), 335–342.

Thiyagarajan, J. A., Mikton, C., Harwood, R. H., Gichu, M., Gaigbe-Togbe, V., Jhamba, T., & Diaz, T. (2022). The UN decade of healthy ageing: Strengthening measurement for monitoring health and wellbeing of older people. *Age and Ageing, 51*, 1–5.

United Nations. (2020). *Session S-F, ed. A/RES/75/131United Nations Decade of Healthy Ageing (2021–2030): Resolution/Adopted by the General Assembly on 14 December 2020.* New York: United Nations.

Visaria, P. (2001). Demographics of ageing in India. *Economic and Political Weekly, 2001*, 1967–1975.

World Health Organization. (2012a). World Health Day 2012-Aging and Health. *World Health Organization.*

World Health Organization. (2012b). Non-communicable Diseases. *WHO Factsheet*.

World Health Organization. (2012c). Me*ntal Health and Substance Abuse, Facts and Figures, Conquering Depression.*

World Health Organization. (2020a). *Data/gho/data/themes/mortality-and-global-health-estimates.* Retrieved from https://www.who.int: https://www.who.int/data/gho/data/themes/mortality-and-global-health-estimates

World Health Organization. (2020b). *United nation's decade of healthy ageing (2021–2030).* World Health Organization.

World Health Organization. (2021). *World health statistics 2021: Monitoring health for the SDGs.* World Health Organization.

World Health Organization. (2015). *World Health Day 2015: Good Health Adds Life to Years.*

Sexual Exploitation of Muslim Naikin Women: A Case Study from Maharashtra, India

14

Malika B. Mistry

Abstract

Sexual exploitation of women is found in all societies all over the world. Sometimes this sexual exploitation of women is undertaken by making use of religion. Devadasi system in India is a phenomenon of sexual exploitation of Hindu women in different provinces of India. They are called by different names in different states, such as Joginis in Andhra Pradesh and Telangana, Jogtis in Karnataka, Bhavin in Konkani, Kalavant in Marathi, and so on. A Devdasi is a young woman dedicated to the temple deity in the village. It is the priest who first sexually uses her. Then she is expected to satisfy the sexual needs of all men in the village who approach her. (Some of the devadasis end up in red light areas in the cities). In fact, a story of Renuka Yellamma has been created in religious terms to validate the above practise. The government has brought out legislation to ban this abhorring practise and rehabilitate these victims. Due to a number of factors, this custom is still in existence. There is no record of how much devadasi population exists in India. Authorities do not collect such data. As we noted, in Maharashtra Devadasis are called Kalavant. "Kala" means art. Who practises "Kala" is Kálavant. Mostly they sing and dance in "tamasha", a popular folk art of Maharashtra. In Marathi cinema, we find "tamasha" songs and dances very often. Another name for Kalavant is "Naikin". Naikins and their male family members are great artistes—singers, dancers and musicians. In early Hindi film industry, many film directors, music directors, actresses hailed from this community. In contemporary Marathi film industry, a number of Marathi film actresses have come from this community. This community is mostly found in Kolhapur and Sangli in Maharashtra which are nearer to Renuka Yellamma's temple at Saundatti in Karnataka. It was quite puzzling for this researcher to know about this aberration in Muslim society i.e. Muslim Naikin women. They are mostly found in Kolhapur and Sangli areas. In literature, hardly any information is available on these women. Therefore, the researcher decided to document about this Muslim community, especially Muslim Naikin women. This is a humble attempt. The objectives of this paper are: (i) To trace the origin of this institution i.e. Naikins among Muslims; (ii) To find their present socio-economic conditions; (iii) To know whether the rehabilitation programmes available for Devadasis are also available to these Muslim Naikin women; and (iv) If programmes are available, to evaluate

M. B. Mistry (✉)
Department of Economics, Poona College of Arts, Science and Commerce, Pune, India
e-mail: drmalika.mistry@gmail.com

S. S. Acharya et al. (eds.), *Paradigm Shifts in Population and Health in India*, Sustainable Development Goals Series, https://doi.org/10.1007/978-981-95-1719-0_14

whether they have been successful in giving dignified lives to these women victims. We are using case-study method. Interviews of these women will be conducted in Kolhapur and Sangli cities. The women will not easily respond because stigma is attached to this institution. Most of them have male partners outside the Muslim community may be because Muslim men do not want to marry them. Our investigation of life of a senior octogenarian Hindi film female artiste who hails from this community revealed that her mother was a Muslim and her father was a Brahmin. She was borne outside the wedlock. She got her daughter married according to Vidhi (Hindu tradition) to a Brahmin film actor. Most of these Muslim Naikin women have a partner called "Ýajman" (host). They are not prostitutes because at a time they have only one partner. If the relationship breaks, a Naikin will find another partner. The study is expected to bring to light very interesting findings and sad/happy stories of these women and their life.

14.1 Introduction

Sexual exploitation of women is found in all societies all over the world. Sometimes this sexual exploitation of women is undertaken by making use of religion. Devadasi system in India is a phenomenon of sexual exploitation of Hindu women in different provinces of India. A Devdasi is a young woman dedicated to the temple deity in the village. It is the priest who first sexually uses her. Then she is expected to satisfy the sexual needs of all men in the village who approach her. (Some of the devadasis end up in red light areas in the cities). In fact, a story of Renuka Yellamma has been created in religious terms to validate the above practise.

The government has brought out legislation to ban this abhorring practise and rehabilitate these victims. Due to a number of factors, this custom is still in existence. There is no record of how much devadasi population exists in India. Authorities do not collect such data. In fact one report prepared for National Commission of Women has made this suggestion. As we noted, in Maharashtra Devadasis are called Kalavant. 'Kala'means art. One who practises "Kala" is Kálavant. Mostly they sing and dance in "tamasha", a popular folk art of Maharashtra. In Marathi cinema, we find "tamasha" songs and dances very often.

Another name for Kalavant is "Naikin". Naikins and their male family members are great artistes—singers, dancers and musicians. In early Hindi film industry, many film directors, music directors, actresses hailed from this community. In contemporary Marathi film industry, a number of Marathi film actresses have come from this community. This community is mostly found in Kolhapur and Sangli in Maharashtra which are nearer to Renuka Yellamma's temple at Saundatti in Karnataka.

It was quite puzzling for this researcher to know about this aberration in Muslim society i.e. Muslim Naikin women. They are mostly found in Kolhapur and Sangli areas. In literature, hardly any information is available on these women. Therefore, the researcher decided to document about this Muslim community, especially Muslim Naikin women. This is a humble attempt.

14.2 Objectives of the Study

The aims of the study are: (i) To trace the origin of the institution of Naikins among Muslims; (ii) To find their present socio-economic conditions; (iii) To know whether the rehabilitation programmes available for Devadasis are also available to these Muslim Naikin women; and (iv) If programmes are available, to evaluate whether they have been successful in giving dignified lives to these women victims. This paper is divided into two sections. In the first section, we try to analyse the situation of Devadasis in India. In the second section, analyse the situation of Muslim Naikin women in Maharashtra by undertaking their case-studies.

14.3 Methodology

The study employed a case-study method. Interviews of these women are conducted in Kolhapur and Sangli cities. The women would not easily respond because stigma is attached to this institution. Most of them have male partners outside the Muslim community may be because Muslim men do not want to marry them. Our investigation of life of a senior octogenarian Hindi film female artiste who hails from this community revealed that her mother was a Muslim and her father was a Brahmin. She was borne outside the wedlock. She got her daughter married according to Vidhi (Hindu tradition) to a Brahmin film actor. Most of these Muslim Naikin women have a partner called "Ýajman" (host). They are not prostitutes because at a time they have only one partner. If the relationship breaks, a Naikin would find another partner. The study is expected to bring to light very interesting findings and sad and happy stories of these women and their life.

I

14.4 Review of the Context

Ditte Hansen, a research scholar and journalist did a study on the devadasis of Sangli. She could readily locate red light districts and the devadasis, or slaves of God, who are primarily members of the Dalit population in the parts surrounding the city of Sangli, which is on the border between Maharashtra and Karnataka.

She wrote her thesis on devadasis, or temple prostitutes. She had always wanted to visit a red-light area to meet and interview authentic devadasis. She had waited many years for this, and it was with a thumping heart that she entered a small house in the centre of a neighbourhood of 500 sex workers. She encountered a group of young women, all of them were sex workers and ranged in age from 18 to 25. Four of them were Devadasis. How does the red-light district operate? The girls must be at least 18 years old before they may work as prostitutes. If this regulation is not observed, the police will appear and cause problems for the entire area.

She was told that the government distributes 56 condoms to each sex worker every week because it was calculated that on average, 8 clients are served every day per sex worker. Unfortunately, when she was there, the government was about to remove this assistance, which would have disastrous consequences for the girls' health and safety. The government also provided buckets for collecting condoms, which was a significant change from the past, when condoms were just dumped on the ground. One item that really startled her and, regrettably, tells a lot about the view on sex and women that permits a continuous series of rapes to take place, was the explanation of the value of having free (but still charged, of course) access to sex workers: The women consider themselves as providing a favour for other women; they believe that they safeguard the safety of the typical woman; if there is no prostitution, a man has the right to go out and "take" whomever he wants. That is, 'your daughter, sister, or mother'. This is a popular belief in Indian society, and it explains why the media reports so many rapes. This is a popular belief in Indian society, which explains why the media reports so many rapes. And all the rapes that go unreported or are too "rural" ("just another Dalit") are far more common.

14.5 The Origins of the Devadasi Tradition

The four girls she met in the small room were devadasis. Her thesis study had led her to a reading and accounting of both the historic tradition, which includes ceremonies, religious beliefs, and foundations found in scriptures and sacred literature, as well as sociological studies from recent years. One of these was "Dalit women speak out—violence against women", which included over 500 testimonials from Dalit women, the majority of whom were devadasis or Joginis. They are goddesses by trade, but they are also prostitutes.

Historically, devadasis were prominent dancers in temples throughout South India, where the tradition started. An inscription from 1014 AD at the Rajarajeshwara temple in Thanjavur, Tamil Nadu, indicates that 400 temple dancers were brought in from all around the area to perform the holy dance, Sadir. They were granted a house, land, and a high level of social standing. Their dancing at temples was viewed as important for bringing the sacred writings to life; they were dancing and reenacting the brahmins' readings, so maintaining religious order.

Later, the sacred marriage of the devadasi (the goddess) and the brahmin (the god) was regarded as beneficial, and myths in sacred literature explain and justify this practice. Later, males may pay to unite with the goddess, which became a sacred union. At least for the man. The women were still respected, and their dance and singing abilities were highly recognized. Then the British arrived, bringing with them a Victorian worldview that saw this ancient behaviour as ugly, barbarous, and absolutely unpleasant. As a result, the dance was eventually split from the devadasis, renamed Bharathanatyam, and is now performed by Brahmin girls. It is one of India's most beloved and well-known classical dances. The last rituals took place formally in the 1960s. Females are now faced with only one option: prostitution.

14.6 The Devadasis in the Red-Light District

The four girls she met were among other devadasis who were revered as goddesses during sexual intercourse yet were treated as Dalits and prostitutes while going down the street. According to an account from the previously described research project, a woman witnessed women encouraging their men to sleep with her (because she was a goddess), but who flung stones at her in public. She was curious about why these four girls were there: did they want it? Were they forced by their families? Were they devadasi descendants? Every one of the four had the same narrative. They were from poor Dalit homes; thus, their relatives had forced them into this trade. Their family depended on their daughters to have sex for money. What about the rituals that distinguished them from the rest of the sex workers in the red-light district? Three of the girls only underwent one rite, the real initiation in which they "married the God (typically Vishnu), which means they cannot become widows or use any of their children's fathers" names for their offspring.

Furthermore, it tells the story of a tradition, which in this case is solely about money. The religious and mythological aspects are no longer present. It's all about getting the girls introduced quickly so they can make money. One girl, however, told her that she had been introduced when she was younger. Her mother had prayed to Renuka Yellamma (the goddess of the devadasis who is also revered by Dalits due to a story that depicts her with a goddess body but a Dalit woman's head) for a boy. She promised that if the desire came true, she would dedicate her daughter to the goddess. So, she did.

Let us grasp this narrative about Renuka Yellamma simply as described by Reddy and Sridevi: "The myth underlying the consecration of girls to the goddess Renuka, wife of sage Jamadagni, goes as follows. Renuka, the consort of Jamadagni, was a pure woman. She was so pure that she could carry water in a newly made pot. She would make one pot every day on the riverbank when she went to gather water. On one of these trips, she noticed a Gandharva couple bathing in the river. She was stunned by the male partner's attractive appearance when she viewed his reflection in the river water. However, due to this claimed violation of her marital vows, her pot broke, and her husband discovered her in the act of "adultery". He decided she had sinned by wanting a man other than her husband. Angered by this piercing of his saintly ego, the sage immediately ordered their 12-year-old son Parsuram to behead his own mother. The son performed as instructed. Jamadagni was pleased with his son's unquestioning obedience and sought to bestow a boon upon him. The astute son begged his father to bring his mother back to life. At this point, the sage noticed a matangi passing past. He decapitated her and put her head to Renuka's body. When Renuka was revived with the body of a holy woman and the head of a matangi, Jamadagni wanted to make apologies for his furious actions. He gifted her with the knowledge that unmarried girls would worship her as their goddess, and these girls would be dedicated to her for the rest of their lives, ready to satisfy all sexual demands put on them by her son Parasuram, who is present in every man. According to Jamadagni, the girls see every man as Parasuram in human form and will readily satisfy his sexual demands without asking for anything in return, including marriage, permanent bonding, or anything in cash or kind. These girls, Jamadagni said, would have no right to refuse a guy, even if he was a leper seeking sexual favours. Their livelihood is based on asking for donations from door to door on Fridays in the name of Yellamma" (2019: 108).

14.7 What a Cruel and Devilish Exploitation of Women in the Name of Religion!

These girls had one thing in common: they were all from Karnataka, a neighbouring state. And, as she discovered, there was a significant difference between devadasis from Maharashtra and Karnataka. Karnataka girls are more likely to become prostitutes. The girls in Maharashtra do not.

14.8 The Male Devadasi

She discovered two gorgeous males dressed in saris. She met Dinesh at 27 and Chandani at 55. In Indian civilization, there is a tradition of hijras, which are males who are either eunuchs, castrated, or gay and dance at the birth of sons, beg, and are considered semi sacrosanct. This description does not apply to these two men. Both go to the temple where she met them, which is a little village temple devoted to Renuka Yellamma. Both go out and 'ask for the goddess'. That means they walk from door to door, sometimes with instruments, sometimes with the large Renuka statue, but always with a begging basket and the words, 'Please give us something with pride'. They bear the mark of Shiva, the God of Destruction and a member of the Trimurti, on their forehead. The offerings are just for the deity and not for themselves. When they are ready for initiation, they marry Renuka's spouse, Jamadagni, and wear a scarlet thread or a see-through mala (beads). Women devadasis wear a yellow thread adorned with three beads. When a man senses that he may be "in need of putting on a sari", he seeks out a guru. That guru calls the family and obtains approval from them.

After that, the man may be schooled in dancing if he wishes, and some male dancers are well-known for this. Others tend to temples and are present at festivals and religious events, bestowing blessings, and executing ceremonies.

The researcher discovered that a transition is occurring; formerly, the rites were done by women devadasis. Now it's time for males. The female devadasis she met with solely reported tending temples, not performing rituals. However, they, like the males, were seen begging, singing, and playing an instrument during religious rituals. Again, male and female devadasis from Maharashtra, rather than Karnataka, do similar chores.

14.9 Being in a Lineage

Other women devadasis she spoke with claimed to be sixth or ninth generation devadasi. However, she did not find any in red light areas. Typically, they were more like "village prostitutes" who had been introduced as children and passed down from mother to daughter due to the family trade. Several of the women weren't prostitutes, but rather begging devadasis, just like the males. Some of them were able to play an instrument intended to praise the deity Renuka Yellamma. So there appears to be a significant difference between being forced by your family to work for money and being descended from devadasis, not to mention the issue of where state you come from.

The girls in the red-light districts were from very poor Dalit households, mostly from Karnataka, who had either been promised to the goddess or had a family in need of money. If a family has two girls, they may "gift" one to the goddess. The tradition associated with the name is not being considered or remembered. It stems from poverty and superstition.

The majority of the women found outside the red-light community were from Maharashtra. They belonged to a lineage of devadasis who continued a trade passed down from their mother, and some had already passed it on to their daughters. Some have had the power and luck to prevent this from happening. The women either go begging, work as village prostitutes, or find a benefactor who will care for them for the rest of their life. Typically, these guys have a "regular family" on the side, but maintain a consistent interaction with the devadasi, perhaps even a romantic one.

14.10 Who Wants to Marry a Devadasi?

The government has taken some action and has started the so-called "devadasi marriages"; a man who marries a devadasi receives Rs. 10,000. Is this a good thing? Maybe. Typically, the women are portrayed as what they are: prostitutes who are "damaged goods". It is all about tradition and culture. Marriage is a significant and essential event in India, and if a woman is unable to find a husband, she is shunned from society and sometimes even her own family. She becomes a burden and a "lesser woman". So, when she marries, she will be able to improve, if not her own, then her children's lives. There must be a transformation in the community. In the lineage situation, the women must cease passing on the tradition. In the case of the red-light district, the focus is on empowering families and Dalit communities. And society's perception of women must alter so that women are not treated as inferior to males, as is the case in many instances. The Maharashtra women had a clear mindset: they wanted change. Unfortunately, the Karnataka women were caught between poverty and superstition. They still lacked the power and resources to establish an escape route. And as long as the sex industry is profitable, it will continue to draw Dalits. And, when combined with age-old religious ideas, it will keep women trapped as sex workers for a long time.

14.11 What Are the Problems Faced by Devadasis?

Harishankar and Priyamvadha (undated) in their study found the following problems faced by the Devadasi women:

- Dedication as devadasis is more common in Hinduism, particularly among the Scheduled Caste population.
- Factors contributing to dedication include gender, lower socio-economic status, caste, education level, family tradition of dedication, and fear of losing the title of "nithyasumangali".
- Some devadasis marry, but this does not resolve their issues. The pair can only live a happy and respectable life if at least one of them works. Otherwise, the marriage may be unsuccessful, sending them back to their former way of life, namely prostitution.
- The primary sources of income for devadasis were begging and prostitution. They cannot be rehabilitated until the government provides alternative forms of income, such as sustainable livelihoods.
- Devadasis are subjected to different types of abuse, including verbal, physical, sexual, sociocultural, and pecuniary.
- State legislation for abolition of the Devadasi system are not that effective due to a number of reasons.
- Governments have implemented a number of projects to rehabilitate devadasis. These schemes include pension plans, housing and land projects, and income-generating enterprises. However, their implementation is inadequate. One explanation could be a lack of or low awareness of the schemes among the devadasis themselves.
- The communities from whom the women are devoted as devadasis should be thoroughly taught about the STDs and AIDS to which the devadasis may be exposed, as well as how antisocial groups may exploit them, in order for the communities to willingly cease this abhorrent practice.

- Devadasis have a distinct musical and dance legacy. As a result, individuals can work as trainers/teachers in various disciplines, gaining both employment and social status.

Tejpal who studied the plight of the devadasis (called Joginis in Andhra and Telangana) has criticised Indian society as follows:

"Even in the twenty-first century, it is disheartening to observe vast sectors of an ostensibly democratic Indian society being affected by uneducated, discriminatory, and unjust practices, such as the Jogini system". The practice has survived in the deep recesses of southern India, taking the lives of women and perpetuating itself in the lives of their children. Poverty, a lack of adequate health care, social marginalization, and systemic caste and gender exploitation are all daily realities for the girls started as Joginis. Fueled by caste, sexism, and ineffective regulation, the immediate future for current Joginis appears gloomy. The Jogini system's existence today should serve as a bold headline for those left behind in the mainstream rhetoric of growth" (2018: 191).

II

14.12 Case Studies

As we noted earlier, in Maharashtra devadasis are called kalavant. Kalavant are naikins. Now let us move to case studies of Naikin women in Sangli and Kolhapur in Maharshtra. First, we shall examine the case studies of Naikin women in general and then move to those of Muslim Naikin women.

14.13 Naikin Women

When I started research on Naikin women it was like travelling in a dark alley. An idea struck to me. I contacted a famous and senior Marathi film actress Miss. A.K. (My husband was a famous Marathi film director. She had acted in his films She has great respect for him.) I explained to her that I am doing research for writing a paper on Muslim Naikin women. She enquired thoroughly why was I interested in this topic. I could convince her that I was doing research to understand this community and know about their lives, problems etc. Then she agreed to share all the information she had with me. Below I will narrate the stories of the Nakin women.

Naikin women and their family members were very talented people well versed in the arts of singing and dancing. In the olden times many famous film personalities in Maharshtra hailed from the Naikin families. Some of them achieved great fame beyond Maharashtra. Their fame reached all of India through the Hindi film Industry. For example, very famous film producers and directors V.S., B.P., music directors like Master V.K. hailed from Naikin families of Kolhapur and Sangli in Maharashtra. Different children of Naikin women had one mother and different fathers. B.P. did not have children. He had owned a film studio in Kolhapur. Some time back he expired. Even today his name is well known in Marathi film industry and in Maharashtra. V.S's wife and daughter were very famous film actresses. His progeny is still associated with film industry. V.K.'s daughter was a famous Hindi film actress.

Naikin women are great artistes of tamasha, a folk dance of Maharashtra. Some examples of these women are M.K., L.G., U.C. and U. Naik. These are famous Marathi film actresses and sometimes they give performances on the stage too. Their children no more have the Naikin background and lead normal lives. For example, Ms. L.G. married a well to do transporter and has got three daughters from him. They are well-educated. One is a dentist. All of them are married and are leading normal lives. The second daughter married a Muslim Shaikh. Naikins are not particular about jati i.e. caste and religion.

14.14 Stories of Muslim Naikin Women

Miss A.K. narrated the following stories of Muslim Naikin women and their family members mostly from Kolhapur. Muslim Naikin women, like their Hindu counter parts, were very famous artists in singing and dancing. (Muslim Naikin women and men often took Hindu names.) A. Patil was a mistress of Kagal Sarcar (Chief of Kagal area near Kolhapur). Her mother was a Muslim Naikin woman. Another well-known Naikin woman as N. Belgaonkar. Their male family members were also great artistes. For example, Balasaheb Mirajkar was a famous Muslim singer. Mammulal Sengaonkar was a famous tabla player. He had a daughter Savarna. She was also an artist. Adamsaheb Rukdikar was another famous tabla player. Abu Wantemulik was another famous artist with Naikin background from Kolhapur. In Miraj next to Sangli city, most of the tambori (a musical instrument) makers are Muslims.

14.15 Case Study of S.L.

S.L. is a famous Hindi film actress who hails from Naikin community of Kolhapur. She would not like to reveal that she is from Muslim Naikin community because stigma is attached to her. Sometime back some writer had mentioned this fact while writing biography of a famous film producer. She was offended. Hence in our paper, we are using only the initials. S.L. is more than 90 years old. She is very beautiful. She had a Muslim mother and Brahmin father. She was born out of wed lock as Naikin women do not marry. They only have a partner called yajman (host). He will financially provide for her. For some reason when he leaves her, she would search for another yajman. S.L. had a urdu name. She went to the famous producer in Kolhapur to join film industry. He was attracted to her beauty specially her beautiful eyes. So, he gave her the name which translates as "beautiful eyes". She has a daughter having a Hindu name. This girl was married to a famous educated and handsome Brahmin Marathi actor. Some time back this actor died due to heart failure. Mother and daughter live together in Bombay in a Brahmin area. The daughter takes best care of her mother.

14.16 Case Study of N. Chiklikar

Miss Chiklikar was extremely beautiful, a great dancer and singer. She acted in Marathi films as a dancer and tamasha artist. She was a contemporary of famous actress A.K. who also hailed from Kolhapur. They were together in the school. Ms. N. had a sister by the name Panna. Both were going to school. When N. was 12 years old, every other day she used to wear a new watch or a new gold chain. A.K. wondered how she could wear such expensive things so often. Many times, she came late to the school. Teachers did not scold her. One day A.K. came to know about the secret of N. wearing the new valuables. N. participated in baithak (sittings of music and dance). She sang melodiously the famous Hindi song 'Dil ka khilona hai toot gaya" (Alas! The toy of heart is broken!) The audience presented the gifts to her for her melodious singing and beautiful dancing. (Naikin's baithaks were famous in Kolhapur. The programmes could be public or private. Private were organized in Kagal, Nippani and Miraj, the nearby areas of Kolhapur.) N. looked older than her age. She too had a Yajman, a Gujarati Hindu gentleman. At age 50, she died due to some disease. People were suspicious about the character of the Naikin women. In Kolhapur, N. lived in a bungalow in Shivaji Park area with her brother. A neighbour who was a Muslim woman was worried whether her husband would be taken away by N. Nothing like that happened. After her death, her brother moved away from that locality.

14.17 Case Study of Ms. Najma

Najma hailed from Kolhapur. She was a Muslim Naikin woman. A Gujarati man Mr. Kapadia from Poona fell in love with her and wanted to marry her. She agreed to the marriage. She came to Poona with him. She changed her religion to Hinduism, took a Hindu name and married him. She had all her relatives in Kolhapur who are Muslims. Sometimes she used to ask her daughter's Muslim friend about Quran. The Muslim friend used to wonder why this Hindu lady was asking about Quran.

It seems Najma had some attachment with her previous religion i.e. Islam.

She had a daughter Priya (earlier Payal) from a previous partner. Her husband accepted her as his own daughter and brought her up lovingly. Educated and got her married. Unfortunately, the son-in-law turned out to be an irresponsible and unfaithful husband. Kapadia had opened an aluminium utensil making factory for Priya's husband. It became a bankrupt business. Priya had two children, a son and a daughter. She went into depression and committed suicide.

Kapadia had a daughter Saumya from Najma. Saumya seeing her sister's fate, decided not to marry. She is 56 now. Yet remains single. Najma died in 2015 when she was 70. Kapadia died before Najma. So Saumya lives in her father's three-bedroom flat. She is B.Com. from SNDT University in Pune. She says she is enjoying her life. Does not have any gainful occupation but sometime back tried her hand at having a boutique. As it was not doing well, she closed the boutique. She attends art of living classes by Sri Sri Ravi Shankar. She had kept her nephew with his with family in her house. As he misbehaved with her, she threw him out. Her niece is happily married.

Najma was Kapadia"s first wife. His parents got him married to a Gujarati woman. He has three sons from his second wife. They have cordial relations with Saumya. Saumya has no property in her name and no source of income. Her step-brothers give her monthly some amount of money which is sufficient for her. When Saumya was advised to ask her brothers to register the flat where she resides in her name for financial security in future, she responded that she has full faith in her brothers, and they will never cheat her.

14.18 Some More Stories of Muslim Naikin Women

One Miss R. coming from a Naikin family fell in love with a Punjabi Hindu film student who was doing Film Direction course at the Film and Television Institute in Poona. Later he married her and moved to Bombay. They have no children. Today he is a well-known film director. Miss R remains a Muslim. She took her two brothers with her to Bombay. One brother assists her husband in film direction. Second one is also involved in helping her husband. She is out of public sight. Though the family was from Naikin community, they could move out of this background and become well established in society. She helped her family members too to settle down in life honourably.

I could find one more family from this background living and well settled in Poona. Mr. Sayyad worked in a corporation. Retired after achieving a high position in the organization. Wife was an academic. She too retired now. They have one son and daughter. Son is an engineer and has settled in USA. Daughter is married. Has no children as she is busy with her career. If you ask them they will refuse their Naikin background. From reliable sources, the researcher came to know about their background.

Case Study of Banoo Babalal Shaikh, a Muslim Naikin Woman from Sangli City

The researcher interviewed one Muslim Naikin woman from Sangli. She got this respondent's contact from Meena Seshu of Sangram organization in Sangli city. Researcher was contacting this lady for nearly 1 month by telephoning her. At the end of March, the researcher visited her in Sangli city at her house and interviewed her in detail. She is bold enough and told that I should use her original name. I had taken an assistant with me. She insisted that the girl should stay with us and listen to her story. She averred that all women have similar struggles and so no need to hide anything from anybody. Below I document her story, her struggles and achievements.

14.19 Childhood

Banoo was the name given to her by parents. Father was Babalal. Surname is Shaikh, a very common surname, from the higher classes of Muslims. i.e. Ashraf category. She said that she is Banoo Babalal Shaikh. This is her permanent name. She never changed it. She is 62 years old (birth year 1959). She was born at Dongergaon village near Mangalveda in Solapur district. When she was 3 years old, her parents migrated to Sangli in search of livelihood.

Her father had married her mother when she was 3 years old. Father was a nephew of her grandfather who had some property. In oder to retain the property within the family, grandfather got his 3-year-old granddaughter to his nephew, who was 16 years old. Her father married another woman of his age to satisfy his marital desires. She finished 2nd standard in Marathi medium. She worked in brick kiln. She used to bring animal fodder from jungle and sell in the market to earn some money. When she was 10 years old, she started working as maid servant at somebody's house. She did dhona-bhandi i.e. washing clothes and cleaning utensils. When she was eleven, she heard orchestra being practised at the neighbour's house. Out of interest, she used to go and observe the orchestra and singing. Somebody there taught her singing. She was included in the shows for singing. Per show she was paid Rs. 2.

14.20 Initiation as Naikin

Banoo wanted to earn more money to the daily needs. One day she met one Khairunnisa who told Banoo to become a Naikin i.e. a Tawaif, learn dancing and singing to earn more money.

This idea appealed to Banoo. She asked Khairunnisa how one can become a Naikin. Khairunnisa, a Muslim Naikin woman, took her to a saint's dargah (tomb) at Nippani. She was married to Raj Baksh, the dead peer (saint). What is the marriage procedure? Mujawar (the priest at the tomb) told Banoo to bring one chadar (a cloth to be spread over the tomb), some flowers, one coconut (nariyal) and one vodhni (big scarf) to cove her head and shoulders. Narial was kept near the tomb. Flowers were spread over the tomb of the saint on the chadar and on the girl on the vodhni over her head and upper body. Also, a thread was tied to her wrist. Then the priest declared that the marriage was done, and she has become doredar (wearing a thread). She was free to do nauch-gana-bajana (dancing-singing-playing instruments). He also declared that she could marry somebody whom she wants during her nauch-gana career i.e. after becoming a Naikin. (Whether the Raj Baksh dargah exists today at Nippani, Banoo does not know).

As a Naikin, she learnt dancing and singing. In Sangli near Sadashiv Talkies in Peth Baug, a Deewan Khana was there. Here Mujra (an Indian dance form performed by Tawaif), singing and dancing was done.

14.21 Livelihood as Naikin

Her father died. Mother was there. She had an elder brother Balu Kondba who became an alcoholic due to bad company. He used to beat up both Banoo and her mother. He married twice. First marriage was arranged and with a Muslim woman. Second time it was a love marriage. He converted her to Islam before marrying her. From the first wife he had two children and from the second wife four children. Banoo took care of both the sisters-in-law, their children and the brother. He died of cancer at the age of 35. Banoo spent about five to six lakhs on his treatment. Mother had asthma. Banoo got her too treated. All this she did by doing mujra.

She was performing mujra and got some money to run her house. Thus nauch-gana became her livelihood. For one song, she was paid one rupee. Later her payment per song was increased to two rupees. Much later she was paid five rupees per song. She lived like this for 16 long years. She was the only Muslim girl in this profession.

14.22 Marriage, Motherhood and Family Responsibilities

When she was 22, she married one Haroon Dawood Shaikh. Proper nikah was performed. After marriage too she continued doing mujra for livelihood. Haroon had garage, cycle shop etc. He was a small businessman. He could have financially supported her. He fell into bad company and became an alcoholic. He lost all his assets. At the age of 25, she begot one son Riyaz. After motherhood too she continued mujra as her livelihood to run the house.

Haroon was already married and fathered two daughters. When he proposed to Banoo he hid this fact from her. Thus, he cheated her. After knowing this fact too, Banoo continued living with him. In fact, Haroon requested Banoo to take both his daughters to learn mujra and become Naikins. Banoo did not want these girls to become Naikins like her. She got them married. Those girls are grateful to Banoo. They respect and maintain good relations with her even today. Haroon developed cirrhosis of liver and died. Then Riyaz was 9 years old. Even today Banoo wears a gold mangal sutra (marriage necklace). In regular terms, she is a widow but in Niakin terms she is Nityasumangali (always married). Except the mangalsutra and ear tops, all other jewellery on her was artificial.

She got her son married to a khandani but illiterate Muslim girl when he was 18 years old. Riyaz has three daughters. Banoo has educated them. First girl completed B.A., second girl S.S.C. and the third completed H.S.C. She got all the girls married early.

She built a seven-room house with her earnings. Recently she demolished three rooms from the house for power company to set up a tower. It is paying her Rs. 15,000 as rent for use of this land. She informed that this is a big amount for her because rent in Sangli is low. She bought a rickshaw for her son. He employed a driver. He also does some work for a political leader in Miraj, the twin town. Per month he adds about Rs. 10,000 to family income. Daughter-in-law is a housewife Banoo also sells bangles at home for extra income. Her house was neat, tidy and well maintained. She has no bank balance.

14.23 As an Entertainer and Entrepreneur

After Haroon's death, Banoo's responsibilities further increased. Now she had to cater to seven members in her family single handedly. Mujra cannot feed so many. So, she decided to start a Lavani (tamasha) Party (company). She employed Usha Naik as her heroine. (Later Usha Naik became a famous Marathi film actress). Her Lavani Party started performing traditional lavani, Patte Bapurao lavani, Honaji Bala lavani. She continued doing this business of entertainment for about 7 years. Along with other artistes, she too sang and danced in the shows. Then her business took a downturn and suffered losses. So, she had to close down her company.

For some time, she stayed at home. No income made it difficult to run her house. So she started selling vegetables which was not enough. Therefore, she wanted to go back to entertainment. She set up Sangeet Party at Sanskriti Kala Kendra in Jaisinghpur, a taluka place near Sangli city. For 10 years, she did this entertainment business of organizing singing and dancing shows. Mostly Hindu girls were employed as the artistes. One Shabnam, a singing and dancing Muslim girl from Aurangabad had joined her Sangeet Party. One Ismail Attar used to beat the drum in her shows. For 10 years she continued this business. The business was declining. During Carona, it became standstill. Last 4 years she has been at home without work. She lamented that she cannot start a new enterprise because she has no capital. Nowadays even to join a Sangeet Party, the girls ask for Rs. 50,000 as advance which she can ill afford to give.

Since 1980, often she was invited to sing songs for Lok Sangeet (Popular Music) programmes at Akashvani Kendra, Sangli. She performed at Delhi, Gwalior and Calcutta. She performed for both Government of India and Government of Maharashtra. Even today her songs are broad cast once in a month on Friday/Monday in the evening. Professionally she is known as Banoo Shaikh Sanglikar.

She gets a pension of Rs. 2250 per month from the Government of Maharashtra as Kalakar Mandhan (artist's honorarium). In the past it was only Rs. 500. This money goes for her medicines. She has knee problem, slip disk, blood pressure. She used to wear five kilo ghungroo on her ankles while doing mujra. She has been dancing for the last 40 years. It has taken its toll on her body. But she is hale and hearty and pulling on. She is thankful to Allah for her independent economic status.

She used to work in Marathi natak (drama). In Moruchi Mavsi (Moru's Aunt) she played the role of maid servant. In Pinjryachi Maina (Maina of the Cage), she played the role of a heroine.

14.24 Her Philosophy

She is a kalakar i.e. artist. Artistes are always young at heart. Her profession taught her this philosophy. No complaints against anybody. She wants to help other artistes. Whenever somebody approached her with some difficulty, she helped them. She married a Muslim gentleman because she wanted to give honourable names to her children. (Today times are very free. Dalit can marry a Brahmin and vice versa. In olden times it was not like that). She gave some new meaning to the words Naikin and Tamasha. Naikin means "Na Yakin" (Na = No, Yakin = Trust, whom nobody trusts. Tamasha (Tamas = Darkness, Asha = Hope, Hope in the darknes). She seems to be creative with her words.

14.25 Why Do Muslim Women Become Naikin?

Her explanation is as follows: In the olden times, kings, sardars, nobles from rajwadas wanted to watch singing and dancing after they were tired. Initially very few women learnt dancing and singing. So, men used to dance. For example, Bal Gandharva, the great singer used to wear saree and sing.

Raja told his Pradhan (Chief) to get some women to sing and dance. Then Muslim women started singing and dancing (This is not correct explanation as we will discuss later.) For Banoo, Tawaif and Naikin are one only. (This is also not correct as we will discuss later). In her view they are dignified. Even today the Naikin women are dignified because they wear six yard or nine-yard saris and then sing and dance whereas film heroines are scantily dressed.

To explain the innocence and dignity of Naikin women, Banoo narrated a story of a Naikin woman and householder woman. There were two neighbours. One was burkha clad and married Muslim woman. Second was Muslim Naikin woman. Through her window, the Muslim woman used to observe the Naikin. Every day many visitors came to Naikin's house. Naikin spoke to them nicely and sometimes they gave her some money and left. Every time she saw a visitor, the Muslim woman threw a pebble in a jar. After a week, the jar was full. She showed this full jar to her husband and told him that the Naikin will go to hell because she is meeting so many men and she will go to heaven because she is pious, was praying five times a day etc. After their death, both of them met God almighty. He sent the Naikin to heaven and the pious Muslim woman to hell. She was infuriated. God told her that she had no business in observing the sinner. All her piety was transferred to Naikin and Naikin's short coming were given to pious woman. The moral is we should not find faults with others and be proud. She followed this philosophy of not calling names to anybody and doing whatever little good one can do to others.

14.26 Religiosity

For Naikins religion does not matter. Banoo informed that one doredar (one to whom the thread is tied) woman can initiate another Muslim woman as Naikin. How is that done? By performing the Pooja (worship) of the Pethi (harmonium). In front of the harmonium, agarbatti (incense sticks), sugar and flowers are kept. A coconut is broken in front of the harmonium. The initiation is over. The researcher informed Banoo that all this is forbidden in Islam as Allah says to worship him alone because he is the creator. Banoo said that she knows but for artistes, it ok because they as artistes have no religion and no caste.

Last 40 years she has been going to one jatra (fair) at Chandgad near Kolhapur. There is a Shiv temple by the name Ravalnath at Chandgad. (The temple is worth two crores of rupees). Naikin applies gulal (red colour powder) on the Murti (statue) of Shiv. Bano has been applying that gulal with all her five fingers on the Shiva statue for the last 40 years. Unless she does that, the procession will not start. It is a four-day programme. On the first day, Bhakti geet (devotional songs) and gazal are sung. Second day same is continued. Third day it is only a two-hour programme. Film songs and film dances are performed. On the fourth day they all leave. Banoo seems to be team leader for this programme. She is paid Rs. 30–40 thousand. She keeps about Rs. fifteen thousand for herself and rest of the money she distributes among all the artistes who have accompanied her. When she was told it was all "shirking" the biggest sin in Islam, she said for artistes it is okay.

14.27 Was She Molested Sexually During Her Career?

Before her marriage, one Bagban, a 65-year-old fruit merchant from Solapur, visited her in Kolhapur and gave a proposal that he would gift her rupees five lakhs and five tola (60 g) gold. She should stay with him in a lodge and allow him to enjoy her. Then he would go back to Solapur and think about the relationship and whether he would like to marry her. Later he may come back and marry her. She refused this proposal and the wealth because she thought it was too risky. If he does not come back and marry her, she would have lost her honour. Later she married Haroon.

It is common that Muslim Naikin women do not marry but have a Yajman from a different community. Why cannot they marry some good Muslim man and settle down? She told the fate of one of her friends, one Miss Rukdikar. She married a good Muslim man. Before marriage he professed love for her. After marriage, he started abusing her, giving her cigarette burns, asking her with how many men did she sleep before her marriage? She was fed up with the harassment and left him. Once again started singing and dancing. She wanted to rehabilitate herself, but the fate was different.

She does not pray because she has not learnt how to perform namaz. She finished reading Quran in Hindi. Her son and granddaughters have learnt namaz. So, they pray. Her son asks her to leave everything now and relax. Banoo says unless somebody picks up her responsibilities she cannot relax.

14.28 Evaluation of Banoo as Naikin

Banoo is a dynamic personality. Quite independent. Has multiple identities—artist, entrepreneur, wife, mother, Muslim woman. She is daring and knows how to bargain. She is self-respecting, risk taking, honest and knowledgeable in her field. All great qualities for a woman on the margin. She struggled and still struggling. She attained a respectable life in society and settled down all her dependents in life with dignity. This is a great achievement for her. This may not be the story of many other Naikin women.

14.29 Discussion

Some scholars and people in general consider tawaifs as prostitutes. According to Booth, tawaif (courtesan) is a dancing girl, a prostitute; a female singer (2007: 1). Other scholars differ with this view. According to Arfeen today even though society at large finds tawaifs as deviant groups who need rehabilitation, the nineteenth and early twentieth-century tawaifs were not sex workers who sold their bodies for making their ends meet or for a standard lifestyle. Kothas in those times were the cultural hubs of that period. These women were powerful and established kothas and ran them efficiently without help of any man. They were definitely not other second sex i.e. secondary or subordinate to men in a male dominated society (2016: 1102). Therefore tawaifs and Naikin women are different.

From this research, what we can understand is this: In the past sufi saints worked to give love and peace among the marginalised and vulnerable communities in different parts of Maharashtra and India. In fact, in Miraj, there is a prominent dargah of a saint. So, when some sufi saint worked with the community of devadasis in Sangli–Kolhapur region, maybe they accepted Islam but continued their profession. Also, the Naikins could not be absorbed into the mainstream Muslim society may be because Muslim men and their families discriminated against them and may be inter marriage was not allowed. This requires further research.

Further, Muslim Naikins have substituted Raja Baksh dargah for Yellamma's temple. They continue worship like activities of Hindu dieties. They do not have much attachment to religion. They are practical people interested in their economic wellbeing.

14.30 Conclusion

It was quite puzzling for this researcher to know about this aberration in Muslim society i.e. Muslim Naikin women. They are mostly found in Kolhapur and Sangli areas. In literature, hardly any information is available on these women. Therefore, the researcher decided to document about this Muslim community, especially Muslim Naikin women. This is a humble attempt.

The objective of this paper are: (i) To trace the origin of this institution i.e. Naikins among Muslims; (ii) To find their present socio-economic conditions; (iii) To know whether the rehabilitation programmes available for Devadasis are also available to these Muslim Naikin women; and (iv) If programmes are available, to evaluate whether they have been successful in giving dignified lives to these women victims.

Our research presently could not trace the origin of this institution in the Muslim community. More investigation is required. From our case studies, we have not found abject poverty among the Muslim Naikin women. Many of them whom we studied look well off. This too requires more research. May be a sample survey needs to be conducted. Whether any programmes of rehabilitation are available for Muslim Naikin women, as of now no programme exists. Banoo wants to follow if any leader is willing to fight for these women's rights. To conclude this is only preliminary research, a beginning. Much more research needs to be undertaken to document about the community of Muslim Naikin women.

Acknowledgements I acknowledge the sincere efforts of Dr. Ajit Kumar Lenka in revising this paper.

References

Ahluwalia, S. (2021). Educating the girl child and promoting equal learning opportunities: A case study of Uttar Pradesh in India. In S. Murtaza & A. U. Khan (Eds.), *Gender and inclusion* (pp. 75–92). Hyderabad: Centre for Development Policy and Practice.

Alam, A. (2021). Politics of economic exclusion: Hitting the belly of Dalit and Muslim workers. In S. Murtaza & A. U. Khan (Eds.), *Gender and inclusion* (pp. 189–198). Hyderabad: Centre for Development Policy and Practice.

Arfeen, A. (2016). The institution of Kotha: A case study of Tawaif-centered films. *Imperial Journal of Interdisciplinary Research (IJIR)*, *2*(4), 1099–1102. http://www.onlinejournal.in

Bano, N., Syed, K., & Ahmed, A. (2021). Socio-economic status of women labour in bangle industry: A case study of Firozabad city (India). In S. Murtaza & A. U. Khan (Eds.), *Gender and inclusion* (pp. 133–144). Hyderabad: Centre for Development Policy and Practice.

Biradar, B. (n.d.). [Review of the book *The courtesan, the Mahatma and the Italian...* by M. S. Pillai]. *The Hindu*. https://www.thehindu.com/books/books-reviews/the-courtesan-the

Booth, G. D. (2007). Making a woman from a Tawaif: Courtesans as heroes in Hindi cinema. *New Zealand Journal of Asian Studies, 9*(2), 1–26.

Dhoundiyal, M. (2021). Pandemic management through a gender lens. In S. Murtaza & A. U. Khan (Eds.), *Gender & inclusion* (pp. 93–100). Hyderabad: Centre for Development Policy and Practice.

Hansen, D. (n.d.). *The Devadasi tradition—Caught between poverty and superstition*. IDSN. https://idsn.org/key-issues/forced-prostitution/devadasi.article/

Harishankar, B. V., & Priyamvadha, M. (n.d.). Exploitation of women as Devadasis and its associated evils. Report submitted to National Commission for Women, New Delhi, 209–225.

Khan, A. U., Mathews, N., & Hussain, N. (2021). How do women vote? And why? In S. Murtaza & A. U. Khan (Eds.), *Gender and inclusion* (pp. 23–48). Hyderabad: Centre for Development Policy and Practice.

Murtaza, S. (2021). Patriarchy and women's oppression in a globalized world. In S. Murtaza & A. U. Khan (Eds.), *Gender and inclusion* (pp. 217–228). Hyderabad: Centre for Development Policy and Practice.

Pande, R. (2021). Equal opportunity for women in the workplace: A myth or reality. In S. Murtaza & A. U. Khan (Eds.), *Gender and inclusion* (pp. 101–122). Hyderabad: Centre for Development Policy and Practice.

Perwez, V. (2021). Dynamic of work culture and working from home: Women professionals reclaiming equal spaces. In S. Murtaza & A. U. Khan (Eds.), *Gender & inclusion* (pp. 123–132). Hyderabad: Centre for Development Policy and Practice.

Reddy, R. Y., & Sridevi, M. (2019). The origin and historical development of Devadasi system in India. *International Journal of Applied Research, 5*(1), 106–109.

Shaikh, R. (2021). Gender bias in India: Attitudes and perceptions. In S. Murtaza & A. U. Khan (Eds.), *Gender and inclusion* (pp. 49–62). Hyderabad: Centre for Development Policy and Practice.

Siddiqui, F. (2021). Equalizing opportunity for marginalised Muslim women through Riba-free microfinance in India. In S. Murtaza & A. U. Khan (Eds.), *Gender and inclusion* (pp. 145–170). Hyderabad: Centre for Development Policy and Practice.

Tejpal, M. (2018). Sexual slavery: A case study of Joginis in South India. *ANTYAJAA: Indian Journal of Women and Social Change, 3*(2), 181–193. https://journals.sagepub.com/home/jws

Uma, S. (2021). Equal opportunity for women at the workplace: Issues and challenges. In S. Murtaza & A. U. Khan (Eds.), *Gender and inclusion* (pp. 1–22). Hyderabad: Centre for Development Policy and Practice.

Vinayan, S., & Sivakumar, D. (2021). Mapping disability in India: The gender dimensions. In S. Murtaza & A. U. Khan (Eds.), *Gender & inclusion* (pp. 171–188). Hyderabad: Centre for Development Policy and Practice.

Ziyauddin, K. M., & Begum, M. (2021). Equal opportunity and social inclusion of minorities. In S. Murtaza & A. U. Khan (Eds.), *Gender and inclusion* (pp. 1–22). Hyderabad: Centre for Development Policy and Practice.

Influence of Domestic Violence on Women's Well-Being and SDGs 15

Sampurna Singh and Sanghmitra S. Acharya

Abstract

Women who have experienced domestic violence or abuse are at a significantly higher risk of experiencing a range of mental health conditions including post-traumatic stress disorder (PTSD), depression, anxiety, substance abuse, and thoughts of suicide. The accruing data reveal strengthening associations between domestic violence on the mental health of women. In India as per National Family Health Survey (NHFS) rounds 4 and 5, it hardly seems larger changes (earlier it was 30% and it reduces to 29.3% respectively) of women have experienced physical violence since the age of 15 years. In fact, during the pandemic, the jobs of women were lost, and they were overburdened with care work at home and lacked support. Families were in a distressful conditions and use of alcohol has increased which trickled down on women in terms of violence. Thus, the evidence shows an increasing case of domestic violence. The increase has pushed the SDGs further and thus, the paper attempts to evaluate the association of alcoholism controlling the nature of husband's and domestic violence further it also explores the awareness level and attitude (coping) in dealing the violence. Further the paper also discusses the impact of violence and alcoholism on achieving the SDGs. The evidence will also be used to examine how the forces circumstances like COVID have affected violence. For this paper NFHS 5 (2019–21) data will be used further to understand the impact of COVID qualitative data collected from men and women in rural and urban slum sites in four cities of India. (Delhi, Hyderabad, Jaipur and Lucknow) thus the research adopted a mixed methods approach.

15.1 Introduction

The Protection of Women from Domestic Violence Act 2005 defines domestic violence as physical, sexual, verbal, emotional and financial abuse of a woman by her partner or relatives living in the same family (Kalokhe et al., 2017) it also includes unlawful dowry demands (Ram et al., 2019). Domestic violence is a public health problem that affects women's physical and mental health (Abramsky et al., 1984). Intimate partner violence (IPV) against women is a significant public health issue globally. It has serious physical

S. Singh (✉)
Senior Researcher, Mindfield Research Services, New Delhi, India
e-mail: sampurna62@gmail.com

S. S. Acharya
Centre of Social Medicine and Community Health, Jawaharlal Nehru University, New Delhi, India

S. S. Acharya et al. (eds.), *Paradigm Shifts in Population and Health in India*, Sustainable Development Goals Series, https://doi.org/10.1007/978-981-95-1719-0_15

and psychological health consequences as well huge economic and social costs. In India as per National Family Health Survey (NHFS) rounds 4 and 5, it hardly seems larger changes (earlier it was 30% and it reduces to 29.3% respectively) of women have experienced physical violence since the age of 15 and 6% have experienced sexual violence in their lifetime. A cross-sectional study involving over 1400 women in the 18 states shows that approximately 39% are victimised because of IPV (Mahapatro et al., 2012). According to another report of Multi-Site Household Survey on Domestic violence in India (ICRW, 2002), domestic violence is high in rural areas, followed by slum areas. Approximately 40–50% of women in rural and urban slum areas reported of physical violence. The study also shows that, in an urban context, the number of reported cases is higher in slum areas than non-slum areas. Some other data set from recent National Crime Records Bureau (NCRB) data of IPC 498A (Cruelty by Husband or his Relatives) also inform that the crime rate under this IPC is about 17 (per one lakh) in India.

Alcohol consumption is increasing day by day in developing countries. As per the World Health Organization, the per capita alcohol consumption in India increased two folds between 2005 and 2016. Alcohol is a risk factor for the occurrence of violent acts because it has direct effects on physical and cognitive performances, contributing to violence by reducing self-control as well as reducing judgment and the ability to recognize signs of danger. It is also acknowledged that alcohol consumption by the male spouse is one of the main contributory factors to domestic violence. Various studies have suggested that alcohol consumption is directly associated with stress and burden in the life of people. Domestic violence due to alcoholism impacts the mental health of women. It also has a direct impact on the upbringing of the children in the family. Domestic Violence not only affects survivors but also their families, in particular children who witness abuse. It impacts their physical and mental health and increases their risk for adult victimization and perpetration. Domestic violence is associated with adverse and long-term health consequences. Emerging research demonstrates the complex relationships between domestic violence, mental health conditions, health-risk behaviors, and other socioeconomic stressors. Domestic violence is widely prevalent and disproportionately experienced by younger, low-income women of color.

The other reason for facing violence by women could be that she is socially and economically dependent on men. Before marriage the major decision in female's life is dependent on their father or brother and after marriage, she becomes dependent on her husband and later on her son. This in turn limits her ability to negotiate with their family and she starts perceiving herself as a burden and bears the frustration in form of violence from different members of the family in silence. Alcoholism and domestic violence became a vicious cycle in the family which also traps the children and, in some cases, the consequences push the families into a vulnerable position from where it is difficult to come out. However, Alcohol use can be both a cause and a consequence of experiencing violence. Although, women who face enormous social, physical and economic stresses along with domestic violence are likely to increase their vulnerability to mental morbidities (Patel et al, 1999).

There is a significant association between domestic violence and mental health. The impact is significant and has long-term health implications. The available literature says abused women had more depressive symptoms as compared to other women (Campbell & Lewandowski, 1997). They are at higher risk of experiencing a range of mental health conditions including post-traumatic stress disorder (PTSD), depression, anxiety, and thoughts of suicide. Whereas lack of coping mechanisms and social support leaves women to stay in distress condition throughout their life. But after marriage, women have very little or no control over their parent's families. She expects support from friends or relatives, as family is considered to be the first point of support. At the institutional level also there are very few organizations to provide support. The fear and uncertainty associated with loss of social and economic instability provide an enabling environment to violence. Women who are uneducated, non-working and dependent on males for their daily needs are more likely to face violence as compared to other women.

Mainly violence is associated with fights between men and women. In the Liberal feminist perspective, it is seen as an act exercised by men who are psychologically deranged over women. Therefore, the occurrence is high in the patriarchal society where all the decision-making is in the control of men. According to Walby (1990), violence cannot be understood without analyzing the patriarchal social structure and different feminist perspectives.

Whereas the Marxist feminist makes a class analysis of violence and argues that the cause of violence lies in the capitalist system, wherein the men at the bottom of the hierarchy exercise violence against women out of 'frustration generated by the circumstances' (Walby, 2000). Thus there are many underlining factors that lead to domestic violence across the world. In the current scenario, it becomes important to understand the associated factors and their correlation. Thus there are different reasons for the violence.

In 2015, all United Nations Member States adopted 17 Sustainable Development Goals (SDGs) which were recognize to end poverty by improving health and education, reduce inequality, and spur economic growth. But due to the sudden pandemic Covid 19 these goals were derailed and a large proportion of population was pushed below poverty line. Lack of food, money and employment effected the health of children and women and increased the stress in family which lead to violence. The evidence shows an increase in the prevalence rate of intimate partner violence (IPV). These rates are higher in the vulnerable populations that includes rural, slum women, belonging to scheduled caste, poor economic class and with lower education.

15.2 Objectives

Thus, this paper attempts to evaluate the association of alcoholism controlling the nature of husband's and domestic violence further it also explores the awareness level and attitude (coping) in dealing the violence. Further the paper also discusses the impact of violence and alcoholism on achieving the SDGs.

15.3 Data and Methodology

The present study uses the fifth round of the National Family Health Survey (2019–21) to understand the current scenario of domestic violence. NFHS is conducted in India in line with the Global Demographic Health Survey (DHS). It is under the stewardship of the Ministry of the family welfare of India (MoHFW), Government of India, which has designated the International Institute of the population sciences (IIPS), Mumbai as the nodal agency for data collection (IIPS 2022). Further, this paper also uses qualitative evidence from other data set which was collected in 2022 from four cities i.e. Delhi, Hyderabad, Jaipur and Lucknow for National Commission of Women (NCW). From each city, 180 women and 30 men respondents were interviewed. For the present paper a mixed-methods approach is used because it allows to validate findings by using qualitative data. Case studies and in-depth interviews in helps to understand the problem and contextualize with society.

15.4 Variable Description

The NFHS includes a few questions on domestic violence and spouse's attitude. For this paper these variables have been categorized.

1. *Intimate Partner Violence (IPV)* Can be broadly divided into three categories
   (a) **Physical IPV:** It was measured by exposure to one or more of these acts by their husband or partner (current or former)—(a) push, shake, or throw something; (b) slap; (c) twist arm or pull hair; (d) punch with his fist or with something that could hurt; (e) kick, drag, or beat up; (f) try to choke or burn on purpose; (g) or threaten or attack with a knife, gun, or any other weapon.

(b) **Emotional IPV:** It was measured by exposure to one or more of these acts by their husband or partner (current or former)
   (a) say or do something to humiliate wife in front of others
   (b) threaten to hurt or harm wife or someone close to her.
   (c) insult the wife or make a wife feel bad about herself.
(c) **Sexual IPV:** It was measured by exposure to one or more of these acts by their husband or partner (current or former)—(a) physically force his wife to have sexual intercourse with him even when the wife did not want to; (b) physically force his wife to perform any other sexual acts she did not want to; (c) force wife with threats or in other ways to perform sexual acts she did not want to.
   The responses were categorized as 'yes' or 'no' for each type of IPV.

2. *Coercive control*
   Coercive control by husband or partner was assessed by six questions where the women were asked if these following applied to their relationship with them—(a) is jealous or angry if she talks to other men; (b) frequently accuses her of being unfaithful; (c) does not permit her to meet her female friends; (d) tries to limit her contact with her family; (e) insists on knowing where she is at all times, and (f) does not trust her with any money. Binary responses we generated for each of the questions and a composite score of 0 to 6 was created to assess the intensity of coercive control of spouse.
3. *Mental Health Indicator*
   The impact on mental health was measured by the Brief Resilience Scale that assesses the ability to bounce back or recover from stressful events. The scale includes 6 items where the individual responds to if they (a) tend to bounce back quickly after hard times; (b) have a hard time making it through stressful events; (c) do not take me long to recover from a stressful event; (d) feel hard for to snap back when something bad happens; (e) usually come through difficult times with little trouble; (f) tend to take a long time to get over setbacks in life.

The responses were taken in Likert scale (**this scale** is a rating scale used to measure opinions, attitudes, or behaviors), and responses were codes as, strongly disagree, disagree, neutral, agree, strongly agree.

15.5 Result and Discussion

Domestic violence has been recognized since 1983 as a criminal offense under Indian Penal Code 498-A. India, shares a big proportion in global burden of domestic violence. The underline cause lies under the patriarchal social structure. Spousal violence is commonly found and the evidences are available through different data sources. Finding from NFHS 5 shows that thirty-two percent of ever-married women aged 18–49 have experienced physical, sexual, or emotional spousal violence. The most common type of spousal violence is physical violence (28%), followed by emotional violence (14%) and 6% of have experienced spousal sexual violence.

For the current analysis, the different types of cohesive behaviour by the spouse are divided broadly into three variables i.e. physical,

Table 15.1 Percentage distribution of women aged 15–49 facing violence

Type of violence	Percentage
Physical IPV	
No	79.83
Yes	20.17
Emotional IPV	
No	89.73
Yes	10.27
Sexual IPV	
No	95.63
Yes	4.37
Total	**65,194**

Note In bold is the total number of women considered for calculation emotional, and sexual IPV. Women aged 15–49 are considered for the analysis from NFHS 5 data. For this analysis the women of age 15 and above are considered because the median age at marriage as per NFHS 5 is 17 years and 23.3% women gets married before attaining the legal age of 18 years. Therefore, the chances of facing the exposure of violence at early age also increases. Table 15.1 presents the percentage distribution of women who have experienced a different type of violence. The finding witnesses that about twenty percent of women aged 15–49 have experienced physical violence, whereas 10% of women have reported facing emotional violence followed by 4% have ever experienced sexual violence in their lifetime. The survey further reveals that more than 50% of women and 42% of men among still believed that a man was justified in beating her wife. Despite this high burden of the problem, beliefs toward the acceptance of violence are common and wide (Yount et al., 2011, Heise et al., 2012). Studies revealed that women's attitude toward and the cultural grants of men's authority to control female behavior are the strongest predictor of domestic violence (Heise et al., 2012). Studies have also showed that more than half of women accept domestic violence. Reasons for justifying were burning food, argues with husband, goes out without telling, neglects children, refuses sex, unfaithful, disobeys and suspects infidelity. Thus, the acceptance of the society makes the problem deep rooted and is hinderance in day today life of families especially women and children.

The NCW data also witness that about 70% of women reported that their husbands have threatened to hurt them. According to the incident of Physical violence, pushed ever and being slapped was reported by about 70% women in all four cities. Slapping was the most common form of violence perpetrated against women. More than 70% women across the cities reported to have been slapped by their spouses. Hyderabad reported lowest (70%) followed by Delhi (76%) and Lucknow (77%), and Jaipur (87%) which reported the highest. Twisting the arm was also reported by more than 50% women in the three cities except Jaipur where it was less than 34% and women reported that their arms were twisted by their respective spouses. Punch and kick was also reported by 58% women in Delhi, which is highest among all the cities, followed by Lucknow (47%), Jaipur (33%) and Hyderabad (20%).

The available data witness an increase in domestic violence cases during the pandemic as males were at home because there was no work going on. The finding from NCW data also indorse an increases in domestic violence cases during the Covid-19. NCW received 5297 complaints of domestic violence in 2020 as compared to 2960 complaints in 2019. The National Commission for Women received 23,722 complaints of crimes committed against women in 2020, the highest in the last 6 years and nearly one-fourth (5249) of the total complaints were of domestic violence. Among states, the highest number of complaints were received from Uttar Pradesh at 11,872 followed by Delhi 2635, Haryana 1266 and Maharashtra 1188. The National Commission for women (NCW) has launched a promotional campaign via electronic and social media to urge female victims of any form of violence to come forward and log the complaint. The present upward trend demands the importance to understand the dynamics of its associated factors. The analysis of which is presented below.

15.6 Association of Background Characteristics and Violence

Sociocultural and economic surroundings determine the metal set up of people as there is no single reason that leads to domestic violence. It is a combination of various sociological/behavioral, religious, and cultural factors that lead to the perpetration of domestic violence. There are many societal norms like dowry, desire to have male child, mobility, poverty etc. attached to domestic violence. Similarly, according to Tsai et al. (2017), poverty, rural residence, gender inequality in schooling and decision making, ethnicity, religion, and exposure to the media were associated with women's attitudes toward domestic violence.

Table 15.2 presents the percentage distribution of women reported experiencing violence by their

Table 15.2 Percentage of women reported experiencing violence by background characteristics

Background characteristics	Percentage
Woman's age	
15–19	1.92
20–24	12
25–29	17.69
30–34	17.92
35–39	19.62
40–44	15.81
45–49	15.04
Marital status	
Married	94.36
Divorced/widowed/separated	5.64
Wealth index	
Poorest	19.18
Poorer	21.34
Middle	20.5
Richer	19.89
Richest	19.08
Woman's education	
No education	28.39
Primary	14.04
Secondary	45.91
Higher	11.67
Woman's employment	
Not employed	70.87
Employed	29.13
Husband's education	
No education	17.85
Primary	14.12
Secondary	53.22
Higher	14.8
Husband's occupation	
Professional/technical/managerial	8.21
Clerical	2.59
Sales	10.54
Services/household and domestic	9.45
Agricultural	33.28
Skilled and unskilled manual	30.2
Other	5.74
Caste	
SC/ST	35.62
OBC	39.68
Other castes	24.7
Religion	
Hindi	75.85
Muslims	12.86
Christians	6.52
Others	4.78
Residence	
Urban	29.73
Rural	70.27
Total	65,194

background characteristics. Women belonging to the poor class are more likely to experience violence. Their experience of physical violence increases with age, from 16% among women age 18–19 to 32% among women age 40–49. The ever been married women have a higher chance to experience violence as come to women who are never-married. The finding from the qualitative data also points that women is more vulnerable because is considered to be a soft or 'suitable target'. In our patriarchal society, girls have always been presented as a burden or a liability for the family and if anything goes wrong from the stereotype, a woman has to face the consequences. A man understands that the societal value of a woman is always less than a man. Taking advantage of these facts, he shows his masculinity by physically harassing his wife. A distressed woman Anamika (name changed), upon asking that why she did not register police complaint against her husband narrated-'*If I lodge a complaint in police or even if I dare to resist his beating, where would I go? He is the sole breadwinner of the family. Who don't get beaten up by husband? He is the one who is feeding us, he can beat us too. Moreover, if police take him to jail he will lose his one day wage and that will cost on the whole family*'.

Women's low education, low employability and economic dependence make them more vulnerable to assault and violence. One of the respondents Sonalika (name changed) said that-'*My husband does not drink alcohol frequently but most of the time he is angry and if he demands anything and I cannot fulfil because of any reason, he start beating me like animals. He beat me so much so that I am not able to get up...'* using her bruised wrist she says-'*... see all my bangles broke... leaving these scars'* Upon asking that why she does not take any help from anyone in such a situation, her reply was-'*Whom should I complaint if my husband whom I am married is culprit who will listen to me? He is the one who takes care of everything, who earns and feeds us. Therefore, I cannot go against him. Sometimes I feel like running away from this house then thought of my kids do not let me do so. I cannot go to my parents' house as I have three more sisters who are yet to be married and my father is a daily wage labourer*'.

The finding from NFHS 5 data presented in Table 15.2 shows that women's experience of violence declines sharply with women's schooling, employment status and wealth. The social status of women determines their status in their family also. By schooling, the percentage of women who report physical violence declines from 39% among women with no schooling to 17% among women with 12 or more years of schooling. Similarly, the experience of physical violence ranges from 38% among women in the lowest wealth quintile to 17% among women in the highest wealth quintile. Women who are not employed are more likely to experience physical violence than women who are employed. have experienced physical violence since the age 15 years.

Finding further shows that schedule caste and other backward class women are more likely to report violence as compared to other class women. More Hindu women are seen reporting violence followed by Muslim, Christen and other class. The experience of physical violence is more common among women in rural areas (31%) than among women in urban areas (24%).

Husbands' education and occupation also has a direct impact on domestic violence. The men with the higher level of education and belong to Professional group are less likely to report violence against women as compared to other occupational group.

15.7 Reasons for Domestic Violence

Overall, 47% of women said that their husband was jealous or angry when they talked with other men. Only 40% of women said that their husband accused them of being unfaithful, 46% of women reported restrictions faced in meeting female friends, 38% of women said that their husband did not allow them to meet family, and 47% women xiii said that their husband insisted on knowing where they are all the time. About 71% women faced humiliation at the hands of the husband. Reported reasons for humiliation were women having an extramarital affair, meeting a friend, and most common was alcohol consumption and arguments that followed after that. The data shows about 75% of women reported that their husbands have threatened to hurt them. Disaggregated picture is evident from Fig. 15.1.

There were a number of reasons reported to cause perpetration of domestic violence. Consumption of alcohol was the most reported reason across the fours cities her the study was conducted. Being poor was the next most reported reason.

15.8 Impact of Alcoholism and Coercive Control on Violence and Family

With the changing lifestyle and stress level consumption of alcohol is increasing day by day. As per the World Health Organization, the per capita alcohol consumption in India increased two folds between 2005 to 2016. Alcohol is a risk factor for the occurrence of violent acts because it has direct effects on physical and cognitive performances, contributing to violence by reducing self-control as well as reducing judgment and the ability to recognize signs of danger (Stewart et al., 2021; Gebara et al., 2015). Alcohol use significantly increases the chances domestic abuse. This is mainly because alcohol can reduce a person's self-control and exacerbate underlying mental health issues, alcohol use can be both a

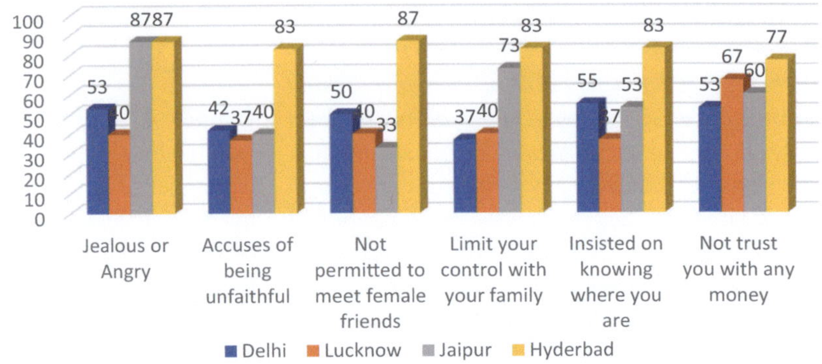

Fig. 15.1 Women's relationship with husband

Table 15.3 Percentage of women reported experiencing violence by husband's charectistics

Husband drinks alcohol	No	46,095 (72.72)
	Yes	17,290 (27.28)
Coercive control	No	37,110 (56.92)
	Yes	28,084 (43.08)
Husband's education	No education	11,640 (17.85)
	Primary	9208 (14.12)
	Secondary	34,695 (53.22)
	Higher	9650 (14.8)
Husband's occupation	Professional/ technical/ managerial	5351 (8.21)
	Clerical	1685 (2.59)
	Sales	6873 (10.54)
	Services/ household and domestic	6160 (9.45)
	Agricultural	21,696 (33.28)
	Skilled and unskilled manual	19,690 (30.2)
	Other	3739 (5.74)

cause and a consequence of experiencing violence (Gadd et al., 2019) (Table 15.3).

The evidences from literature documents strong relationship between alcoholism, domestic violence and their interplay which impacts individuals' mental health and wellbeing. Literature also acknowledges' that women disproportionately bear the health and psychological burdens of violence. Domestic violence directly impacts on children health in the family (Fig. 15.2).

15.8.1 Association Between Alcohol Consumption and Different Type of Violence

Alcohol induce violence was very high in the study area. The finding shows that around 78% of women faced any form of domestic violence across the four cities. The physical form of violence was around 59.6%, emotional violence was 73% and sexual violence was 34.7%. The highest prevalence of domestic violence was in Jaipur (100%), followed by Lucknow (80%), Delhi (76.9%), and Hyderabad (70%). The relationship of violence with social support and empowerment shows a significant association: i.e. with decreasing social support the chances of facing domestic violence increase by 83% (OR: 1.83; $p < 0.01$), and with lower empowerment the chances of facing domestic violence increases by 14% (OR: 1.14; $p < 0.05$).

15.9 Domestic Violence, Coping Mechanism and Mental Health

Women's reports of controlling behaviours by their husband decline with age. Very low proportion of women seek help, NFHS 5 data shows that only 14% of women who have experienced physical or sexual violence by anyone have sought help to stop the violence. Help seeking is much more common among women who have experienced both physical and sexual violence (26%).

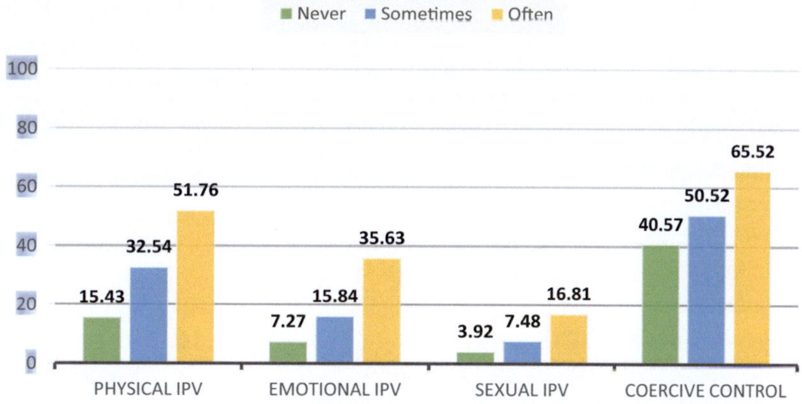

Fig. 15.2 Frequency of alcohol consumption

Otherwise they bear the violence in silence and they accept it as their destiny Help seeking to stop the violence does not vary much by other characteristics. The most common source of help was the woman's own family (61%). The second most common source for help was the husband's family (29%). Seventeen percent of women sought help from a friend. Among institutional sources of help, the most common is police (6%), followed by a social service organization (3%). Only 2% each have ever sought help from a doctor or medical personnel or a lawyer.

Finding from the survey carried out in four states shows that more than 90% of women from Jaipur and Hyderabad tried to seek help, followed by Delhi (66%) and Lucknow (30%). The study registers that domestic violence is very much socially structured and is part of the patriarchy mind-set. A subtle understanding was prevalent among the entire respondent that a woman need a man for survival. This perception was so strong among the women that while interviewing them many of them mentioned the following several times in varying words and expressions-

> I am married to him and now he is everything to me.
>
> Well… once married, he has the right to beat me up….
>
> So what if he beats me…? He feeds me too…

Women lacked self-esteem to the extent that they could not imagine their life without their husband and they are under constant fear. Financial deprivation was one of the common practices followed by man to have control over the woman. Women complained that whatever their husbands earned, they spent on alcohol and gave very little or no money for the household expenses. This was one of the common reasons that most of the women were stressed and malnourished. Another important reason was character assassination. Even if a woman smiles while talking to anyone, she was tagged as a woman of bad character and hence becomes a victim of violence.

For coping, the majority of women rely on their own families for any help. Very few women knew about the 181 helpline number and tried seeking help from this number. More than 90% women for Jaipur, 70% women from Hyderabad and 42% women reported about they sought help form their own family. Lower percent of them seek help form outside family that is neighbor, social service organization, doctor personal and police. Among the sampled women, very few had reported about tried of any medical treatment to cope up with domestic violence. Below is the story of a women who has been the victim of domestic violence and have tried to seek help. For the privacy reason the name as been changed, in word of Mona…

Case Study Ex1—Mona's Story of Alcohol Use, Domestic Violence and Mental Health

Mona is 24 years old. She is currently married but stays at her parent's home because of domestic violence caused by husband. She is native of Delhi and has stayed in Munirka village for the past 23 years. She studied in government school until 11th class. Then she got married at 17 years of age. She started working as a house maid but is currently unemployed due to pandemic. She belongs to the general category, stays in a pucca rented house which has a pit toilet and residential water facility. She is a victim of domestic violence. Her husband is jealous when she talks with other men, accuses her of being unfaithful and does not allow her to meet her friends. He often humiliates her in front of others, threatens to hurt and harm her and sometimes insult her and make her feel bad about herself. She has faced extreme form of physical and sexual violence which includes having been pushed, shaked off, twisting of arm and pulling of hair, being slapped, punched on face, being kicked and dragged and attempt to choke her throat and burn her. She has also been forced to perform unwanted sexual acts. As a result of domestic violence she has faced cuts, bruises, deep wounds and broke her bone. To seek help she called the police but police had not been of any use. They did not file her complaint. She seek help from her mother but her family is violent against her. Her brother frequently beats her up. Her children have witnessed domestic violence and she fears that his children may behave in the same manner with other women. They may become very fearful and silent. Mona said that the primary reason for domestic violence is alcohol consumption by husband and brother and her husband gets angry over small things leading to extreme violence. Her husband drinks alcohol regularly and spends more than his monthly earnings on purchase of alcohol. She thinks that selling alcohol should be banned as it leads to violence and creates money related problems

To those who had knowledge about mental health problem/disorder, from them information about different mental health problems was collected. Depression was largely acknowledged among women, 97% women of Lucknow followed by Delhi (76%) and 30% from Jaipur and Hyderabad followed by restlessness. Thus, the intersection of alcohol use, domestic violence and mental health is non-linear and cyclic. Alcohol use may get triggered by mental health (stress and depression), which may lead to violence. Or violence may lead toward alcohol which may in turn cause stress and depression.

15.10 Impact of Domestic Violence on SDGs

For achieving the SDGs, we require balancing three dimensions of sustainable development: economic growth, social inclusion, and environmental protection. Health is influenced and interlinked with all three dimensions. Health, education and poverty are also influenced by the mental condition of the person. Mental well-being depends on the living conditions of a person. During pandemic there was increase in the domestic violence cases. The situation worsened as women could not go out due to lockdown from their abusive situations and were repeatedly facing abuse. Their health and overall living conditions were impacted. Children were forced to drop out of school and people from the informal sector did not have the opportunity to work. They were pushed toward poverty. Pandemic had an impact in the implementation of the public health measures. Health facilities did not provide the routine facilities as they were busy dealing with the emergency services. The current analysis of key health indicators shows a decline in performance, especially for the poor population residing in slums and rural area. They were also forced to live in unhygienic conditions which could be a cause of many health issues. Thus, the goal of achieve gender equality and empower all girls and women was impacted.

The other reason for the violence against women is the gender inequality, due to which women suffer at different level. She does not have access to decent work and face occupational segregation and gender wage gaps. In many situations, they are denied access to basic education and health care and are discriminated. This inequality begins from the birth of a girl child.

However, adolescent girls, young women, women belonging to ethnic and other minorities, trans women, women working in the sex industry, women refugees and migrant workers, and women with disabilities, face a higher risk of different forms of violence. Evidence also suggests that unless we end violence against women/girls we won't be able achieve SDG 5 which aims toward achieving gender equality and empowering all women and girls. The achievement of goal 5 will enable and accelerate progress on all SDGs and by ending violence against women and girls globally, we will be able to achieve 14th and 17th Sustainable Development Goals.

15.11 Conclusion

There is sufficient literature that documents the prevalence of high domestic violence rate and have also identified various reasons. The relationship between alcoholism, domestic violence and their interplay that impacts upon an individuals' mental health and wellbeing is also well known. Literature supports the fact that married men with a history of violence have higher rates of alcoholism when compared to their non-violent counterparts. Studies report rates of alcoholism of 67% and 93% among wife batterers (Zilberman & Blume, 2005). It is also acknowledged that children growing up in the domestic abusive atmosphere, watching alcoholic fathers ignore their primary needs of the family, beating up their mother face severe emotional trauma and are more likely to grow up abusive in nature.

For prevention, there is need to chance the mindset of the people and start treating women/girl with equality. Female is considered as a secondhand citizen, so she is abstained or discriminated from the basic right of food, education, employment etc. She is brought up in a family in a week form and hence becomes a victim and faces different forms of violence. The whole situation demands interventions for women and children. In school there is a need for counsellors addressing mental health issues and separate shelter homes are required for children not going to school. It is believed that investing in women is like investing in the family. So, there is need for creating awareness on gender equality at a grass-root level, starting from the family level. Poverty and inequality are also the root cause of violence. But the preventive measures-addressing poverty and inequality-the root causes, remain inadequate.

Violence is preventable, investing in, and prioritizing the prevention of violence against women and girls is critical for achieving positive social, economic and political outcomes. Intervention and policies for awareness and prevention are urgently need. Therefore, the government needs to equips itself to treat causes of inequality against women. Beside this community-level training/awareness is required so that women are more aware of domestic violence. All health practitioners should be trained on aspects related to domestic violence, its physical and mental health impact. At grass root level there should be regular awareness campaigns through radio, television, newspapers, and magazine. As poverty, inequality and violence are interlinked and plays an important role in achieving the SDGs, so the domestic violence must be treated as a serious public health issue.

References

Abramsky, T., Watts, C. H., Garcia-Moreno, C., Devries, K., Kiss, L., Ellsberg, M., Henrica Anthony, G. (1984). *The constitution of society: Outline of the theory of structuration*. Berkeley. ISBN 978-0520052925. OCLC 11029282.

Campbell, J. C., & Lewandowski, L. A. (1997). Mental and physical health effects of intimate partner violence on women and children. *Psychiatric Clinics of North America, 20*(2), 353–374.

Ethiopia, U. W. (2016). *Shelters for women and girls who are survivors of violence in Ethiopia National Assessment on the Availability, Accessibility, Quality and Demand for Rehabilitative and Reintegration Services*. Addis Ababa.

Gadd, D., Henderson, J., Radcliffe, P., Stephens-Lewis, D., Johnson, A., & Gilchrist, G. (2019). The dynamics of domestic abuse and drug and alcohol dependency. *The British Journal of Criminology, 59*(5), 1035–1053.

Gebara, C. F. D. P., Ferri, C. P., Lourenço, L. M., Vieira, M. D. T., Bhona, F. M. D. C., & Noto, A. R. (2015). Patterns of domestic violence and alcohol consumption among women and the effectiveness of a brief intervention in a household setting: A protocol study. *BMC women's health, 15*(1), 78.

Heise, L. L. (2012). *Determinants of partner violence in low and middle-income countries: Exploring variation in individual and London School of Hygiene and Tropical Medicine*

ICRW. (2002). *Men, masculinity and domestic violence in India.* Summary Report of Four Studies.

International Institute for Population Sciences (IIPS) and ICF. (2017). National Family Health Survey (NFHS-4), 2015–16: India. Mumbai: IIPS.

International Institute for Population Sciences (IIPS) and ICF. (2021). National Family Health Survey: Fact sheet (NFHS-5), 2019–21: India. Mumbai: IIPS.

Kalokhe, A., Del Rio, C., Dunkle, K., Stephenson, R., Metheny, N., Paranjape, A., & Sahay, S. (2017). Domestic violence against women in India: A systematic review of a decade of quantitative studies. *Global Public Health, 12*(4), 498–513.

Mahapatro, M., Gupta, R. N., & Gupta, V. (2012). The risk factor of domestic violence in India. *Indian Journal of Community Medicine: Official Publication of Indian Association of Preventive and Social Medicine, 37*(3), 153.

Patel, V., Araya, R., De Lima, M., Ludermir, A., & Todd, C. (1999). Women, poverty and common mental disorders in four restructuring societies. *Social Science and Medicine, 49*(11), 1461–1471.

Ram, A., Victor, C. P., Christy, H., Hembrom, S., Cherian, A. G., & Mohan, V. R. (2019). Domestic violence and its determinants among 15–49-year-old women in a rural block in South India. *Indian Journal of Community Medicine: Official Publication of Indian Association of Preventive and Social Medicine, 44*(4), 362.

Stewart, D. E., MacMillan, H., & Kimber, M. (2021). Recognizing and responding to intimate partner violence: An update. *The Canadian Journal of Psychiatry, 66*(1), 71–106.

Tsai, A. C., Kakuhikire, B., Perkins, J. M., VořechovskaÂ, D., McDonough, A. Q., Ogburn, E. L., et al. (2017). Measuring personal beliefs and perceived norms about intimate partner violence: Population-based survey experiment in rural Uganda. *PLOS Medicine, 14*(5), 1002303.

Walby, S. (1990). *Theorizing patriarchy.* Blackwell Publishers Ltd. Oxford, UK. Cambridge USA (p. 20). https://pib.gov.in/Pressreleaseshare.aspx?PRID=1657678)of 'ministry of Women and Child Development' on September 22, 2020.

Walby, S., & Myhill, A. (2000). *Reducing domestic violence… What works?*

Yount, K. M., Halim, N., Hynes, M., & Hillman, E. R. (2011). Response effects to attitudinal questions about domestic violence against women: A comparative perspective. *Social Science Research, 40*, 873–884.

Zilberman & Blume. (2005). Domestic violence, alcohol and substance abuse. *Brazilian Journal of Psychiatry, 27*(Suppl 2), S51–S55.

Spirituality, Democracy, and Social Well-Being

16

Anubhuti Jambhulkar

Abstract

This chapter explains the interlinkage between democracy and social well-being through the lens of spirituality. Indian society since historical times has been plagued by 'graded inequality' premised on caste, a governing feature of Indian social life. Hence there is no singular social but multiple socials in India. A defining feature of this graded inequality is isolation, segregation and enforced exclusion on one hand and an absence of fraternity and social endosmosis on the other. Social being reciprocal, the location and construct of self becomes an important category in understanding how the social gets constituted in categories like nation, religion, caste consciousness and finally democracy in the Indian context. Given the diversity of Indian society, the social is deeply embedded in the religious. Thus, religion is an important vantage point to understand the very experience of social and how it shapes and reshapes Indian democracy. Suffering as an experience often gets relegated to diseases, disorders, pathologies, etc. However, suffering happens to be a phenomenon universally experienced by every individual whether healthy or diseased. Hence, the study of suffering, what constitutes the 'social' in suffering and thus social well being as an antidote become crucial and relevant in contemporary times. In recent times, there has been a surge in the anti-conversion laws in India based on rhetoric of nationalism. But in spite of numerous attempts of secularization of the public sphere, Indian consciousness still continues to be dominated by religion. Hence, the study of phenomena of religious conversion acquires an added relevance in contemporary times. Nationalism in its truest spirit ushers in a democracy when the sanctity and dignity of individual personality is respected and upholded in the truest sense of the term. Fraternity becomes a means to that end. The Indian Preamble proposes, "Fraternity, assuring the dignity of individual and unity and integrity of the nation". This chapter explains the interlinkage between spirituality, *Maitri* and social well being vis-a-vis democratic triad of liberty, equality and fraternity.

16.1 Introduction

As a lived experience, suffering is often equated with diseases, disorders, and pathologies, ultimately resulting in the medicalisation of human body. However, suffering is universally experienced by every individual/sentient being whether healthy or diseased, depending on the social locale

A. Jambhulkar (✉)
Doctoral Fellow, Centre of Social Medicine and Community Health, Jawaharlal Nehru University, New Delhi, India
e-mail: anubhutijambhulkar@gmail.com

S. S. Acharya et al. (eds.), *Paradigm Shifts in Population and Health in India*, Sustainable Development Goals Series, https://doi.org/10.1007/978-981-95-1719-0_16

in which the individual is located, thereby making it a universal ontological fact of our existence both as biological and social beings. Hence, study of suffering, what constitutes the 'social' in suffering and thus social well-being as an antidote to it becomes crucial and relevant in contemporary times in the study of public health, more so in the Indian context, given its highly stratified nature. "Research into social suffering is addressed to a wide assemblage of both spectacular and ordinary occasions when human dignity is violated and people come to some kind of grief and harm; but, in every instance, an emphasis is placed upon the ways in which such events are experienced by individuals as social forces and cultural phenomena" (Wilkinson, 2005). Seen in the light of what Wilkinson emphasises, the social and cultural determinants of suffering then become the locale to understand the phenomenology of suffering and caste. Offering a critique of the biomedical model, Frank notes, "Suffering is the subversive voice in the biomedical discourse; it is central amongst all the things that do not fit. Social science and biomedical discourse perpetuate this censoring when they reduce suffering's embodied locality to extra local categories that organize responses. Clinicians informed by such discourse respond not to the person who suffers but to the person viewed as an instance of a type of suffering that the text has taught the professional to recognize" (Frank, 2001) The construct of self is a central factor in understanding both the ontology and epistemology of suffering as a lived experience. Moreover, the social construct of self helps decipher both the ontological as well as the epistemic nuances of experience of the self. The self is inextricably linked to consciousness. Caste as a consciousness, manifests itself in inflicting the social with layers of inequality, discrimination and most importantly violence, not just physical but also psychic amongst the many other social ills. Religious conversions have been occuring since historic times and have been sought as an alternative to overcomes structures of oppression across the world. Ambedkar's mass conversion to Buddhism dated 14th October 1956 is often documented as one of biggest religious conversion in the history of Social Movements in India.

In the recent times, there has been a surge in the anti-conversion laws in India based on rhetoric of nationalism. But despite numerous attempts of secularisation of the public sphere, Indian consciousness still continues to be dominated by religion. Hence, the phenomena of religious conversion acquires added relevance in contemporary times. Ambedkar's contribution to social well being vis-a-vis the ideals of democracy and spirituality find very little mention in the domains of public health. This chapter attempts to understand Ambedkar's perspective on social well being. Spirituality is an essential facet of human existence as it makes life fulfilling and meaningful. In the caste system, Dalits were deprived of spirituality and religiosity both. For example, not being permitted to enter temples, not being allowed to hear, and recite the religious scriptures, not being allowed to take part in rituals and ceremonies. The only function of the Dalit self and mind in Hindu social order was to serve those above. This deprived them of their own essence and human sanctity. Ambedkar considered religion as a torchbearer of hope in human life. Since, Hinduism denied this to Dalits, Ambedkar's quest for religious conversion began in search of a spirituality which on one hand could make life fulfilling and on the other could impart substance and spirit to the social coexistence of Dalits with fellow members of society, thereby offering prospects of both individual and social well-being.

16.2 Situating the Phenomenology of Graded Inequality, Conflict, and Suffering

As per Ambedkar, the Hindu social order is based on the doctrine of "graded inequality" in which castes "stand one above the other in an ascending scale of hatred and descending scale of contempt" (Ambedkar, 1987, p. 48). Hence, there is no one singular social but multiple socials in India. He further differentiates between inequality and graded inequality. He further notes that inequality does not have a capacity of self-preservation while graded inequality possess because in the social system of inequality, all those in lower stratum can integrate as an independent unit and overcome inequality while in case of graded inequality, no strata are as underprivileged as those except those in lowermost rungs of the hierarchical pyramid of caste and varna system (*Ibid.*). Thus, the resultant defining features of this graded inequality were social isolation, segregation and enforced exclusion on one hand and a complete absence of fraternity and social endosmosis on the other. Social being reciprocal, the corporeal situatedness and social construct of self then become a very important category in understanding how this very social gets constituted in categories like nation, religion, caste consciousness and finally democracy in the Indian context. The self in Indian sociality lives in a dialectic of secular and religious ideals. "The practical instincts of man do not yield to the secular ideal if the two are in conflict. This means that a religious ideal has a hold on mankind, irrespective of an earthly gain. This can never be said of a purely secular ideal" (*Ibid.*, p. 23). Given the diversity of Indian democracy, the social is embedded in the religious. Thus, religion becomes an important vantage point to understand the very experience of social and how it shapes and reshapes Indian democracy. For Ambedkar, the essence of religion implied life and preservation of life which gets constituted in sharing of vital life experiences like birth, death, marriage, puberty, as well as sharing of food, partaking in rituals, etc. with fellow individuals (*Ibid.*). Graded inequality denied the sharing of these very vital life experiences amongst different caste groups and thereby made the sociality devoid of sentiment of fraternity which could foster the spirit of goodwill for all. In addition to it, graded inequality also prescribed restitutive coercive laws for those who dared to break these rules codified by Hindu religious scriptures. This made self in the Hindu social order individualistic and an isolated self whose ultimate purpose of life was the transmigration of soul. In the philosophy and *praxis*[1] of Buddhism, the social is an embodiment of the experiential which ought to transcend individualised atomistic existence and metamorphose itself to a radical merger with whole existence through the *Maitri* paramita. It is through *Maitri* that Ambedkar seeks reconstruction of society through the annihilation of caste consciousness that degrades the dignity and sanctity of human personality to its lowest ebb. One of the most degrading manifestations of caste was the coercive practice of untouchability.

"The impact of non—touching is on both the brahmin and the Dalit—both of them cannot fulfil the act of touching but they have different phenomenological experiences of the same. In the case of former, it could be associated with psychological feelings of revulsion, power, rejection and so on, whereas in the latter it is associated with feelings of humiliation, shame and so on" (Sarukkai, 2009). It is here that the ontology of Dalit self acquires the empirical ground to understand the social suffering arising from the practice of caste making caste the most prevalent and humiliating form of social conflict in Indian society. The body hence constitutes the most immediate possibility for locating the construct of self, more so in the context of untouchability as a physical and a sentimental manifestation of practice of caste. However, this physical material self is directed by the consciousness of mind and it is here that social self emerges by the interaction of consciousness, body and finally the social environment where the corporeal and experiential self is situated. Thus, we can say that the very foundation of the essence of self is the experience of social. In the Hindu social order, the Dalit self is located outside of the Varna system called as Avarna which in the language of Ambedkar (1989) made them "unfit for human association" (p. 93). Being unfit for human association implied that being denied the opportunity of sharing vital life experiences like joys and sorrows, birth and death, marriage, and conjugality with the fellow members of society including the denial of sharing of territorial spaces. The most natural outcome

[1] There have been many interpretations of usage of the word 'praxis'. However, in my usage of the term, I imply it to mean a self-conscious action with an *aditthana* to bring about a temperamental and behavioural change to overcome structures of oppression by moral means.

of this was not just physical segregation but also psychic and sentimental segregation which disabled one human from generating the feelings of empathy and compassion for another human as his fellow being having the universal corporeal organic existence. It is in the light of this that I seek to locate the practice and consciousness of caste as a form of social conflict and an experience of social suffering.

Elaborating about the religious and attitudinal behaviour of Hindus towards the Untouchables, Ambedkar (1989) says that the former's behaviour towards the latter is that of "moralistic unconcernedness" (p. 99) which made the Hindus to discriminate and segregate the untouchables from the rest of the society. The absence of moral unconcernedness lead to social isolation and fragmentation of social space. Since the social space is constituted not just as spatially but also sentimentally; it reduced the untouchables as locales of suffering rendering them unfit for human association. This moralistic unconcernedness of Hindus was a result of graded inequality, since Hinduism formulated it as a divine schema of religious governance, thereby making it a sacrosanct duty of every Hindu to uphold it, no matter whether it is just or unjust. Hence Hinduism failed to become a religion of principles. Ambedkar distinguishes rules and principles saying that rules are to be followed as a duty, whether they are good or bad but principles are yardsticks which enable an individual to distinguish between good and bad (Ambedkar, 1979). This rule-based moralistic unconcernedness, devoids the Hindu self the freedom to develop a temperament of fellow-feeling for the untouchables and promotes garnering the spirit of animosity, for every person who is not a member of that Hindu self's own caste. Finally, it is this moral unconcernedness which strips the mind of Hindu self from any sort of public conscience. "*Public Conscience* was the term that Dr. Ambedkar employed to capture the ideas surrounding the individuals who constitute our social life more generally. By public conscience, he referred to 'conscience which becomes agitated at every wrong, no matter who is sufferer' and 'leads an individual to join the struggle to remove the wrong'. Public Conscience was conditioned upon 'fellow feeling', the phrase that Dr. Ambedkar had used to describe *fraternity* (Rathore, 2020, p. 109). Seen in this light, this absence of the spirit of public conscience could never lead to destruction of the caste system and untouchability from within the praxical framework of Hinduism, despite numerous attempts of removal of caste by Hindu Social Reform Movements. It is here that one can locate the birth of Buddhism as a religious doctrine which promotes this very public conscience in Ambedkar's schema, thereby making the Buddhist self, consciously develop a dispositional moralistic concernedness in contrast to Hindu religious doctrine.

A minute reading of the biographical sketch of Buddha until the process of his enlightenment as enunciated by Ambedkar in his seminal text *The Buddha and His Dhamma* sheds light on a few important findings of great relevance in this context. One, that Gautama (prior to enlightenment) left his home in order to avert the conflict between Sakyas and the Koliyas on sharing of waters of river Rohini and not due to seeing old man, sick man, etc. Two, after getting the news of peace amongst the Sakyas and Koliyas, Buddha did not return back to his householder life. The news of peace between the two conflicting camps made Buddha contemplate and realize two things: One, that (Ambedkar, 1992), "the problem of war is essentially a problem of conflict. It is only a larger part of the problem" and two, that "the conflict between nations is occasional. But the conflict between classes is constant and perpetual. It is this which is the root of all sorrow and suffering in the world" (pp. 57–8). Buddha described this phenomenon of suffering as "social conflict."

16.3 Transforming Subjects of Fragmented Social Order to Citizens Governed by a Democratic Republican Polity

Graded inequality comes with a repressive apparatus of humiliation and violence ultimately resulting in suffering which in turn necessitates

Indian democracy to look at the prospects of fraternity and social endosmosis. Role played by the human consciousness in the socio-cultural and political life of individuals is an important factor which constitutes democracy as a social experience. For Dewey, the triad of democracy becomes practical only when the distinction between secular and religious ceases to exist. For Durkheim, religion is the chief force which promotes social cohesion in society. In this context Durkheim (1995) says, "The principal features of collective life have begun as none other than various features of religious life, it is evident that religious life must necessarily have been the eminent form and, as it were, the epitome of collective life. If religion gave birth to all this is essential in society, that is so because the idea of society is the soul of religion. Thus, religious forces are human forces, moral forces" (p. 421). Thus, seen from a Durkheimian Perspective, a moral community could emerge from the springboard of religion. Ambedkar had deep concerns for developing a moral community where the relationship of one individual with another ought to be based on respect and empathy. In his text *On the Jewish Question (2014) (1844)*, Marx divides the true development of human consciousness into two-fold life. One being life in a political community that is where man is a species being and thus a communitarian being, while the second being life in civil society, where man is a secular being, a private individual in himself. As per Marx, when man is a species being, he is deprived of his real individual life and hence is bound to experience an unreal or false universality. He ultimately reduces the Jewish Question to the "conflict" between species being and the spiritual being and thus emancipation of state from religion is not real emancipation for man as per him. For him, the ultimate human emancipation is possible when an individual species being ends the separation between social and political power. In the context of Indian society, Ambedkar takes a totally unique turn wherein as per him, in the dialectics of religious and secular ideals, it is always the religious ideals which hold a sway over the Indian mind. Hence for him, a civic religion based on a common civic morality could usher in psychological unity amongst the masses of one of the most diverse nations of the world. Thus, Ambedkar sees nationalism as a psychological sentiment capable of both positive and negative consequences. Ambedkar (1990) sees "forgetfulness" of bitter relations of past and reconstitution of new bonds of solidarity based on the premise of ethicality and fraternity. It is the radical disposition to have compassion and love even for one's foe, an important aspect of the ontology of fraternity and Maitri.

As per Verderame, Marcel Mauss centres the idea of nation within the framework of social cohesion. "Social" for him then becomes a manifestation of individual experiences on one hand and link between physical, psychological, psychic, and sociological aspects on the other, finally manifesting itself in a totality of social facts whereby individual and social are no longer separate. Thus, this "completeness matures entirely only if nations, as has said, become democratic at every level." Thus, for Mauss, social is reciprocal and nation is interlinked to this reciprocal. As per Ambedkar (1990), "For nationality to flame into nationalism two conditions must exist. First, there must arise the "will to live as a nation." Nationalism is the dynamic expression of that desire. Secondly, there must be a territory which nationalism could occupy and make it a state, as well as a cultural home of the nation" (p. 39). Thus, Ambedkar perceived the idea of nation as a socially constructed space premised on psychological unity of masses evolved by interaction amongst the individuals who constitute it. As per Garza (2014), "for Ambedkar, a nation was a living soul or a spiritual principle constituted by the common possession of a rich heritage of memories; and by the actual desire of the population to live together and to preserve the memories of common sacrifice, joys, victories, and sorrows. Ambedkar noted that the sharing of common past was dependent on forgetfulness and historical error. That is, past antagonism, religious or political, needed to be contained or forgotten as they could endanger the image of a unified community." Garza further reiterates that for Ambedkar, space was an entity emerging from the interactions between the individuals who constitute it as well as it was a social determinant which in turn also decided and directed the behaviour of individuals who constituted it. The Indian Constitution envisages [1]"fraternity" as the foremost goal imparting solidarity to the social life of Indians. On 25th November 1949 in the Constituent Assembly Ambedkar said, "a political democracy cannot last unless at the base of it lies social democracy. And what does a social democracy mean? It means a way of life which recognizes liberty, equality, and fraternity as principles of life" (CAD, 1949). Thus the political in the Indian democracy is essentially governed by the social. In the democratic triad of liberty, equality and fraternity, liberty and equality can be ushered through law. But for fraternity, there can be no law. Hence, fraternity is more of a social construct. Sociologically, fraternity could be seen as a social action which strengthens social ties and attempts social cohesion in society.

16.4 Conversion as a Reconstructive Ethic: Realising Fraternity in Substance and Spirit

Religious conversion was a well contemplated and conscious decision to enter humanity by the praxis of Dhammic morality aimed to recover the lost self which was devoid of its own essence, under the servitude of caste. Right at the outset of conversion, many accusations were levelled on Ambedkar by his opponents, after the Yeola declaration where Ambedkar proclaimed that he shall not die as a Hindu. These accusations included, conversion for reaping political dividends, material gains, conversion not being faith based, etc. However, Ambedkar refuted each one of them and this can be seen in his two texts *Away from Hindus* and *What Way Emancipation?* where he not only refuted these false accusations but also elaborated the reasons for his decision to convert. In his speech, *What Way Emancipation?* Ambedkar (1979) says, "nothing but spirituality is the base of my conversion" (p. 144). Along with this, he also explains how he has no political benefit to reap from conversion to Buddhism. So, we can say that conversion to Buddhism was a spiritual praxis of Ambedkar's moral ontology. So, we naturally arrive at a question then why Ambedkar preferred Buddhism only and not any other religion and at first place why conversion. In this context of Ambedkar and his conversion, Stroud (2017) says, "If Ambedkar sought social endosmosis, why did he give a call for exit from Hinduism? The call for conversion to Buddhism is not a call to break away from interacting with others in Indian society, it is a call to break away from thinking about these individuals and oneself using categories of caste. The new orientation of Buddhism allows for social experience in and around others to have a new egalitarian meaning and potential". For Ambedkar, conversion to Buddhism meant a radical re-conception and reorientation of the Dalit self, transitioning from a life of dejection, humiliation, and absence of dignity to reclaiming a life of happiness, dignity, and respect for the sanctity of human personality. In sum, it implied realising one's own humanity. Thus, for Ambedkar, the principle of morality and spirituality were two grounds to base his praxis of conversion.

Hinduism and its psycho-socio-cultural apparatus premised on strict adherence to caste sanctified by Hindu religious scriptures reduced it a religion based on rules where it was the religious duty of every Hindu to uphold the structure of caste. Contrary to it, Ambedkar found Buddhism to be a civic religion whose central tenet was morality and relation of human to human, where the pivot was not God or revelation or scripture but human mind and righteousness which made it, a religion based on principles. Along with this, other factors for Ambedkar choosing Buddhism for conversion include the indigenous origin of Buddhism. The other religious alternatives also consisted of presence of caste, emphasis on rituals, orthodoxy, etc. In the context of explaining the subject matter of religion and distinguishing it from that of Dhamma, Ambedkar (1987) writes *"The purpose of dhamma is to reconstruct the world and not to find origin of universe"* (p. 322, emphasis mine). This he says so because almost every religion preaches morality. But Ambedkar was not satisfied with mere morality. He desired a morality which was both sacred as well as universal and put it to the touchstone of reasoning by contemplating that in the process of morality becoming social, does morality acquire an anti-social element because if that happens it leads to isolation and thus embodies anti—social spirit which was detrimental to the process of social cohesion based on temperamental and attitudinal change. The morality of Hinduism was caste and hence it failed the test of being sacred and universal. For example, caste as codified by coercive and violent sanctions in laws of Manu and other Hindu religious scriptures. Practice of caste made and is still making the triad of democracy fragile in India. Ambedkar's conversion to Buddhism was on one hand an act to annihilate the very consciousness of perceiving every individual from the lens of caste and on the other a moral praxis of cultivating the spirit of mutual respect for sanctity of human personality and fraternal concord for everyone, for Ambedkar sought social endosmosis, which was the hallmark of a free social order.

Often when it comes to scholarships on religious conversions, especially the ones to Buddhism, it gets relegated to an act for political emancipation. However, in Ambedkar's own words (1979), "castes cannot be abolished by inter-caste dinners or stray instances of intercaste marriages. The caste is a state of mind. The teachings of Hindu religion are the root cause of this disease… For annihilating castes and untouchability from amongst untouchables, change of religion is the only antidote" (p. 130). Ambedkar's conversion to Buddhism aimed at ushering in a new cultural paradigm based on the ideal of universalizing fraternity by the praxis of maitri. In various Buddhist schools of thought, Maitri paramita is seen as a spiritual practice of cultivating loving-kindness and goodwill for every living being on earth by the means of training of mind, which is an important aspect of Ashtanga Marga. However, it does not imply developing individualism because here the individual becomes more radically and actively social through development of universal belongingness because it is premised on the principle of anatma (no-soul). Thus, the Buddhist theory of no-soul at first instance dismantles the other-worldly self on one hand and attempts to create an impermanent everchanging self radically more collective through maitri paramita. In Ambedkar's opinion, in the triad of democracy, fraternity was that principle which in spirit and substance sustained liberty and equality. He says, "The word fraternity is not an adequate expression. The proper term is what Buddha called Maitri. Wherein lie the roots of fraternity without which democracy is not possible? Beyond dispute, it has its origin in religion" (Ambedkar, 1987). In Ambedkar's schema, religion was very essential to human existence, one because the individual is not just a biological organism but also a social being having thoughts, emotions, and values and two, because preservation of social life was the chief function of religion. Moreover, Ambedkar separated religion from theology as according to him, religion was associated with rites, rituals, observances, practices, etc., while theology implied an entity which was just secondary to religion. Ambedkar perceived religion as a social force for the spread of common good and hence he delved deep into doctrines of every religion before arriving at a decision of choosing the religion for conversion. Examples of conversion to Buddhism exist even during Buddha's time where it was always non-coercive, aimed to usher in a temperamental change in mind of the convert. For example, the conversion of the dreaded bandit, Angulimala. Angulimala's name prior to becoming a dreaded criminal was *Ahimsaka.* When he had gone to his Brahmin teacher's centre, he excelled in all his endeavours. Out of jealousy, his fellow colleagues falsely accused him of having an illegal relationship with wife of his teacher and this prompted his teacher to ask him a guru-dakshina of one thousand human finger which made a deadly transition of Ahimsaka to Angulimala. When nine hundred and ninety-nine people were killed by him and just one more finger was left to be cut, Buddha met *Angulimala* and tried to persuade him morally. The example of *Angulimala* also highlight how caste and its cultural apparatus (Example: Guru Dakshina in this case) stripped the person from goodness inherent within him and made him a criminal for no fault of him. Not just this, it also shows how caste blinded him without even make him recognize the heinous crime he was committing on name of guru-dakshina. Just when Anglimala tries to attack Buddha, Buddha says to him, "The good in you is not yet dead. If you will only give it a chance it will transform you" (Ambedkar, 1957, p. 205). This example elucidates how Buddha's model of conversion was one of to bring about a dispositional change in the mind of the convert, without a pinch of coercion and basing it on principle of virtue and loving kindness.

Conversion to Buddhism for Ambedkar also implied adopting new ways of thinking, acting, behaving, and engaging oneself socially. It is evident from the writings of Ambedkar that conversion emphasised adopting a new life. For example, Dalits were earlier made to pick up dead animals, especially the cows and buffaloes. In the absence of food, Dalits began eating these animals. Further, they were forced to remain relegated as members of the working class with no avenues of social mobility. This made them vulnerable to many diseases and the social stigma associated with caste ensured that no one would dare to touch their bodies, leave aside even understanding the health issues which they suffered along with tormentous humiliation of the ascriptive status of being Dalit. Dalit women were not allowed to cover their upper body parts as a practice of caste, leave aside getting educated or taking other important life decisions. Ambedkar had asked his followers to give up all these humiliating and uncivil practices. In one of the addresses delivered to the Dalits, he urged them to buy two pairs of clothes for themselves, one for labourial work and two for occasions other than those of labouring. Being the father of whole community, he was very much concerned about women of his community. Ambedkar had even visited Kamatipura, the red light area of Bombay and urged the Dalit women sex workers to give up the profession and live a life of dignity and morality. We also find that at another instance he tells them that even if they have just one pair of dress, still they should make it a point to wash it and only then wear it. He was also an ardent advocate of family planning, welfare, and control. The practicing aspects of Buddhism were Sila,[2] Ashtanga Marga[3] and Paramitas[4]. Further, these Buddhist ideals also affirmed to the democratic triad of liberty, equality, and fraternity. Thus, Buddhism presented a strong amalgamation of morality and democracy which had the capacity to liberate the everyday sociality from bondages of injustice and lawlessness.

16.5 Universalising Fraternity through Maitri

In Buddhist social theory, suffering is the base on which the Four Noble Truths are grounded. In understanding the construct of self and suffering, the role of consciousness is a pivotal, for it shapes and reshapes our experience of everyday social life. However, Buddhist thought is not just limited to suffering and its causes. It also talks about dukkha-nirodh[5] that is overcoming suffering by following the Majimma Patipada,[6] thereby also laying a philosophical ground for understanding social wellbeing by the lens of Buddhism. For Ambedkar (1987), the human personality was quintessentially "sacred" and needed "a proper climate for development" (p. 99). Ambedkar sought the sacred in the Buddhist ethic of Maitri and the proper climate for development in social democracy. Alleviation of suffering, the

[2] Sila implies moral temperament to abstain from doing wrong.

[3] Ashtanga Marga implies the eight-fold path preached by Buddha consisting of Right views, Right aims, Right Speech, Right conduct, Right livelihood, Right perseverance, Right mindfulness, and Right contemplations.

[4] Paramitas in Buddhism refer to the ten perfections/virtues to be strived for namely panna (wisdom), sila (moral temperament), Nekhamma (renunciation of pleasures), Dana (giving/donating without expecting anything in return), Virya (energetic action), Khanti (forbearance), Succa (upholding truth), Aditthana (resolute determination to reach the goal), Metta (fellow-feeling for all), and Upekkha (detachment, not indifference).

[5] Dukkha-nirodh refers to the cessation of suffering.

[6] Majhimma Patipada is term in Pali which Buddha used to explain Middle-path that is avoidance of two extremes of pleasure and self-mortification and developing and sustaining equanimity of mind in every circumstance.

quest for fraternity, dignity, social democracy and most importantly a common civic morality based on principled religion have thus been a dominant stream of thought in the writings of Ambedkar, whether it is on the Indian nation in general or the Dalits as a community in particular. It is evident from his writings, right from his autobiographical notes titled *Waiting for a Visa* from where emerges the experiences of young Ambedkar based on casteism and caste induced suffering on account of humiliation, ultimately culminating to denial of very existence of dignity of untouchables to his magnum opus *The Buddha and his Dhamma* where he seeks not just dignity but also an emancipation and social change through the Buddhist way of life based on principles of morality, respect for dignity and fraternal goodwill for every living being on earth. Buddhist social thought theorises a movement from suffering to emancipation and maitri is one such democratic means. In philosophy of Buddhism, consciousness (vinnana in Pali) is a pivotal factor to ground experience as a realm of social. But consciousness is just one of the experiential aggregates, others being matter, sense-perception, and mental factors resulting from lived experience. In various Buddhist schools of thought, *Maitri* paramita is seen as a spiritual practice of cultivating loving-kindness and goodwill for every living being on earth by the means of training of mind, which is an important aspect of Ashtanga Marga. However, it does not imply developing individualism because here the individual becomes more radically and actively social through development of universal belongingness because it is premised on the principle of Maitri and anatma (no-soul). Hence the Buddhist self in Ambedkar's discourse is one who is socially engaged in striving to uphold the moral order of the universe with conscious efforts.

Ambedkar proposed a morality which was both sacred as well as universal. He tested the notion of morality by understanding that in the process of morality becoming social, does it acquire an anti—social element because if that happens it leads to isolation and thus embodies anti—social spirit in itself. Caste was the morality of Hindu social order and hence it failed the test of being sacred and universal. For example, caste as codified by coercive and violent sanctions in laws of Manu. Also, until morality is not made universal and sacred, there cannot be growth of individual beings and progress of society. Elaborating on social conflict, he quotes Buddha: "a society which rests upon the supremacy of one group over another irrespective of its rational or proportionate claims inevitably leads to conflict. The only way to put a stop to conflict is to have common rules of morality which are sacred to all" (Ambedkar, 1957, p. 325). While distinguishing between dhamma and morality, Ambedkar writes, "What is the remedy? The only remedy lies in making fraternity universally effective. What is fraternity? It is nothing but another name for the brotherhood of men which is another name for morality. This is why the Buddha preached that Dhamma is morality and as Dhamma is sacred so is morality" (Ibid.). Dhammic Morality in the form of sila whether one is a Buddhist or not was both sacred as well as universal because sila was about bringing about an attitudinal and temperamental change which could make the sociality grounded on righteousness and thus wellbeing. Soon after enlightenment, when the five parivrajakas requested Buddha to expound the insight that he gained through enlightenment. Buddha told them about his path which he called as the Dhamma whose pivot was the right relation between human and human. He further postulated that the world is full of suffering as humans are living in sorrow, misery and poverty and removal of this suffering was the only purpose of his dhamma. He thus anchors his dhamma on two principles, one, giving recognition to existence of suffering and two propounding a methodology for the removal of that suffering and for him this methodology was a threefold path based on purity, righteousness, and virtue. By purity, he meant sila; by righteousness, he meant the ashtanga marga and by virtue, he meant the ten paramitas. Maitri is one of the ten paramitas.

16.6 Towards Social Well-Being

Right in the preface of Annihilation of Caste (1979), Ambedkar describes caste as a sickness of Hindus and says,"their sickness is causing danger to the health and happiness of other Indians" (p. 26). In one of his writings titled *Frustration*, Ambedkar makes a phenomenological comparison between the Untouchables and Jews. He opines that the case of experience of untouchables is one of utmost frustration to the extent that they are not even able to realize the true essence of their own selves. He places Jews in a contrast to Untouchables because though a frustrated lot, yet they could arise from their sufferings like a phoenix rises from the ashes. As per Ambedkar (1993), the Jews could overcome their frustration and sufferings due to what he terms as a "*plus condition of mind and body*" (p. 734) which arose from two chief sources; one, their reliance on God (covenant) as a source of mental power and two their favourable social environment. As per Ambedkar, the untouchables suffered frustration because they lacked this very condition because the Hindu social order breeded an unpropitious social environment characterized by a lack of social endosmosis, social well-being and a complete absence of fraternal concord and goodwill amongst fellow members of the Hindu social order. "This plus condition of body and mind is also the result of Social Environment, if the Environment is propitious. In a society where there is exemption from restraint, a secured release from obstruction, in a society where every man is entitled not only to the means of being, but also of *well—being*, where no man is forced to labour so that another may abound in luxuries, where no man is deprived of his right to cultivate his faculties and powers so that there may be no competition with the favoured, where there is emphasis of reward by mento, where there is *goodwill towards all*" (Ibid., 735). While elaborating on Hindu social order, Ambedkar locates two disastrous features as the base of Hinduism. One, social and religious inequality and two, a complete degradation of human personality. For Ambedkar, the social order to ensure well—being of every citizen ought to be one based on democratic triad of liberty, equality and fraternity and the Hindu social order was a complete denial of the same. Fraternity for him was both a *necessary and a natural moral sentiment* which ought to be cultivated just like any and every other physical condition of human existence. Ambedkar's conversion to Buddhism dated 14th October 1956, was one such attempt to usher in this plus condition of mind and body and to cultivate this natural moral sentiment of fraternity. Ambedkar (1989) further states, "Religion emphasizes, universalizes social values and brings them to the mind of the individual who is required to recognize them in all his acts in order that he may function as an approved member of the society. But the purpose of religion is more than this. It spiritualizes them" (p. 409).

The praxis of Maitri thus presents the most immediate and radically fraternal space which could in turn enable every individual who constitutes it to establish a social relationship with every other being as one's own kindred based on principles of quality and loving kindness, thereby attempting to reconstruct the fragile Indian society as a democracy based on social endosmosis. Ambedkar's conversion thus aimed towards creating a holistic model of social well-being.

References

Ambedkar, B. R. (1979). *Annihilation of caste with reply to Mahatma Gandhi* (Vol. 1). London: Government Central Press.

Buswell, R., & Lopez, D. (2014). Angulimala. In *The Princeton dictionary of buddhism* (p. 149). Princeton University Press.

Cháirez-Garza, J. F. (2014). Touching space: Ambedkar on the spatial features of untouchability. *Contemporary South Asia, 22*(1), 37–50. https://doi.org/10.1080/09584935.2013.870978

Dewey, J. (1927). *The public and its problems* (p. 188). Swallow: Swallow University Press.

Dewey, J. (2008). *The early works, 1882–1898: 1882–1888. Early essays and Leibniz's new essays concerning the human understanding* (Vol. 1). New York: Southern Illinois University Press.

Durkheim, E. (1995). *Elementary forms of religious life*. Berlin: The Free Press.

Frank A. W. (2001). Can we research suffering? *Qualitative Health Research, 11*(3), 353–362. http://qhr.sagepub.com/content/11/3/353
Marx, K. (2014). *On the Jewish question* (pp. 137–150). London: Routledge.
Moon, V. (Ed.). (1957). *Dr. Babasaheb Ambedkar writings and speeches* (Vol. 11). London: Government of Maharashtra.
Moon, V. (Ed.). (1987). *Dr. Babasaheb Ambedkar writings and speeches* (Vol. 3). London: Government of Maharashtra.
Moon, V. (Ed.). (1989). *Dr. Babasaheb Ambedkar writings and speeches* (Vol. 5). London: Government of Maharashtra.
Moon, V. (Ed.). (1993). *Dr. Babasaheb Ambedkar writings and speeches* (Vol. 12). London: Government of Maharashtra.
Moon, V. (Ed.). (2003). What way emancipation? In *Dr. Babasaheb Ambedkar writings and speeches* (Vol. 17, Pt.3). London: Government of Maharashtra.
Sarukkai, S. (2009). Phenomenology of untouchability. *Economic and Political Weekly, 44*(37), 39–48. https://www.jstor.org/stable/25663542
Stroud, S. R. (2017). The rhetoric of conversion as emancipatory strategy in India: Bhimrao Ambedkar, pragmatism, and the turn to Buddhism. *Rhetorica: A Journal of the History of Rhetoric, 35*(3), 314–345. https://doi.org/10.2307/26378087
Verderame, D. (2014). The "Social" as reciprocity: Marcel Mauss and the idea of nation. In *Classical sociology beyond methodological nationalism* (pp. 117–151). Brill.
Wilkinson, I. (2005). *Suffering: A sociological introduction.* Berlin: Polity Press.

Part V
Conclusion

Conclusion: Bridging the Social Inequalities in Health

17

Sanghmitra Acharya, Sampurna Kundu, and Sampurna Singh

The preceding chapters present an evident interlinkage between population, development, and health. The book clearly illustrates that health depends on the propensities of population and development of the systems which are associated with it. The current SDGs also aims to ensure good health and well-being at all ages (Goal 3). The Indian public health care delivery system, initially was designed for infectious and parasitic diseases, has now evolved with the shift towards non-communicable, degenerative diseases. The book has highlighted the importance of health system in accommodating the diverse and increasing population and its health needs. The hospital bed-based approach reinvigorates the system, aiming to meet World Health Organization bed-population norms. This involves increasing hospital beds in existing institutions and creating new ones to achieve a balanced distribution. The approach emphasizes the importance of health facilities in proximity of the people for efficiency and effectiveness. This is specifically important for access to services for antenatal, delivery, post-natal and child care, which can help in reducing child mortality and enhance maternal health. India has progressed in reducing gender disparities in mortality rates, particularly in early childhood; over the past seven decades. It highlights the persistent challenges in achieving equal opportunities for survival.

Although India has made progress in reducing mortality, it still faces challenges in achieving equal opportunities for overall and childhood survival. The contributors also highlight the gender-specific changes in life expectancy at birth and mortality decline at younger ages. India has achieved the under-5 mortality rate as per MDG and is expected to achieve the SDG before 2030. India's progress in reducing child mortality is faster than global trends, with a reduction in its share of global child deaths from one-fifth in 1950 to 14% in 2020. Additionally, the country's lower female to male death ratio suggests further improvement in female mortality. Besides this, over the past three decades, India has also seen significant improvements in household living conditions and socio-economic indicators, including access to basic amenities,

S. Acharya (✉)
Centre of Social Medicine and Community Health, School of Social Sciences, Jawaharlal Nehru University, New Delhi, Delhi, India
e-mail: sanghmitra.acharya@gmail.com

S. Kundu
Postdoctoral Research Fellow in Epidemiology, Faculty of Health and Life Sciences, University of Exeter, UK, Exeter, United Kingdom
e-mail: sampurna34@gmail.com

S. Singh
Senior Researcher, Mindfield Research Services, New Delhi, India
e-mail: sampurna62@gmail.com

S. S. Acharya et al. (eds.), *Paradigm Shifts in Population and Health in India*, Sustainable Development Goals Series, https://doi.org/10.1007/978-981-95-1719-0_17

increased literacy rates, and higher levels of women owning bank/post office accounts. These improvements have significantly impacted the lives of women and girls, through ensuring better education, employment, decision-making, and access to services.

Gender does not solely affect health outcomes, but it interacts with other social determinants. Gender-biased practices, such as, forced marriages, dowry, son preference and sex selective abortions, have a negative impact on female population. India's gender-governed society, where men control most institutions, have higher access to resources like food, healthcare, and education. Poverty, social class, religion, caste, and place of residence also influence child health outcomes. However, while it is suggested that more female participation in the labor force is likely to reduce bias against girls in India, it would require to be triangulated with the decision-making process. The study by Ram et al. (present volume) establishes that India's full immunization coverage has improved and gender gaps have reduced, contributing to a reduction in childhood mortality and the adoption of the vision of 'Decade of Vaccines', in the Global Vaccine Action Plan.

The government has announced ambitious schemes like 'Poshan Abhiyan', 'Swatchta mission', 'Sarva Shiksha Abhiyan', and 'Naari Shakti', but translating these promises into reality requires a nuanced understanding of implementation issues. Prioritizing young children as 'right' holders is crucial, as their rights are low-cost and affect their education. Mass awareness campaigns, sensitivity towards frontline workers, representation from minority communities, and more grassroot level facilities like Anganwadi centers in marginalized localities can help in addressing discrimination. This would enable creating a strong protective environment which is essential for programmatic intervention. Supporting migrant children is crucial. However, the gap between what the ICDS program is expected to deliver and what actually gets delivered needs to be minimized and redesigned to include the migrant children. The institutional setup does not recognize the long working hours, harsh working conditions, and inadequate social support systems of migrant workers. The sedentary bias of the ICDS program should be revisited, and successful experiments by NGOs should be scaled up by the government. Making underserved neighborhoods better is also necessary, as they face differential needs such as safe water deficit, open defecation, and poor hygiene. A balanced approach towards development of poor neighborhoods without pushing residents to the brink of invisibility is the need of the hour. Inclusive policies for migrant workers should be considered, as voting rights are not portable and migrant workers are politically insignificant.

The book also discusses innovations like, mobile health centers (MHCs), that can provide primary care in underserved areas and during pandemic crises. They can be deployed to address population needs. Health digitalization impacts frontline workers. Nutritional anemia among adolescents is a major public health concern in developing countries. Food diversification and integrated nutrition intervention programs can reduce IDA prevalence. The digitization of work has shifted Anganwadi workers' goals to numerical targets and statistical data, leading to confusion about their nature of work. The top-down approach of policy implementation with inadequate time training has made data entry and collection secondary to the work they do, affecting their understanding of care work. This research highlights the need for better training and policy implementation. The ICDS program has expanded into Poshan Abhiyaan and Poshan 2.0, adding community-based events and Jan Andolan for holistic nutritional awareness. However, this has increased job responsibility, slow compensation, and paperwork. Workers are expected to organize community events, but these interactions are dependent on apps and dashboards. The informal and volunteer nature of the job makes it difficult for workers to participate in decision-making processes. They are not included in the consulting and feedback process. The government advocates for real-time monitoring to address data gaps in health system delivery, but this data-driven governance also highlights the importance of the lowest-level workers, such as Anganwadi workers, in achieving program success in a neoliberal era.

Recently, community health workers in India like ASHA has been recognized by WHO and won the Global Health Leaders Award, which indicates the strong role of community health workers in meeting the health needs at grassroot levels (Asthana & Mayra, 2022).

India faces a significant unmet medical need, despite attempts towards universal healthcare coverage (Dubey et al., 2023). Socioeconomic factors contribute to this issue, with unmet need widening despite overall decline. Barriers to healthcare acceptability disproportionately affect the poor, particularly in rural areas, younger age groups, and backward regions. Despite increased investment in health infrastructure, rural areas still lack access to healthcare. Addressing these barriers requires state-specific policies and trained community health workers to improve healthcare delivery efficiency. A multisectoral policy approach is needed to address geographical heterogeneity and ensure equity in healthcare access.

Anemia remains a significant public health concern in developing countries, especially among reproductive-age women, especially adolescent girls. A healthy diet can protect against nutritional anemia, particularly in India, where adolescent girls face the highest prevalence. The book highlights the future reproductive health issues in India, highlighting the need for comprehensive gynecological care and adequate knowledge for women. Current public healthcare services focus on pregnancy and maternal health, but addressing women's health in all aspects is crucial. Less educated women may avoid hysterectomy due to fear or ignorance, while private hospitals may exploit their lack of knowledge. A comprehensive study on hysterectomy and its impact on women's health is essential for achieving Sustainable Development Goals. The main contributor to the rural–urban differential is the number of pregnancies, wealth, social-group, and lifestyle factors. Undergoing hysterectomy is not mandatory for all cases; unless it is extremely life-threatening which need to made aware of along with other gynaecological morbidities. Measures are needed to ensure suitable and treatment options availed among the respective age groups which are accessible, affordable and of better quality.

Further, the book focusses on the importance of school health and hygiene, focusing on the provision of WASH facilities, proper sanitation practices, and well-maintained toilets. It highlights the alarming issue of girls' dropout rates due to insufficient toilet facilities and the challenges they face in managing menstrual hygiene. The initiatives of international organizations, government programs, and the role of NGOs in addressing health and hygiene challenges in schools is imperative. The role of hygiene education in fostering healthy growth and development for future generations is critical. The study by Lenka and Chanchal (present volume) reveals that water supply and sanitation issues exist at different levels in both areas due to various factors such as economic, political, socio-cultural, educational, administrative, structural, technology, lack of awareness, and environmental factors. The water supply is often 'short-lived', causing households to travel long distances to collect it. The drinking water is of poor quality and contaminated with bleaching powder, making it unsuitable for drinking, cooking, and bathing. Toilet facilities are lacking, and many households use buckets for water. Sanitation workers are not regular, and many households are unaware of government sanitation schemes. Therefore the need for improved access to water and sanitation services particularly for those who provide these services (Acharya, 2023).

As regards well-being, there is an intersection of environment, mental health, and spirituality. the conservation of habitats is a priority, and discourses surrounding it must shift to address environmental issues. Emerging concepts like critiquing neo-liberal policies, affirming political ecology theory, well-being perspectives, and ecofeminism can frame a more inclusive agenda. These concepts question the economic-driven development paradigm, which leads to environmental mishaps, poverty, and social corrosion. Political ecology recognizes the climate crisis through a gendered lens, as women are considered marginalized to the food system, leading to faulty pregnancies, undernourishment, and higher mortality rates. Collective responses to climate change are crucial.

India has launched various programs and schemes to support the elderly population over a period of time. The Integrated Programme for Senior Citizens (1992), National Action Plan for Senior Citizens (1992), National Social Assistance Programme (1995), National Policy for Older Persons (1999), National Initiative on Care for the Elderly (2004), Maintenance and Welfare of Parents and Senior Citizens Act (2007), and National Programme for the Healthcare of the Elderly (2011). These initiatives aim to address the physical and social dependency of the elderly population, ensuring a healthy aging environment in India.

As the book explores some specific excluded communities, the Muslim Naikin women, a group found in Kolhapur and Sangli areas, emerges as an area of interest. Paradoxically it has remained a topic with limited literature which reflects on their economic and sexual exploitation. Their socio-economic conditions and sexual violence against them need more in-depth analysis. The scarcity of literature imposes restrictions in evaluating the effectiveness of rehabilitation programs for these women. Domestic violence still being quite prevalent is a significant issue. Alcoholism adds another dimension to domestic violence impacting mental health and well-being. Married men with a history of violence have higher alcoholism compared to non-violent counterparts. Children growing up in abusive environments, witnessing alcoholic fathers ignore their family's needs, face severe emotional trauma and are more likely to grow up abusive. To prevent violence, it is crucial to change mindsets and treat women and girls with equality. Given the social norms, women are often considered second class citizens, deprived of basic rights like food, education, and employment, despite improvement in certain development indicators. Interventions for women and children, such as counseling and separate shelter homes, are needed. Poverty and inequality are also root causes of violence, but preventive measures remain inadequate. Investing in and prioritizing violence prevention is critical for achieving positive social, economic, and political outcomes. Governments, community-level training, and regular awareness campaigns are needed to address these issues. Domestic violence must be treated as a serious public health issue, as poverty, inequality, and violence are interlinked and play a significant role in achieving the Sustainable Development Goals.

The idea of holistic health goes beyond the conventional biomedical model, ushering in biopsychosocial framework. Thus, the book concludes on the note that how spirituality can promote social well-being. In 1979 book, Ambedkar argues that the Hindu social order breeds an unpropitious environment, lacking social endosmosis, social well-being, and fraternal concord. The social order should be based on democratic values of liberty, equality, and fraternity, which are universally recognized and spiritualized. Ambedkar's conversion to Buddhism in 1956 aimed to cultivate this natural moral sentiment and establish a social relationship with others based on principles of quality and kindness.

17.1 Concluding Remarks

Population, health and development are interlinked via a series of factors. Population dynamics, health infrastructure, health system, health services, development process, broadly, are intertwined and influence each other. The constituents of population dynamics-fertility, mortality and migration are known to affect the health of the population. Development inputs in the health sector affect the population health too. There are regional disparities in the distribution of healthcare facilities, with urban areas having better access than rural regions, for instance. While India has made strides in improving its healthcare infrastructure, yet the challenges persist. The Disease Burden of communicable diseases such as malaria, tuberculosis, and waterborne diseases still pose significant challenges. Non-communicable diseases (NCDs) like diabetes and cardiovascular diseases are on the rise, contributing to the double burden of diseases.

Constant efforts have been made by the government to improve maternal and child health, but issues like high maternal mortality rates and malnutrition persist, especially in some states. The government has implemented various immunization programs to protect against preventable diseases, targeting children and pregnant women. Covid vaccine is the newt addition in this endeavor. There have been Public Health Campaigns to showcase the strategies and plans for various health conditions and hygiene requirements ranging from maternal and child health, immunisation and sanitation. India has launched public health campaigns to address issues such as sanitation, hygiene, and family planning to improve overall health outcomes. Campaigns to create awareness about open defecation, handwashing, menstrual hygiene, small family norms, contraception, spacing of the births have been a constant element in the population concern of the country.

The constant efforts to lower the population growth is evident from the campaign messages like-'Chhota parivaar, sukhi parivaar'; 'Hindu, Muslim, Sikh, Isaai, chhote parivaar mein sabhi ki bhalaai' which were floated by the state. These, however, did not specify the number of children as part of the 'small family'. Therefore, gradually with no or insignificant reduction in population growth, 'bus do ya teen bachche, hote hai ghar mein achche'; 'agla bachcha abhi nahin, teen ke baad kabhi nahin' suggestively stipulated the ideal number of children to be borne as three, during the decades that followed the inception of the family planning programme in the country in 1956. During the 1960s and 1970s the small family norm instructed not more than three children. But subsequently, the shift to 'hum do hamare do'; 'ek ke bad abhi nahin, do ke baad kabhi nahin', lowered the family size to two children. This perhaps has been the most fervent campaign in the history of population concern the world over. The campaigns for health and development have been at an advantage of the changed media formats with more visual and social platforms available. The influencers ranging from the cinema personalities to the political leaders on the print, visual and auditory media have been campaigning for thc 'clcan India mission', universal immunisation programme etc. Interestingly, there is a connect which is visible in cleanliness, health and development, for instance, through these campaigns. Ensuring healthy living conditions, through access to education, employment and housing are feasible for fewer children than more, reflecting the larger connect between the SDGs-1, 3, 4, 5, 6, and 10 particularly.

As regards development, an important indicator is Economic Growth. India has experienced significant economic growth, leading to an expansion of the middle class. However, income inequality remains a concern, with stark disparities between urban and rural areas and privileged and under-privileged. Efforts have been made to improve literacy rates, and there has been progress in increasing school enrolment. However, challenges like dropouts and quality of education persist. Although, infrastructure development, with projects aimed at improving transportation, energy, and communication networks is continuing, visible gaps are vying for attention. Urbanization is also a prominent trend causing urban primacy in some cities enabling them to become medical primate centres too. The inequality is affecting the access to health and other development resources. Poverty alleviation programs, including social welfare schemes, have been implemented to address the needs of marginalized communities. However, poverty remains a significant challenge in the face of the inequalities.

Initiatives like Digital India aiming to increase internet access and technology adoption, especially in rural areas have made strides in digitalization across sectors especially health. Rapid industrialization and urbanization have led to environmental challenges, including air and water pollution. The government has initiatives to address environmental concerns and promote sustainable development. Digital improvisations have helped in addressing the environmental concerns too.

It is important to note that progress is not uniform across the country, and data suggests that different states face different challenges and successes. They have different development regimes, population compositions and health infrastructure. There could be changes in policies and programs too. It has been found out that SDG1(No Poverty) is associated with all other SDGs. Reducing poverty is found to be statistically linked to favoring the progress of SDGs 3 (Good health and well-being), 4 (Quality education), 5 (Gender equality), 6 (Clean water and sanitation), and 10 (Reduced inequalities). Therefore, different initiative with different degree and kind of interventions will be required to meet the SDG goals. The present volume attempts to weave together the papers from different vantage points in establishing this association.

References

Acharya, S. S. (2023). *Sustainable sanitation in Swachh Bharat: What we owe to the cleaning brigade*. Academic Publication.

Asthana, S., & Mayra, K. (2022). India's one million accredited social health activists (ASHA) win the global health leaders award at the 75th world health assembly: Time to move beyond rhetoric to action? *The Lancet Regional Health—Southeast Asia*. https://doi.org/10.1016/j.lansea.2022.100029

Dubey, S., Deshpande, S., Krishna, L., & Zadey, S. (2023). Evolution of government-funded health insurance for universal health coverage in India. *The Lancet Regional Health—Southeast Asia*. https://doi.org/10.1016/j.lansea.2023.100180

Annexure 1

Trends in life expectancy at birth (LEB, in years), per 1000 live births infant mortality rate (IMR) and under-5 mortality rate (U5MR) for male and female, world and India (1950–2100)

Year/period	World						India					
	LEB (in years)		IMR (per 1000 LB)		U5MR (per 1000 LB)		LEB (in years)		IMR (per 1000 LB)		U5MR (per 1000 LB)	
	Male	Female	Male	Female	Male	Female	Male	Female	Male	Female	Male	Female
Panel: 1950–2020												
1950	44.6	48.4	147.0	140.0	228.7	219.4	42.6	40.8	177.2	185.9	276.3	291.8
1960	46.0	49.4	137.9	132.4	220.1	214.8	45.9	44.5	154.8	162.2	236.4	249.4
1970	54.2	58.1	101.0	96.1	150.6	144.1	48.9	47.6	139.0	144.8	208.7	218.9
1980	58.2	62.9	82.7	78.2	120.2	114.6	53.5	53.7	112.7	118.1	163.7	172.9
1990	61.5	66.5	66.5	62.7	95.2	90.4	57.9	59.5	87.5	92.5	122.3	130.4
2000	64.1	68.9	54.7	51.8	77.4	73.7	61.8	63.6	64.9	71.2	87.0	96.6
2010	67.6	72.7	38.5	35.7	52.8	49.2	65.3	68.6	43.2	47.4	55.3	61.2
2020	69.4	74.8	29.9	26.6	39.7	35.5	68.6	71.8	26.3	26.9	32.3	33.1
Panel: 2023–2100												
2030	72.0	77.2	26.1	21.3	35.9	29.6	72.0	75.6	19.5	17.5	24.3	22.0
2040	73.5	78.6	22.5	17.1	31.4	24.2	74.0	77.9	13.9	11.5	17.4	14.6
2050	74.8	79.8	19.9	14.2	27.8	20.2	76.0	79.9	10.1	8.2	12.6	10.4
2060	75.9	80.8	17.8	12.2	25.0	17.3	78.0	81.6	7.7	6.5	9.6	8.2
2070	77.0	81.8	15.7	10.4	22.0	14.7	79.9	83.1	5.9	5.3	7.3	6.7
2080	78.0	82.7	14.0	9.0	19.5	12.6	81.8	84.5	4.6	4.4	5.6	5.6
2090	78.9	83.5	12.6	8.0	17.3	11.1	83.5	85.8	3.7	3.8	4.5	4.8
2100	79.9	84.3	11.3	7.2	15.3	9.8	84.9	87.0	3.1	3.3	3.7	4.1

Source UN World Population Prospects, 2022

S. S. Acharya et al. (eds.), *Paradigm Shifts in Population and Health in India*, Sustainable Development
Goals Series, https://doi.org/10.1007/978-981-95-1719-0

Annexure 2

Trends in levels of initiation of breastfeeding, pre-lacteal feeding, exclusive and age-appropriate breastfeeding, feeding/dietary practices, immunization, and prevalence and treatment seeking behaviour for diarrhoea, fever, and symptoms of acute respiratory infections among male and female children, India (1992–93 to 2019–21)

Indicator	Male children					Female children				
	1992–3	1998–9	2005–6	2015–6	2019–21	1992–3	1998–9	2005–6	2015–6	2019–21
Breastfeeding practices										
Newborn was initiated breastfeeding within one hour of birth (%)	9.4	16.1	23.2	41.5	41.5	9.2	15.8	23.1	41.5	41.3
Newborn received a pre-lacteal feed (%)	–	–	57.6	21.1	16.1	–	–	57.7	21.0	14.9
Children below 6 months exclusively breastfed (%)	41.4	46.2	47.0	56.1	63.2	45.3	47.4	45.8	53.7	64.3
Children below 2 years received age appropriate breastfeeding (%)	55.7	57.6	68.4	66.3	63.7	56.7	58.8	66.9	65.2	62.7
Food/dietary practices for children aged 6–23 months										
Fed solid/semisolid food (%)	56.5	67.4	85.0	74.9	74.8	56.2	69.0	84.4	75.3	74.4
Fed milk/other milk products (%)	45.0	53.8	56.3	52.2	53.9	41.1	50.6	52.8	50.1	52.4
Fed a minimum diverse food (%)	–	–	12.8	19.6	23.6	–	–	12.8	20.1	23.5
Fed minimum meal frequency (%)	–	–	40.8	36.5	38.4	–	–	41.0	35.3	39.3
Fed a minimum acceptable diet (%)	–	–	8.5	9.7	11.5	–	–	8.1	9.4	11.3

(continued)

S. S. Acharya et al. (eds.), *Paradigm Shifts in Population and Health in India*, Sustainable Development Goals Series, https://doi.org/10.1007/978-981-95-1719-0

(continued)

Indicator	Male children					Female children				
	1992–3	1998–9	2005–6	2015–6	2019–21	1992–3	1998–9	2005–6	2015–6	2019–21
Children aged 12–23 months who were fully immunized (%)	36.7	40.4	45.3	62.1	76.9	34.1	38.3	41.2	61.9	75.9
Prevalence and treatment for diarrhoea among children										
Prevalence of diarrhoea (%)	10.3	19.4	9.5	9.5	7.6	9.8	18.9	8.4	8.9	7.0
Sought advice/ treatment (%)	67.1	71.8	69.0	77.8	76.7	63.4	69.3	66.9	75.6	75.6
Sought treatment within a day (%)	–	–	41.2	54.5	54.5	–	–	37.3	54.4	54.7
Sought treatment from public health facility (%)	24.0	20.1	19.1	22.9	30.7	25.7	18.8	16.9	25.0	31.8
Sought treatment from private health facility (%)	71.8	73.0	77.5	71.2	67.1	68.8	72.8	80.0	68.3	65.9
Prevalence and treatment for fever among children										
Prevalence of fever (%)	21.1	30.3	15.4	13.4	13.7	19.4	28.5	14.2	12.4	12.6
Sought advice/ treatment (%)	75.5	56.4	78.9	81.7	80.4	69.5	50.1	75.5	80.1	79.1
Sought treatment within a day (%)	–	–	46.7	58.5	59.3	–	–	43.9	57.3	57.4
Sought treatment from public health facility (%)	23.6	19.5	14.7	21.9	26.7	23.8	17.4	15.9	23.8	27.9
Sought treatment from private health facility (%)	72.8	73.8	83.9	72.7	70.8	71.6	73.9	81.8	70.5	69.1
Prevalence and treatment for symptoms of ARI among children										
Prevalence of ARI (%)	7.1	20.7	6.0	2.9	3.0	5.9	17.9	5.6	2.5	2.5
Sought advice/ treatment (%)	79.9	73.2	77.4	87.6	57.4	76.2	68.0	71.9	82.6	54.8
Sought treatment within a day (%)	–	–	39.4	59.9	39.4	–	–	39.3	54.7	37.3
Sought treatment from public health facility (%)	23.3	20.7	15.1	22.1	27.9	25.9	18.7	10.3	23.0	28.4
Sought treatment from private health facility (%)	73.8	71.9	83.7	73.5	69.5	69.1	71.8	87.8	71.9	67.6

Annexure 3

Description of socio-economic, feeding practices and maternal and child health care utilization indicators estimated from the five rounds of National Family Health Survey (1992–93 to 2019–21)

Indicators	Definition
Population living in urban areas (%)	Percentage of population (household members) living in the urban areas
Households with improved source of drinking water (%)	Percentage of households using an improved source of drinking water
	Improved source includes: Piped into dwelling, piped into yard/plot, piped to neighbour, public tap/standpipe, tube-well or bore-well, protected well, protected spring, rain water, tanker truck, bottled water
Households with basic sanitation service (%)	Percentage of households using any improved toilet facilities, that is not shared with other households
	Improved sanitation includes: Flush to piped sewer system, flush to septic tank, flush to pit latrine, flush-don't know where, ventilated improved pit latrine, pit latrine with slab, composting toilet
Households using open defecation (%)	Percentage of households using no facility/bush/field
Women aged 15–49 years ever been to school or can read full or part of sentence (%)	Percentage of women respondents aged 15–49 years who ever attended school, and others who can read all or part of a sentence given
Households with one or more women aged 15–49 years completed 10 or more years of education (%)	Percentage of women respondents aged 15–49 years who have completed schooling up-to 10th standard or above

(continued)

S. S. Acharya et al. (eds.), *Paradigm Shifts in Population and Health in India*, Sustainable Development Goals Series, https://doi.org/10.1007/978-981-95-1719-0

(continued)

Indicators	Definition
Total Fertility Rate (TFR, average number of children per woman)	The average number of children a woman would have by the end of her childbearing years if she bore children at the current age-specific fertility rates. Age-specific fertility rates are calculated for the 3 years before the survey, based on detailed birth histories provided by women
Median age at first marriage among women aged 20–49 years	The median age in years when women (20–49 years) first lived with a spouse or consensual partner
Proportion of women aged 20–24 years married before age 18 (%)	Percentage of women aged 20–24 years married before the completion of 18 years of age
Currently married women using any modern contraceptive method (%)	The percentage of currently married women aged 15–49 years who were currently using any modern method of contraception
Currently married and non-pregnant women using any modern spacing method (%)	The percentage of currently married and non-pregnant women aged 15–49 years who were currently using any modern method of contraception for spacing between the births
Ever married women aged 15–49 years sterilized after having one or two daughters only (%)	Percentage of ever-married women aged 15–49 years who opted for either of the birth-limiting methods (female sterilization, male sterilization) after they has either only one or only two daughters
Ever married women aged 15–49 years who were anaemic (%)	Percentage of women aged 15–49 years with any anaemia (mild, moderate, severe)
Children under-5 years who were anaemic (%)	Percentage of children age 6–59 months with any anaemia (mild, moderate, or severe)
Children under-5 years who were stunted (%)	Percentage of children under 5 years of age whose height-for-age z-score is below minus 2 (−2.0) standard deviations (SD) below the mean on the WHO Child Growth Standards (moderately or severely stunted)
Children under-5 years who were wasted (%)	Percentage of children under 5 years of age whose weight-for-height z-score is below minus 2 (−2.0) standard deviations (SD) below the mean on the WHO Child Growth Standards (moderately or severely stunted)
Children's birth size and weight	
Children who were smaller than average size at birth for gestational age (%)	Percentage of live births in the 5 years preceding the survey who have average or larger size at birth, by mother's estimate of baby's size at birth
Children who weighed less than 2.5 kg at the time of birth (%)	Percentage of live births in the 5 years preceding the survey weighed at birth reported as less than 2.5 kg
Maternal and child health service utilization	
Women who registered their pregnancy in first trimester (%)	Percentage of married women aged 15–49 years with a birth in the last 5 years who received antenatal care in the first trimester of their pregnancy
Women who received antenatal care from skilled provider (%)	Percentage of women aged 15–49 years with a birth in the last 5 years receiving antenatal care from a skilled provider for the most recent birth
	Skilled provider includes: Doctors, Nurse/midwives, ANM/midwives

(continued)

(continued)

Indicators	Definition
Women who received full antenatal care (%)	Percentage of married women who had at least four ANC visits, at least one tetanus toxoid (TT) injections, and consumed 100 or more iron-folic acid (IFA) tablets/syrup during her pregnancy
Institutional births out of all births (%)	Percentage of live births to women aged 15–49 years in the past 5 years delivered in a health facility
C-section births out of all births (%)	Percentage of live births to women age 15–49 in the 5 years preceding the survey delivered by caesarean section
Mothers or child received one or more postnatal check-up within 48 h of birth (%)	Percentage of mother or children who have received any postnatal check-up/visit at institution or at home within 48 h of the delivery
Children aged 12–23 months who were fully immunized (%)	Percentage of children age 12–23 months who received all basic vaccines at any time before the survey according to either vaccination card or mother's report
	Full basic vaccination includes: 1 dose of BCG; 3 doses of DPT; 3 doses of polio vaccine (excluding polio vaccine given at birth); 1 dose of Measles/MCV
Breastfeeding Practices	
Newborn was initiated breastfeeding within one hour of birth (%)	Percentage of last-born children born in the past 2 years who started breastfeeding within one hour of birth, regardless of whether the children are living or dead at the time of the interview
Newborn received a pre-lacteal feed (%)	Percentage of last-born children born in the past 2 years who were ever breastfed and who received a pre-lacteal feed in the first 3 days after birth
Children below 6 months exclusively breastfed (%)	Percentage of last born children under 6 months who are alive and living with mother are being exclusively breastfed (nothing else in the 24 h preceding the interview)
Children below 2 years received age appropriate breastfeeding (%)	Percentage of youngest children under 2 years who are living with their mother who are age-appropriately breastfed:
	If the child is under 6 months—exclusively breastfed
	Child aged 6–23 months—who are breastfed and given solid or semi solid in the 24 h preceding the survey
Food/dietary practices for children aged 6–23 months	
Fed solid/semisolid food (%)	Percentage of last-born children aged 6–23 months, who are alive and living with their mother are fed solid/semisolid foods (excluding dairy products)
Fed milk/other milk products (%)	Percentage of last-born children aged 6–23 months, who are alive and living with their mother are fed tinned milk/formula/fresh milk/cheese, yogurts or other milk products (excluding breastmilk)

(continued)

(continued)

Indicators	Definition
Fed a minimum diverse food (%)	Percentage of last-born children age 6–23 months who are living with the mother, are fed a minimum dietary diversity of 5 out of 8 food groups fed during the day or night preceding the survey
Fed minimum meal frequency (%)	Percentage of youngest children age 6–23 months who are living with the mother who are fed minimum meal frequency of:
	(a) 2 or more solid or semi-solid or soft feeds for breastfeeding children age 6–8 months, or 3 or more solid or semi-solid or soft feeds for breastfeeding children age 9–23 months; or
	(b) 4 or more solid or semi-solid or soft or milk feeds for non-breastfeeding children age 6–23 months
Fed a minimum acceptable diet (%)	Percentage of youngest children age 6–23 months who are living with the mother who are fed a minimum acceptable diet based on minimum dietary diversity and minimum meal frequency they are fed during the day or night preceding the survey:
	(a) Breastfed children—minimum dietary diversity and minimum meal frequency
	(b) Non-breastfed children—minimum dietary diversity but excluding the dairy products category (4 out of 6 groups) and minimum meal frequency and 2 or more milk feeds
Prevalence and treatment of acute illness (diarrhoea, fever, symptoms of ARI)	
Prevalence of diarrhoea/fever/symptoms of ARI	Percentage of children under age 5 who were reported to have any diarrhoea/fever/symptoms of ARI at any time in last 2 weeks preceding the survey
Sought advice/treatment (%)	Percentage of children under age 5 with diarrhoea/fever/ symptoms of ARI at any time in the 2 weeks preceding the survey for whom advice or treatment was sought from a facility
Sought treatment within a day (%)	Percentage of children under age 5 with diarrhoea/fever/ symptoms of ARI at any time in the 2 weeks preceding the survey for whom advice or treatment was sought the same or the next day
Sought treatment from public health facility (%)	Percentage of children under age 5 with diarrhoea/fever/ symptoms of ARI at any time in the 2 weeks preceding the survey for whom advice or treatment was sought from a public health centre or provider (including NGO/charity/ trust run hospital and Anganwadi/ICDS centre)
Sought treatment from private health facility (%)	Percentage of children under age 5 with diarrhoea/fever/ symptoms of ARI at any time in the 2 weeks preceding the survey for whom advice or treatment was sought from a private health centre or provider (including private pharmacy)